Movement Disorders of the Upper Extremities in Children

Jörg Bahm

Editor

Movement Disorders of the Upper Extremities in Children

Conservative and Operative Therapy

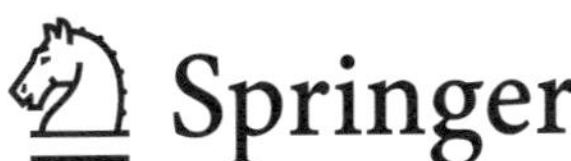 Springer

Editor
Jörg Bahm
Section for Plexus Surgery of the Department for Plastic,
Hand and Burn Surgery
University Hospital
Aachen
Germany

ISBN 978-3-030-53624-4   ISBN 978-3-030-53622-0   (eBook)
https://doi.org/10.1007/978-3-030-53622-0

This Springer imprint is published by the registered company Springer Nature Switzerland AG
The registered company address is: Gewerbestrasse 11, 6330 Cham, Switzerland

Contents

Introduction

Jörg Bahm

1.1 Definitions

Movement disorders of the upper extremity are usually related to congenital or acquired impairment of neuromuscular function of the musculoskeletal system.

Primary muscle damage cannot be surgically improved and therefore is not discussed here. A distinction is made between nerve damage within the peripheral nervous system, including the conductive pathways and that of the brain, which is usually associated with spasticity.

It is important to make a clear distinction between the various clinical features and to explain essential basic concepts: We assume that the basic anatomy and physiology of the nervous system and the musculoskeletal system are known by the reader [1] and we refer the reader to Kummer [2] for biomechanics and to further literature in the appendix.

Typical movement changes in the newborn can be seen, for example, in the context of a *lack of oxygen during birth* (hypoxic brain damage inducing a spastic movement disorder of one or both upper extremities, eventually also involving the lower extremities), in a *birth-associated nerve injury to the neck* (damage to the brachial plexus—infantile plexus palsy) or a complex neuro-orthopaedic disorder such as *arthrogryposis* (arthrogryposis multiplex congenita, AMC; upper and/or lower extremities affected; usually but not exclusively on both sides). Of course, there are also rare neurogenic disorders of the spinal cord neurons (e.g., spinal atrophy), but they cannot be treated surgically and are not considered here.

All the above-mentioned clinical entities happen in the newborn and infant and become apparent through the one-sided or two-sided conspicuous *movement disorder* (especially when comparison with a normal contralateral limb is possible); *sensory changes* are rarely measurable at this age.

The following discussion describes the characteristics of the individual diagnoses.

Clinical characteristics of major upper extremity movement disorders in children
- *Spasticity*: central nervous origin, especially hypoxia
- *Flaccid weakness or paralysis* indicates a lesion of the peripheral nervous system (PNS):

J. Bahm (✉)
Department of Plastic, Hand and Burn Surgery,
Section for Plexus Surgery, University Hospital,
Aachen, Germany
e-mail: jbahm@ukaachen.de,
jorg.bahm@belgacom.net

© Springer Nature Switzerland AG 2021
J. Bahm (ed.), *Movement Disorders of the Upper Extremities in Children*,
https://doi.org/10.1007/978-3-030-53622-0_1

examination of dermatomes and myotomes lead to a localization of the disorder
- Unilateral/bilateral involvement; eventually including lower extremities
- neurogenic vs. myogenic damage
- Tangible "mechanical" cause (shoulder dystocia, traffic accident, open injury, palsy associated with a tumour)

Every motion disorder of the upper extremities that we are considering is related to the nerves and that is why we first distinguish between *central nervous* (brain) or *peripheral lesions*.

The *central nervous system* (CNS) can be damaged by a lack of oxygen during birth (peripartal anoxia in cerebral palsy), a disorder of blood circulation (bleeding, thrombosis) or a tumour of the pyramidal tract. In most cases, this is accompanied by speed-dependent muscle spasticity.

In addition, there are many causes of damage to the *peripheral nerves*, ranging from the spinal cord neurons to the radicles, the spinal nerves, the plexus itself and the common trunk nerves (Kline et al. [3]; Fig. 1.1). These peripheral lesions are accompanied by a more or less pronounced muscle palsy of characteristic muscles (myotomes).

Traumatized nerves *degenerate* distal to the site of injury, whereby the distal axon portion dissolves into the basic structures thus preparing the *regeneration* process by newly sprouting regeneration cones. The target muscles wither, atrophy (*denervation amyotrophy*) and switch to a basal action pattern, the electromyographically detectable spontaneous activity. They then rebuild only when the newly regenerating nerve fascicles reach them again via the motor end plate and restart muscular contractile activity. Then practice and patience are necessary in order to achieve a good functional level again, including also a sound interaction with the other muscles and the restoration of central control.

1.2 Clinical Manifestations (Neurological-Orthopaedic)

What is conspicuous at any age is first of all the appearance, the posture of the extremity in comparison to the healthy opposite side (Fig. 1.2).

Let us therefore first look for changes in the basic attitude: for example, an internal rotation of

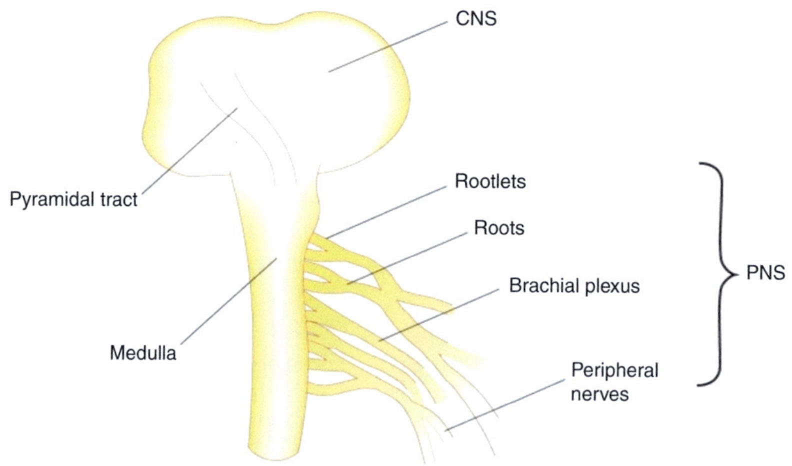

Fig. 1.1 Sites of damage to peripheral nerve tracts

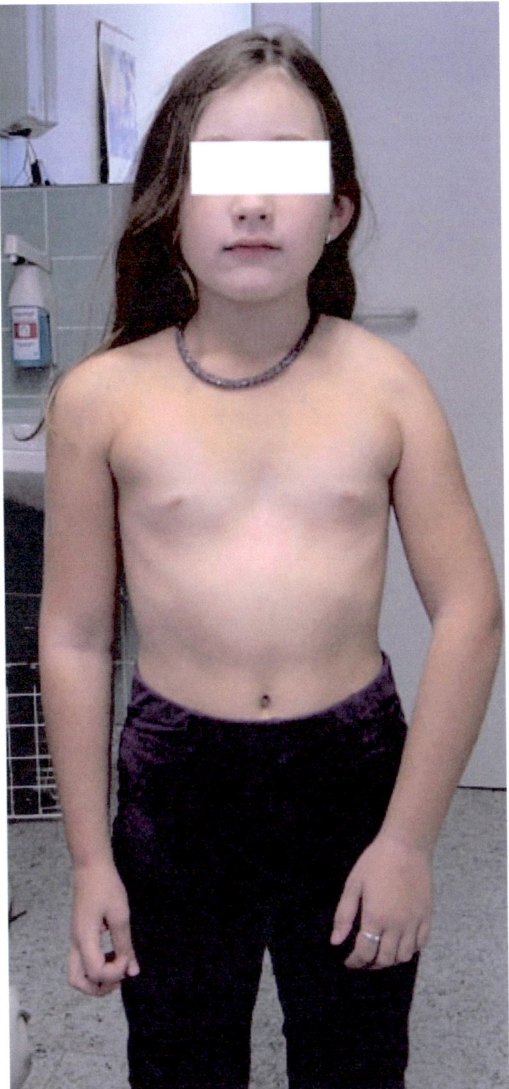

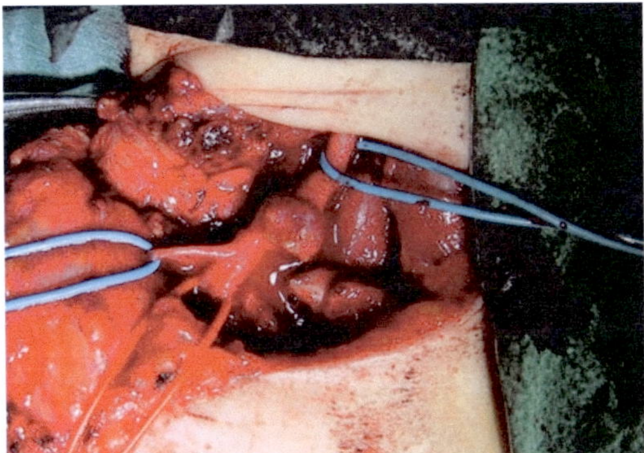

Fig. 1.3 Cocontractions: mixed reinnervation of antagonists by traumatic neuromas

1.2.1 Spontaneous Motor Skills

They are often reduced in extent and strength, where amyotrophy might not be visible in the newborn due to increased subcutaneous fat tissue. Both when the child is lying and sitting, the contrast to the healthy arm is noticeable; and the problem zones can easily be determined and a distinction can be made between upper and complete paralysis, for example.

1.2.2 Cocontractions

With pronounced proximal nerve lesions, reinnervation in neuromatous areas (where the individual regenerating minifascicles mix) leads to mixed reinnervations, either among like-minded muscles (agonists) or with opponents (antagonists). If the proximal nerve is now activated, a signal is generated that is simultaneously sent to the opponents across the lesion (Fig. 1.3) and thus simultaneously activates opposing muscles.

The result is a movement that begins slowly, like a "stiffened" movement, which then comes to a standstill with increasing effort: the arm part remains "stuck" halfway along the movement path.

By means of a surface electromyogram (sEMG) registered in parallel on both antagonists, this coactivation can be very well documented and then the effect of botulinum toxin injected into the antagonist can be observed

Fig. 1.2 Posture comparison healthy—affected extremity

the shoulder, an angulated elbow, a pronated or supinated forearm, a dropped or laterally deviating wrist, fist or flabby fingers.

Arms that are severely affected are not included in the body scheme at all and are discarded (the so-called *neglect*), since insufficient afferent information probably does not convey sufficient self-awareness about that limb to the CNS. Sometimes the babies bite into the affected arm or move it with the other upper extremity as if it were a foreign body.

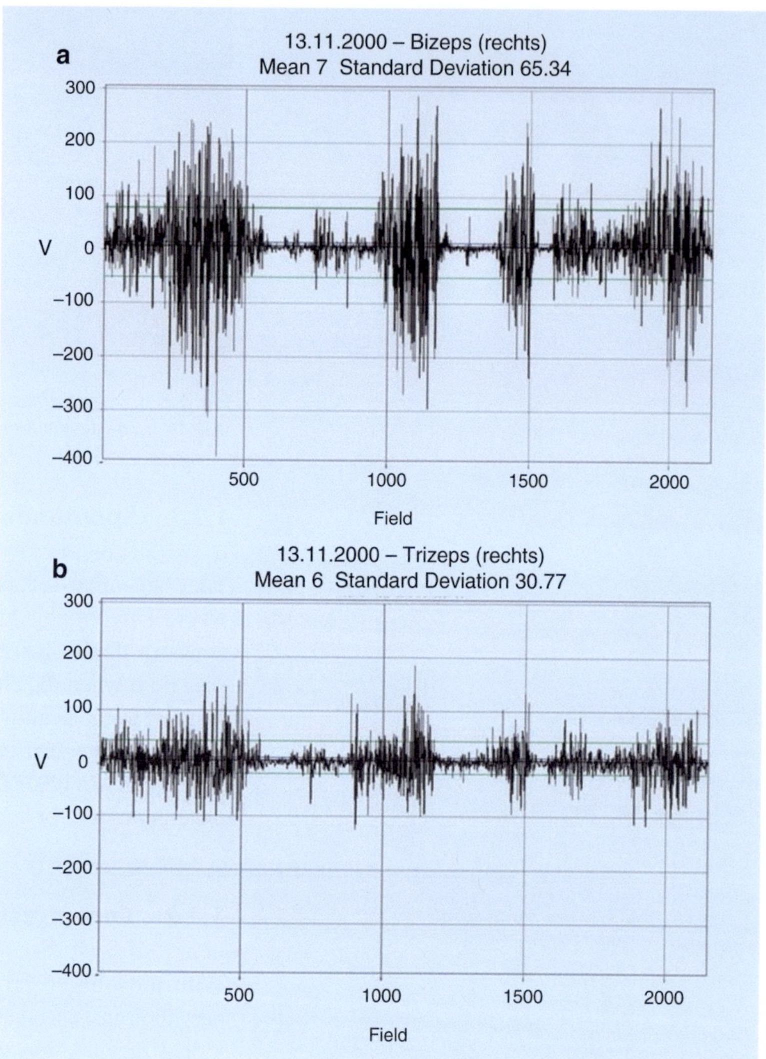

Fig. 1.4 (a, b) Coactivation of musculus biceps and triceps visualized in the surface electromyogram

within the framework of therapy, also over time (Bahm et al. [4]; Fig. 1.4).

Of course, not all cocontractions are pathological, since we have to position our arms in certain postures in space, hold them against gravity, and this is only possible by simultaneously activating different antagonists. However, *pathological* cocontractions can, however, considerably disrupt common movement patterns, for example, within the scapulohumeral rhythm running at the shoulder level, or very visibly during elbow flexion, thus preventing a typical hand-to-mouth movement, even though each muscle is well developed and responds individually to the neu-

ral stimulus. The electromyogram (EMG) of the individual muscle is also not pathological; the pathophysiology only becomes visible when looking simultaneously at the EMG patterns of both antagonists (Chap. 6).

1.2.3 Spasticity

In central nervous disorders, the reflex pathway is usually disturbed in a way that a spontaneous pathological myotonus, the so-called spasticity, develops. This is not a global phenomenon but is only found in certain muscle groups, which then considerably influence and change the movement pattern.

Spastic phenomena are also speed-dependent, so that the examiner and physiotherapist are required to move the affected joints very slowly and progressively against the spastic contracted muscle.

Due to the increased, non-antagonized build-up of strength, spasticity rapidly leads to considerable joint contractures and growth changes in joints and bones, so that orthoses and corrective interventions (botulinum toxin, myotomy, tenotomy or musculotendinous slide or release) must be performed very early in order to balance or maintain at least elementary movement patterns.

Morphologically, the spastic musculature shows a connective tissue infiltration over time; ultrastructural changes of the sarcomere are also discussed.

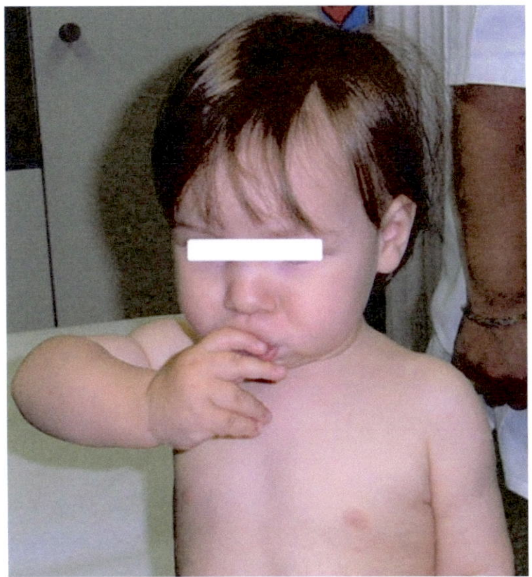

Fig. 1.5 Trumpet sign

1.2.4 Compensation Movements

The learning programme of the usual age-dependent movement patterns (excellently described by Vojta [5]) is disturbed by all these phenomena and the maturing brain certainly receives a number of "error" messages which it tries to compensate dynamically. The toddler very quickly develops compensatory movement patterns by supporting weaker, normally developed muscles or by replacing impossible chains of movement with bypass movements (e.g., the hand-to-mouth movement typical of a trumpeter when there is no strong biceps muscle and no active external rotation of the shoulder, Fig. 1.5).

Compensation can disappear over time when the weak muscles regenerate or are assisted by muscle transfers. Some disturbances, like those affecting unconscious compensatory movements such as the swinging of the arms during running, are only "caught up" during puberty; for years parents have been worried that the arm is parked along the body during the race in a posture that is

reminiscent of the original state of paralysis and therefore worries the relatives again and again.

In the case of severe paralysis, and in particular paralysis which is inadequately treated at the beginning, the compensation patterns, which can include the entire upper body, become a permanent supplementary feature of the movement sequences (Fig. 1.6).

There is a fear of a secondary scoliosis because of the incorrect posture of the trunk.

1.2.5 Accompanying Symptoms

The following questions arise:

- Are the other extremities affected?
- In the case of severe plexus palsy, is the ipsilateral hemidiaphragm paralysed (damage to root C4 and the phrenic nerve)? This is associated with repeated respiratory infections or even life-threatening ventilatory deficiency.
- The Claude Bernard-Horner syndrome (Fig. 1.7) (ptosis of the upper eyelid, myosis of the pupil, enophthalmia) related to complete

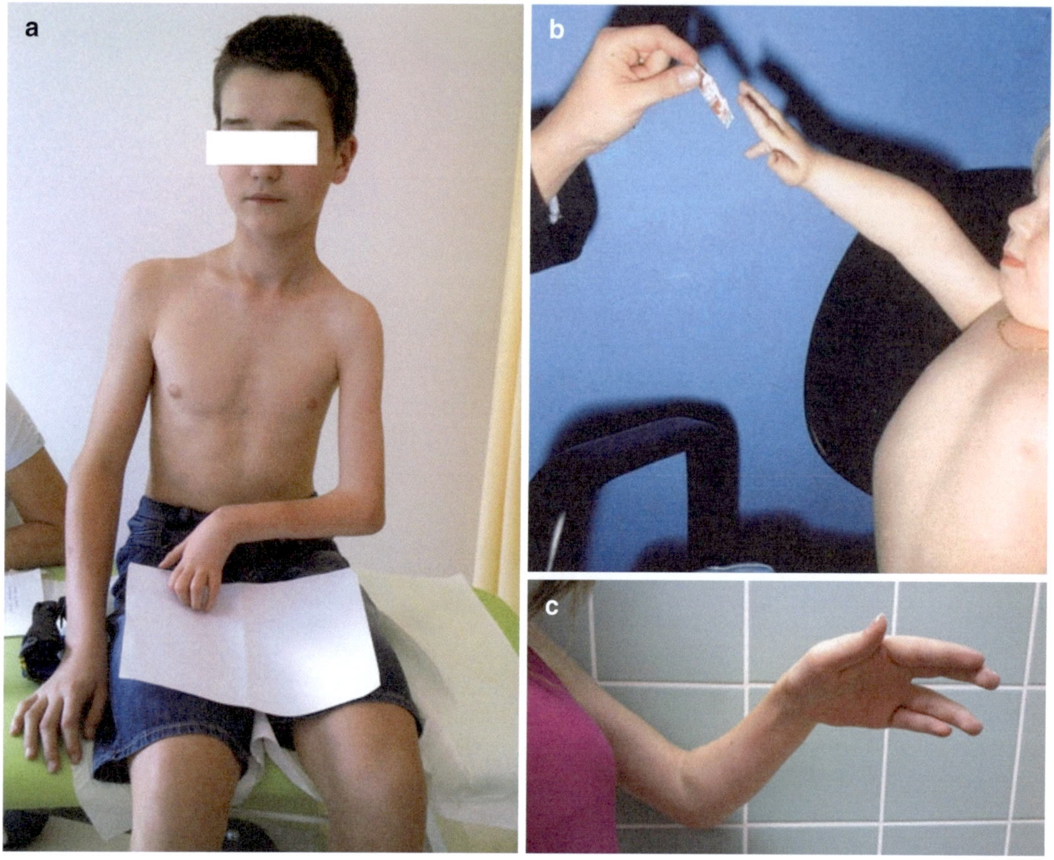

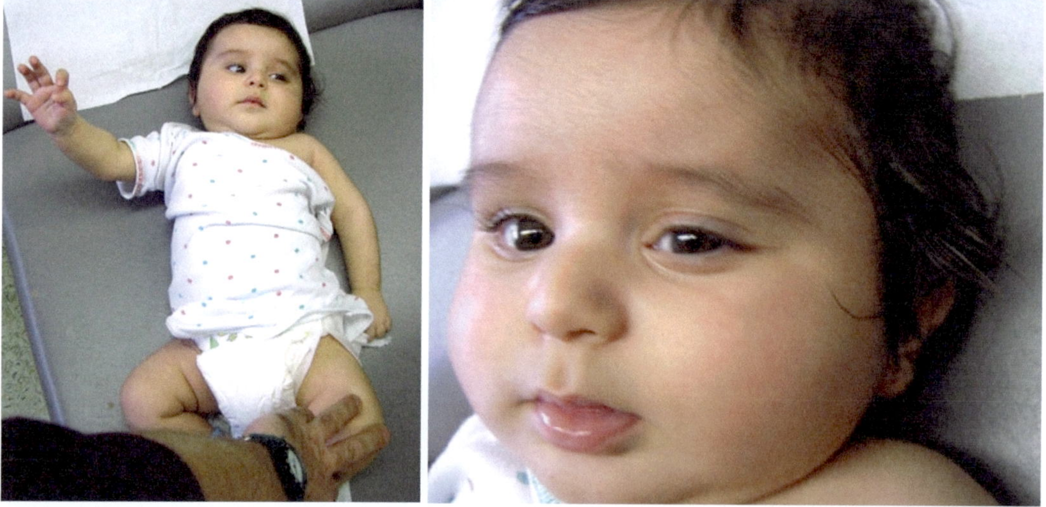

Fig. 1.6 (**a–c**) Compensating movements of the trunk to improve the muscle weakness at the shoulder (**a, b**); joint contractures (**a, c**)

Fig. 1.7 Claude Bernard-Horner-Trias in severe damage of the root Th1 with concomitant injury of the sympathetic nervous system (myosis, ptosis, enophthalmia)

plexus palsy, may indicate severe injury to the spinal nerve Th1.

1.2.6 Repeated Examinations

All these characteristics must be studied again at intervals of several months and the development must be documented (Chap. 4), as this is where the main arguments for surgical indications and the evaluation of therapeutic success lie.

We see the infants first every 2–3 months, after neural reconstructions every 6 months, later once a year until the growth of the body is completed or until the symptoms are relieved.

1.3 Significance for our Social Living

Children and adolescents with movement disorders of the upper extremities meet different social actors in different age groups and above all ignorant and, unfortunately, often intolerant peers, who react differently to the visible and function-changing body image changes and thus trigger increasingly disturbing perceptions in the adolescent, who originally experienced themselves as an infant in their own way as intact. These problems might accumulate in school age and during puberty.

We briefly outline the problems that lie ahead:

- *Preschool age*
  - Adaptation of toys, scooters and bicycles; participation in water sports and swimming courses
  - Integrative kindergarten places, coordination of physiotherapy within the kindergarten or outside
  - Understanding of teachers and friends, family members
  - Parallel involvement of parents with forensic and legal issues
- *School*
  - Adaptation of sports activities and their grading; inclusion

- Self-esteem, acceptance of the changed body image, social interaction with classmates
  - Discussion of the causality of changes and therapy options
  - Parents' position in decision-making processes (from caring to self-determination)
  - Teenagers experience themselves in front of the mirror and in front of their peers: they want to be inconspicuous
- *Education, level of physical disability*
  - Choice of education, restrictions
  - Curriculum vitae describing (or not) the degree of disability
  - Position regarding competitive sports and professional activities
  - Development of a long-term perspective
- *Occupation and social life*
  - Long-term physical stress at work
  - Load-dependent pain
  - Periods of incapacity for work
  - Possible late damage: shoulder complaints, early joint wear and tear
- *What about the parents?*
  - Guilt on the part of pregnant women?
  - Further desire to have children and planning childbirth?
  - Integration of the concerned child into the family community. Legal processing over 10 years and more
  - Demands on existing social services

References

1. Schünke M. Topographie und Funktion des Bewegungssystems. Stuttgart: Thieme; 2000.
2. Kummer B. Biomechanik–Form und Funktion des Bewegungsapparates. Köln: Deutscher Ärzteverlag; 2005.
3. Kline DG, Hudson AR, Kim DH. Atlas of peripheral nerve surgery. Philadelphia: Saunders; 2001.
4. Bahm J, Meinecke L, Brandenbusch V, Rau G, Disselhorst-Klug C. High spatial resolution electromyography and video-assisted movement analysis in children with obstetric brachial plexus palsy. Hand Clin. 2003;19:393–9.
5. Vojta V, Schweizer E. Die entdeckung der idealen motorik. Pflaum München. 2009.

History of Reconstructive Operations

A. Gohritz and M. Langer

2.1 Introduction

Muscle and nerve transfer operations are fascinating procedures in reconstructive surgery, as they can restore irreparably lost motion sequences. The function of paralysed or destroyed muscles can be restored either by shifting healthy tendon-muscle units (muscle transfer) or by using dispensable donor axons (nerve transfer) from the surrounding area.

Main Indications for Muscular or Nerve Transfer Surgery Include:

- **Lesions of the lower motoneuron**
  - Peripheral nerve injury of the upper extremity
    Brachial plexus, axillary nerve, suprascapular nerve, long thoracic, musculocutaneous nerve
    Radial, medianus, ulnar nerve, combined lesions
  - Peripheral nerve injury of the lower extremity
    Lumbosacral plexus, femoral nerve, sciatic nerve, tibial nerve, peroneal nerve
  - Diseases of the peripheral nervous system, for example, Charcot-Marie-Tooth syndrome, Hansen disease (leprosy), poliomyelitis, Guillain-Barré syndrome
- **Lesions of the upper motoneuron**
  - Spinal cord injury (at the cervical level, tetraplegia)
  - Traumatic brain injury (TBI)
  - Cerebrovascular insult (stroke)
  - Cerebral palsy
- **Destruction of the muscle-tendon-unit**
  - Direct tissue trauma (e.g., crush, rupture, burn, electrical injury)
  - Ischemia (compartment syndrome, Volkmann contracture)
  - Inflammation (especially rheumatoid arthritis)
  - Tumour (e.g., malignant soft tissue tumours)
- **Congenital malformations**
  - Hand and foot anomalies with missing muscles or anomalies of the tendon insertions

Historical observation shows that many of today's standard operations for movement disorders of the upper extremities can be traced back to concepts developed by mostly German-speaking surgeons and orthopaedic surgeons between the end of the nineteenth and the beginning of the twentieth centuries, gained pri-

A. Gohritz
Department of Plastic, Reconstructive and Aesthetic Surgery, Hand Surgery, University Hospital Basel, Basel, Switzerland

M. Langer (✉)
Department of Trauma, Hand, and Reconstructive Surgery, University Clinic Muenster, Muenster, Germany
e-mail: langer.martin@ukmuenster.de

© Springer Nature Switzerland AG 2021
J. Bahm (ed.), *Movement Disorders of the Upper Extremities in Children*,
https://doi.org/10.1007/978-3-030-53622-0_2

marily from the treatment of epidemic poliomyelitis and gunshot wounds in the First World War.

This historical review provides insight into the development of surgical restoration of lost nerve and muscle function, especially in brachialis plexus lesions. It presents some important protagonists from the time between 1880 and our time, with focus on the German-speaking countries.

2.2 Development of Operative Orthopaedics at the End of the Nineteenth Century

The historical development of modern reconstructive orthopaedics and surgery for movement disorders of the upper extremity takes place during an extremely turbulent time and reflects contemporary historical events and technological, social and political changes.

In the second half of the nineteenth century, apart from mechanical therapies (with the help of apparatus) and dynamic treatments (massage and physiotherapy), surgical treatment increasingly arises in orthopaedics. Surgery could in many cases significantly reduce the time, effort and cost of treatment, for example, by surgically severing contracted tendons in clubfoot or torticollis instead of stretching them over months and years as usual. The cutting of the Achilles tendon, reintroduced by G. F. Louis Strohmeyer (1804–1876) in 1831, was a ground-breaking example here. New techniques, such was arthrodeses, tendon grafts or later nerve procedures are introduced.

2.2.1 Scientific and Technological Conditions

At this time, new possibilities for diagnosis and surgical therapy of numerous diseases were created by scientific findings in physics, bacteriology, physiology and pharmacology. The decisive factor for the evolution of extremity surgery, however, was the introduction of a safe **pain management** in the middle of the nineteenth century and later the effective **avoidance of**

Table 2.1 Requirements for the development of modern extremity surgery and tendon and nerve transfer surgery at the transition from the nineteenth to the twentieth century

Prerequisites/technology	Type of procedure
Anaesthesia	Gas anaesthesia: nitrous oxide 1844 (Wells), ether 1846 (Morton and Warren), chloroform 1847 (Simpson) Peripheral nerve anaesthesia: cocaine infiltration 1892 (Schleich), finger block 1888 (Oberst) Intravenous regional anaesthesia 1908 (Bier)
Asepsis (sterility)	Hand hygiene 1847 (Semmelweis), rubber gloves 1894 (Halstead), disinfection of the operating field with iodine tincture 1908 (Grossich)
Antisepsis (bacterial reduction)	Carbolic spray 1867 (Lister), steam sterilization 1892 (by Bergmann and Schimmelbusch)
Bloodlessness	Rubber bandage 1854 (Esmarch)
Special diagnostics of nerve injuries	Nerve stimulation to differentiate between motor and sensitive fibres (ca. 1910), cervical myelography (1947), electromyography (1948), action potentials of peripheral nerves (1949), histamine test (1954)
Medical information exchange, especially between USA and Europe	Facilitated travel opportunities, increased number of medical journals/reports at congresses, emergence of major well-known centres with international visitors

wound infections (Table 2.1): "Antisepsis and asepsis led to a complete renewal of surgery and, after centuries of hospital wound infection, transformed the surgical departments into places that could be entered in the hope of leaving them alive again" [1].

Now it was possible that complex operations be carried out with a justifiable risk, e.g. joints opened, bones sawed through and straightened, muscles and tendons transferred, and nerves sutured. Surgeons and orthopaedists succeeded in performing procedures that were previously considered impossible, which were refined with increasing experience and after analysis of the clinical results. Another important factor was the rapidly increasing flow of medical information due to easier travel and the increasing number of scientific publications in journals and at congresses. Beginning with the turn of the century, there was a lively exchange of ideas and experiences among European and American surgeons, not only during congresses, but also during hospitalizations in the operating theatre. New ideas were quickly clinically tested, and joyful medical experimentation were hardly restricted, not least because the idea of medical liability does not yet existed [2].

2.2.2 Historical and Social Influences

Contemporary historical events and social and political changes also had a strong influence on the progress of surgical function restoration, as will be illustrated by examples that primarily affect the German-speaking countries (Table 2.2).

2.2.2.1 Epidemic Occurrence of Poliomyelitis

The industrialization changed the incidence of many diseases. Poliomyelitis epidemica anterior acuta (polio) is a viral infectious disease that affects the muscle-controlling nerve cells of the spinal cord and leads to death or permanent paralysis. The orthopaedist Jakob von Heine (1800–1879) from the Black Forest presented the clinical picture in 1840 in his book "Beobachtungen über Lähmungszustand der unteren Extremitäten und deren Behandlung" ("Observations on paralysis status of the lower extremities and their treatment"), and in the second edition of 1860 he coined the term "spinal poliomyelitis". By the end of the nineteenth century, polio was spreading at an alarming rate, presumably as a paradoxical consequence of improving hygiene and the resulting decline in (dirt-induced) autoimmunization, so that it was classified as an epidemic disease around 1880. Mostly children between the ages of 3 and 8 years were affected, less often also adolescents or persons into adulthood. From about 1910 onwards, regional epidemics were observed every 5–6 years in Europe and the USA, affecting thou-

Table 2.2 Contemporary historical events with relevance for the development of functional surgery

Year	Events relevant for the development of functional surgery
Since about 1880	Poliomyelitis epidemics in the USA and Europe (previously only endemic occurrence) with frequent subsequent paralysis, especially in children and adolescents
1883	Introduction of health insurance (1883), accident insurance (1884) and pension and disability insurance (1889) by Otto von Bismarck in Germany
1906	Germany-wide recording of all physically handicapped persons—"Reichskrüppelzählung" (German Reich Cripple Count)
1914–1918	First World War with typical gunshot wounds of trench warfare—millions of war wounded
1920	"Prussian Cripple Care Act" (entitlement of every physically disabled person up to the age of 15 to get free treatment and education)
1939–1945	Second World War
1960s to 1980s	Increase in motorization, especially with motorcycles, helmet duty, increased survival of (polytraumatized) patients with severe nerve injuries

sands of people and mainly leaving behind children with physical sequelae.

2.2.2.2 Introduction of New Insurance Systems (e. g. in Germany by Bismarck in 1883)

As a political innovation at the end of the nineteenth century, politicians felt compelled to respond to the needs of the ordinary population—not so much out of compassion as to calm down radical and socialist influences. In 1883, Reich Chancellor Otto von Bismarck introduced new statutory insurance systems, primarily aimed at workers. His motives were political in nature, he wanted to avoid social unrest and to withdraw the influence of the church and labour unions with his own voluntary insurances. "My thought was to win the working classes, or should I say, bribe them, to see the state as a social institution that exists because of them and wants to care for their well-being" [3]. This required a substantial improvement in the medical care of the population, any sick or injured person could now claim medical treatment. Even long-term treatment was possible if, for example, injuries were recognized as an occupational accident.

2.2.2.3 Recording of the Physically Handicapped in the German Reich ("Cripple Count") 1906 and "Prussian Cripple Care Act" (1920)

The next decisive stage was the so-called "**Cripple Care**" from which "war orthopaedics" and later "peace orthopaedics" develops. The central event of this development was the registration of all physically disabled people in the German Reich on 1 October 1906, known as the "Reichskrüppelzählung" (Cripple Count). "Cripple" was not a pejorative term then, it simply meant a physically handicapped person.

The orthopaedist **Konrad Biesalski** (1868–1930) (Fig. 2.1) noted the high number of physically handicapped children as a school doctor. He saw the main task of his specialist area in the "research and treatment of the pathological conditions of the musculoskeletal system under socio-biological indication" [4]. For him the "cripple" (physically handicapped) was not a helpless and frail "sick" and thus objects of the church's care for the poor. He defined him as a curable sick person to whom a special "care" must be devoted with the aim of reintegrating him or her socially and professionally into society: "The cripple is to become employable, in short, a taxpayer from a pauper, a parasitic to a productive one, a social member of human society from an antisocial one. If this is achieved through sufficient welfare facilities, many millions of cripples who are unable to work will be released for other purposes every year, and just as many millions […] will be earned anew through the work of the cripples who have been made fit for work" [5].

Biesalski enforced this nationwide survey for the benefit of disabled people—and in the interest of orthopaedic physicians. Planning and evaluation were inadequate and the number of children and adults declared to be "in need of care" are far

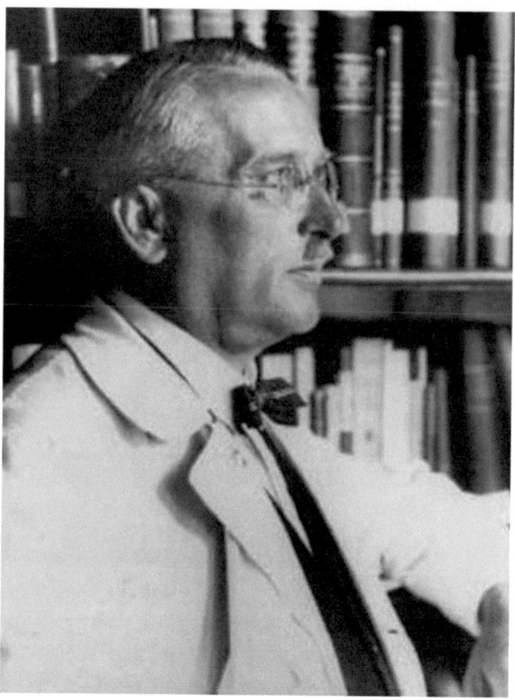

Fig. 2.1 In 1906, Konrad Biesalski (1868–1930) initiated the nationwide registration of all physically disabled persons (so-called "Reichskrüppelzählung"). Its aim is to empower those affected: "…to turn a charity recipient into a taxpayer". This was achieved by means of a socio-medical concept consisting of medical, pedagogical and vocational measures (cripple care), which today can be regarded as the basis of modern rehabilitation and care for the disabled [6]

exaggerated. The real data were withheld from the public in order not to jeopardize the development of the new care branch. The propagated figures suggested a blatant imbalance between the excessive demand for orthopaedic therapy and the negligible supply of it. The suffering of the physically handicapped and the desire to save on social expenses became a convincing argument for the expansion of orthopaedics throughout the country: the importance of the subject is greatly increased overall, and in 1924 orthopaedics becomes a compulsory subject in medical training [6]. This takeover of surgical tasks is not always welcomed: "The orthopaedists are robbers and take the surgeons one field of work after the other—and Fritz Lange is the worst", said the surgical professor in Munich, Erich Lexer (1867–1937), about his orthopaedic colleague [7].

Thanks to public attention, government grants and a high willingness of the population to donate, further large orthopaedic clinics could be built within a short period of time. Famous examples are the Oskar Helene-Heim in Berlin (run by Biesalski himself) or the Staatliche Orthopädische Klinik in Munich (under Fritz and later his nephew Max Lange). Almost all renowned orthopaedic clinics owe their foundation to the Krüppelfürsorge, the "detour via the home for cripples" [8]. Patient accumulation in these large orthopaedic treatment centres enabled the testing and establishment of innovative surgical methods [6].

After the First World War, despite the greatest financial problems, the "Prussian Cripple Care Act" was passed on 6 May 1920, which brought the breakthrough to orthopaedics and rehabilitation medicine. It granted every child up to the age of 15 the right for free orthopaedic treatment, schooling and vocational training, which was unique in the world.

All this would hardly have been possible without the numbers manipulated by Biesalski himself, the results of the Reichskrüppelzählung appear from today's point of view as "lie for a good purpose" [6].

2.2.2.4 Treatment of the Injured Extremities of the First World War 1914–1918

Since the beginning of the First World War and even afterwards, surgeons and orthopaedists had to deal with the treatment of the typical injury consequences of trench warfare. At the outbreak of war, 111 clinics and counselling centres were available throughout Germany for the care of injured soldiers ("war cripples"), which were set up as a result of Biesalski's initiative [5]. The treatment concepts developed in "cripple care" were successfully transferred for "war orthopaedics" to treat the paralysis patterns following nerve and muscle destruction as a result of gunshot wounds.

More than four million disabled persons remained on the German side, while in 1924 more than 650,000 war-disabled persons with a 25% reduction in earning capacity were still entitled to benefit from a pension.

During the First World War, there were many innovative developments in the field of orthopaedic technology, but also in surgical methods. This applied above all to muscle replacement operations on the upper extremities (Table 2.3): "While before the war tendon transfers for wrists and finger joints had not gone beyond sparse experiments, tendon plasties for irreparable radial paralysis can now be counted among the most grateful operations in orthopaedic surgery", wrote Perthes in 1922 [9].

2.3 Historical Development of Tendon and Muscle Transfers

2.3.1 Early Pioneering Work

At the end of the nineteenth century, muscle paralysis was almost exclusively the late consequence of poliomyelitis. A complicated apparatus supply was mostly used for the stabilization of the paralytic floating joints. For example, for the unstable shoulder caused by paralysis (Fig. 2.2) a construct consisting of belts and a shoulder ring was recommended, on the inside of which three inflatable cushions were attached "so that the joint can be given the necessary support without causing pressure on nerves or vessels" [29]. These bandages and apparatus were expensive and unaffordable for the thousands of sufferers, so that here the "cheaper" (and more effective) methods, such as joint stiffening or muscle transfers surgery, were used.

The surgeon **Carl Nicoladoni** (1847–1902) from Graz was the first to publish the idea of restoring the function of a paralysed muscle by shifting an adjacent healthy muscle in 1880. He replaced the function of the triceps surae by transferring both peroneal tendons—albeit with limited success due to separation of the tendons [31]. Previously, Tillaux (1869) and Duplay (1876) had already shifted tendons, but in the case of irreparable extensor tendon injuries. Muscle transfer operations were initially performed much more often on the lower extremity than on the arm and hand. The reason for this was the typical paralysis pattern of poliomyelitis, which is the main

Table 2.3 Development of tendon transfer surgery

Year	Describer, origin	Work/technique
1869 1874	Tillaux, France Duplay, France	Tendon transfers for extensor tendon defects
1880	Nicoladoni, Austria	First tendon transfer in case of polio-induced foot deformity (peroneal tendons on triceps surae)—only short success, recurrence due to separation of the tendons
1891	Hoffa, Germany	"Lehrbuch der orthopädischen Chirurgie" (Text book of orthopaedic surgery)—first standard work of orthopaedic surgery
1894	Drobnik, Poland	Extensor tendon replacement surgery on the hand in partial radial palsy (poliomyclitis)
1897	Franke, Germany	Extensor tendon transfer for complete radialis palsy
1897	Rochet, France	Tendon transfer and release on forearm and hand in spastic hemiplegia
1899	Codivilla, Italy	Fundamental studies on tendon transfer in the lower and upper extremities in poliomyelitis and cerebral palsy, e.g., tibialis posterior transfer, early opponensplasty (flexor digitorum superficialis of little finger), recommends early mobilization
1902	Vulpius, Germany	"Tendon transplantation and its use in the treatment of paralysis", Deltoideus-pro-triceps replacement
1903	Reiner, Austria [10]	Tenodesis (partial arthrodesis)
1910	Vulpius, Germany [11]	"The Treatment of Spinal Poliomyelitis"
1913, 1920, 1924	Vulpius and Stoffel, Germany [12]	"Orthopaedic surgery" (3 editions)—standard indications and techniques for muscle transposition, e.g., Brachioradialis-pro-extensor carpi radialis
1914	Henze and Mayer, USA	Studies on tendon adhesions, especially with the use of alloplastic material (silk strings)
1916	Biesalski, Germany	Triceps-to-biceps transfer
1916	Mayer, USA [13]	Biceps-to-triceps transfer
1916 1919/1920	Schmidt, Germany Lexer, Germany	Latissimus transfer as biceps replacement
1916	Biesalski, Germany Mayer, USA	"Physiological tendon transplantation"—techniques of tendon transfer, tendinous and periosteal fixation
1916/1921	Jones, England	New techniques for tendon replacement, especially PT-ECRB (today's standard surgery for wrist extensor replacement)
1917 1918	Schulze-Berge, Germany	Pectoralis major transfer for biceps replacement
1918/1919	Steindler, USA [14]	Biceps replacement by proximalization of the forearm muscles
1918	Perthes, Germany	"Four tendon plasty" with extensor tenodesis at the wrist during restoration of radial nerve function
1921	Huber, Germany [15]	Opponensplasty with abductor digiti minimi muscle—today mostly used in thumb hypoplasia
1922	Bunnell, USA	Atraumatic technique, bloodlessness with tourniquet, tendon grafts (Palmaris longus, FDS, toe extensors), nerve suturing/reconstruction before muscle transfer, fat grafts as sliding tissues, tendon redirections (pulleys)
1922	Starr, USA	Basic rules for tendon transfers, division of donor muscles
1943	Sudeck, Germany [16]	Simultaneous nerve reconstruction and simplified tendon transfer in radial palsy ("inner splint")
1944, 1948	Bunnell, USA [17]	"Surgery of the Hand"—basics of modern hand surgery, in 2nd ed. 1948: first functional reconstruction for C6 tetraplegia

Table 2.3 (continued)

Year	Describer, origin	Work/technique
1946	Merle d'Aubigné, France [18]	Classic technique for radialis replacement (pronator teres to extensor carpi radialis brevis, flexor carpi ulnaris to extensor digitorum communis, palmaris longus to extensor pollicis longus)
1949	Littler, USA [19]	Function reconstruction in combined nerve lesions on the hand with tendon transfer and arthrodesis
1952	Brand, USA	"Reconstruction of the Hand in Leprosy"—motor (and sensitive) reconstruction for leprosy
1956	Pulvertaft, England [20]	Interlacing technique to the tendon suture
1957	Zancolli, Argentina	Zancolli lasso plasty surgery for intrinsic hand muscle paralysis
1960, 1962	Boyes, USA [21, 22]	Selection of the donor muscles, counts 58 different methods of radial nerve palsy, new idea: FDS 4-transfer
1967	Saha, India	"Surgery of the Paralyzed and Flail Shoulder"
1967	Zancolli, Argentina [23]	Re-routing of the biceps tendon to correct supination contracture
1968/1979	Zancolli, Argentina [24]	"Structural and Dynamic Bases of Hand Surgery"—functional reconstruction in peripheral nerve and plexus lesion, cerebral palsy and tetraplegia
1970	Tamai, Japan [25]	Microsurgical transplantation of functional muscle tendon units
1985	Brand, USA	"Clinical Mechanics of the Hand"—biomechanics of muscle function and transposition, influence of muscle architecture on muscle transfer surgery
1979	Moberg, Sweden	"The Upper Limb in Tetraplegia"—basics of arm and hand function reconstruction, classification, international meeting on tetraplegia surgery
1985	Steinau and Biemer, Germany	Muscle transfer surgery after extremity preserving resection of malignant soft tissue tumours
1992	Lieber, USA [26]	Influence of the muscle architecture of forearm and hand muscles on muscle transfer surgery
1994	Ninkovic, Austria [27]	Simultaneous neuro-musculo-tendinous transfer (gastrocnemius transposition with microsurgical nerve connection to peroneal nerve in case of drop foot)
2002	Lieber, USA and Fridén, Sweden, [28]	Experimental studies on optimal muscle tension (including laser diffraction) and influence of muscle architecture
2010	Fridén, Sweden	Alphabet operation for single-step reconstruction of active flexion and passive extension of thumb and fingers and intrinsic hand function in tetraplegia, early mobilization possible after stable side-to-side tendon sutures

cause of paralysis and which rarely rises to the upper extremity [32]. The Polish paediatrician Drobnik transferred this idea to the upper extremity in 1894 and restored the extensor functions in partial radial palsy (polio) [33].

Felix Franke (1860–1937), a surgeon from Braunschweig, performed a tendon transfer operation in 1897 in a complete radial nerve palsy. He transferred the tendons of the flexor carpi ulnaris muscle to the finger extensors and of the flexor carpi radialis muscle to the abductor pollicis muscle and extensor carpi radialis brevis muscle, as well as a tenodesis of both radial wrist extensors. He thus could "rightly claim that there is no more incurable radial paralysis as long as at least the median nerve and ulnar nerve are not paralyzed" [34].

Alessandro Codivilla (1861–1912), director of the Rizzoli Orthopaedic Institute in Bologna, conducted fundamental studies on tendon transfers in the lower and upper extremities in poliomyelitis and cerebral palsy and recognize important principles such as the distinction between paralysed and muscles which are only atrophic due to inactivity and the ideal of a balance between agonists and antagonists. He described the first opponensplasty (by means of FDS 5) and recommended postoperative early mobilization of the transferred muscles [35, 36].

Oscar Vulpius from Heidelberg (1867–1936) (Fig. 2.3) was one of the first to scientifically examine muscle transfer operations in his 1902 work

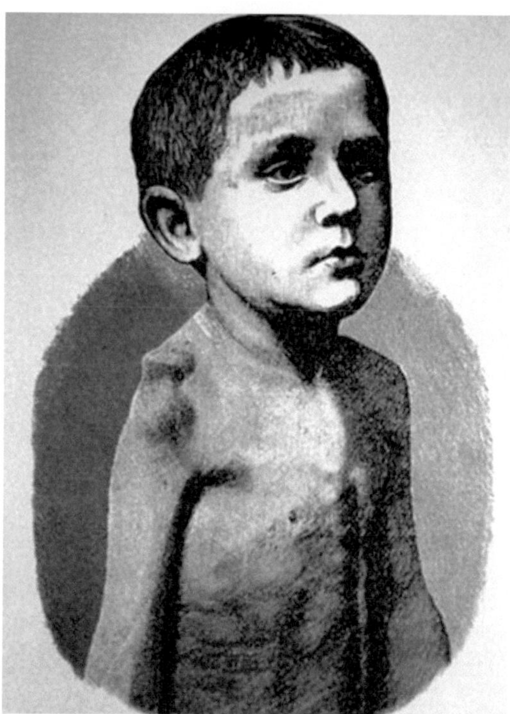

Fig. 2.2 Typical "floating shoulder" as a result of polio-myelitis: "If these muscles become functionally incapacitated for any reason, the capsule loses its tension, but the arm sinks, following its weight and the pull of the internal rotators, as far down as the slack capsule allows. The weight of the arm now constantly pulls on the atonic capsule and is thus able to stretch it significantly. But this destroys the function of the joint, and the result is a floating joint."… "The whole arm is dangling from the flaccid capsule…. Likewise the use of the hand is very limited by the hyperpronation of the forearm" [29, 30]

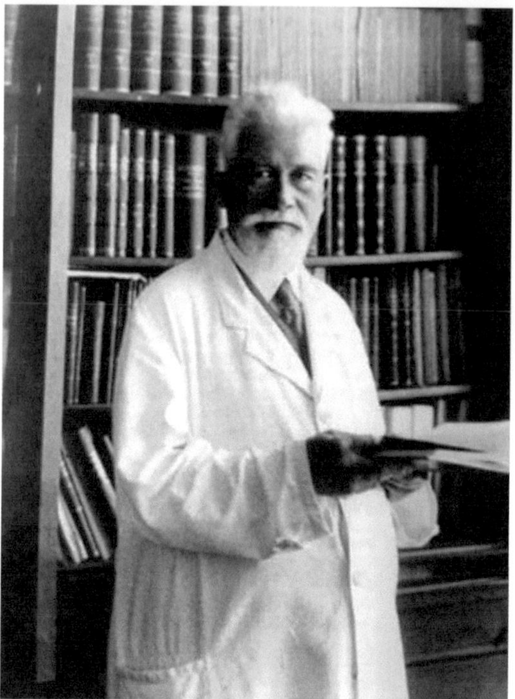

Fig. 2.3 As early as 1900, Oskar Vulpius (1867–1936) intensively studied the idea of tendon transfers for paralysis of the extremities, its surgical techniques and follow-up treatment. His admonishing words are still valid today: "Anyone who reaches for a knife to perform an orthopaedic operation thus assumes the moral obligation to carry out the after-treatment in an exact manner. Those who cannot meet this demand due to a lack of special talent, inclination or time, or who lack the necessary facilities, should correctly keep their hand off the knife." (Courtesy of the archive of the Vulpius-Klinik Bad Rappenau)

"Die Sehnenverpflanzung und ihre Verwertung in der Behandlung der Lähmungen" (Tendon Transplantation and Their Use in the Treatment of Paralyses). His focus was on the treatment of the consequences of polio, which mainly affected the lower extremity, but he also gave numerous case descriptions of tendon grafts on the upper extremity. It was a comprehensive presentation of the cases published so far, with own experiences and comments. Vulpius described twelve cases of tendon transfers in extensor injuries and nine cases of flexor tendon injuries in the hand, including four cases of radial palsy. Interestingly, he already used a braiding suture technique, as it was later utilized by **Guy Pulvertaft** (1907–1986). The respective passage in the text shows his deep understanding of tendon physiology: "Where the strain on the tendons is particularly strong, where a sufficiently long immobilisation of the operated extremity is not ensured, where the nature of the tendon gives reason to fear that the tendon sutures will be pulled out, one can place one or the other looped suture between the button sutures. The crossing tours of the suture may, of course, cover only a part of the tendon in order not to endanger its nutrition [37, 38]".

In 1913 (Part 1, 1911), Vulpius and his attending physician **Adolf Stoffel** (1880–1937) published their work "Orthopaedic Surgery", unrivalled for almost 40 years, with numerous standard techniques of muscle transfers which are still valuable today, in current paralysis patterns (Fig. 2.4). The second important basic work, with experimental and clinical studies, was completed as early as the summer of 1914, but

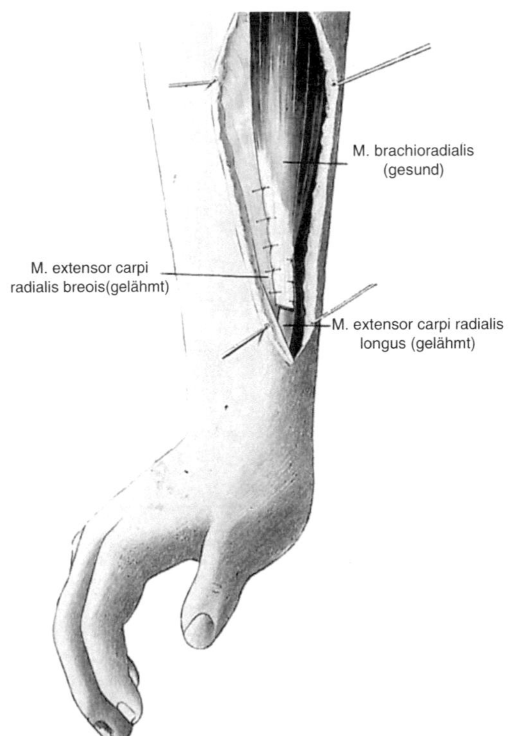

Fig. 2.4 Vulpius and Stoffel provided the first description of the restoration of wrist extension by transposition of the healthy brachioradialis muscle onto the paralysed radial wrist extensors, extensor carpi radialis longus et brevis. Today, this method is classically used for the reconstruction of a passive key pinch reconstruction in individuals with high tetraplegia (functional group 1). (From: [8])

was not published until 1916 due to the start of the war—"Physiological tendon transplantation", written by Biesalski and his assistant **Leo Mayer** (1884–1972) [39] from the USA. They are investigating experimentally and clinically the different possibilities of tendon transfer and fixation.

2.3.2 Period of the First World War

Due to the enormous number of cases during the First World War, orthopaedic surgeries for the treatment of paralysis after nerve injuries were gaining enormous importance, with the focus shifting from the lower to the upper extremity.

At the end of his book, Biesalski reports on "Clinical experiences after completion of the manuscript":

Since the manuscript of the book was already finished in August 1914, during the 2 years that have passed since then, there has of course been ample opportunity to apply the physiological tendon transplantation to the large paralysis material of my clinic, in which so far more than 300 individual tendon transplantations have been performed. Subject to later critical publication, it can already be generally said today that the successes were very satisfactory, even surprisingly good in some cases, and that in the rare cases where failures occurred, technical mistakes were also regularly proven. Also with spastic paralyses, tendon transplantations were carried out more frequently than earlier with good success… With war injuries, tendon transplantations were often carried out on the hand … [40].

Muscle and tendon transfers functioned even better than after poliomyelitis, as in comparison an "excellent substitute" of non-paralysed donor muscles was available. Biesalski himself took over a military hospital department in Berlin, where he was assisted by a single assistant to look after the 500 soldiers accommodated there. Nerve and tendon plasties, the therapy of infectious complications of the central nervous system, bones and joints occupied the largest part of their work. The hospital in Zehlendorf, which has up to 300 beds, was supervised by Biesalski's research assistant, the American Leo Mayer, until the USA entered the war in spring 1917 [5]. A large number of the surgical techniques still used today were developed between 1914 and 1920 (Table 2.3).

2.3.3 1920s to 1930s

In many countries, orthopaedics is making enormous progress by treating war-wounded patients. After the end of the war, Stoffel [41] summarized his experiences:

Despite the fact that poliomyelitis, the main source of tendon operations in peace, hardly ever produces any work for the military hospital, interventions on the muscle tendon tract are often on the list of operating theatres…. The new explosive ordnance often causes exceptionally severe soft tissue injuries. Over a longer distance, several adjacent tendons and muscles are torn apart, often to form a mush. The suppuration that soon begins destroys further parts of the tendon substance. If the unusual functions are of a highly important nature, they must be replaced at all costs. The present way of fighting means that injuries are more frequently observed on the upper than on the lower extremity. Injuries of the hand and fingers equipped with numerous tendons still predominate here, which require strongest help like no other member. Creating a useful working hand is therefore one of our most urgent tasks.

Borchardt wrote in 1922 [42] in the Handbook of Medical Experiences in the World War: "I consider it a malpractice not to draw the attention of the injured to the possibility of surgical treatment".

In Great Britain, **Sir Robert Jones** (1857–1933) tries and tests new techniques for tendon replacement, above all the today classical method for wrist extensor tendon transfer in radial palsy by transposition of the pronator teres muscle to the extensor carpi radialis brevis muscle (Jones 1916, [43]).

Sterling Bunnell (1882–1957), Captain of the US Army Medical Corps, treated countless war injuries on the front lines in France and concentrated his entire interest on reconstructive hand surgery: ground-breaking and new are the tendon and nerve transplantations he performed to bridge defects after severe hand trauma, special pull-out wire sutures for tendon reconstructions and dynamic splints in the after-treatment [44]. In his works published between 1918 and 1922, he propagated, among other things, atraumatic tissue treatment, operations in bloodlessness with tourniquet, use of free tendon grafts and primary nerve suture, and reconstruction before undertaking muscle replacement operations. He thus laid the foundations of modern hand surgery, before his book "Surgery of the Hand" was published in 1944 (2nd edition in 1948), which also included the experiences of the Second World War. Marc Iselin (1898–1937) from Nanterre wrote in 1938 the work "Chirurgie de la Main", which was later translated into several languages. From 1941 onwards, he was almost exclusively engaged in hand surgery, including functional reconstructive surgery.

Important Principles for Tendon Transposition According to Bunnell (Published 1918–1922):
– Bloodlessness in the operative field achieved by tourniquet
– Atraumatic surgical technique
– Fatty tissue as a gliding aid for tendons
– Preservation/creation of tendon redirections (pulleys)
– Avoidance of central palmar incisions to avoid contractures
– Free tendon grafts (Palmaris longus, FDS or toe extensors)
– Careful progressive splinting to improve contractures
– Preparation of the wound bed in case of scarring by tissue flaps
– Early, but not exaggerated, motion exercises
– Opponensplasty with flexor carpi ulnaris muscle as donor muscle (redirected via the os pisiforme).
– Principle of "one tendon—one function"
– The principles of primary nerve suture and reconstruction to be observed
– Epineural suture, fine silk threads, significantly better results with distal nerve sutures
– Attention to sensibility and its significance for the hand function

2.3.4 Second World War (1939–1945)

The Second World War again caused countless gunshot wounds to the upper extremity, especially the radial nerve. Starting with the "Viersehnenplastik" (four-tendon-plasty) according to Perthes [45], German authors tested different variants with tenodesis of the wrist and force transmission by muscle transfers to all finger tendons of the extensor side. Instead of the tenodesis that eliminated wrist flexion, an attempt was made to achieve active hand extension by shifting the flexor carpi radialis muscle, the brachioradialis muscle or the palmaris longus muscle. In 1943, Paul Sudeck (1866–1945) described a "single-tendon plasty" with the flexor carpi ulnaris muscle transfer simultaneously with the radial nerve reconstruction in order to immediately restore stability and function to the patient by "internal splinting" without an external orthosis—a simple and effective technique that has proven beneficial in special indications until today. In 1944, Bunnell's book "Surgery of the Hand" was published, which became the official textbook of the US Army and found worldwide recognition.

2.3.5 Post-War Period

After the Second World War, pioneers like **Marc Iselin** (1898–1987), **Robert Merle d'Aubigné** (1900–1989) and **Raoul Tubiana** (1915–2013) in France, **Guy Pulvertaft** (1907–1986), **Douglas Lamb** (1921–2001) in Great Britain, and **Paul Brand** (1914–2003), **William Littler** (1915–2005) and **Daniel Riordan** (1917–2002) in the USA developed a variety of different techniques [46]. **Joseph Boyes** (1905–1995) collected a total of 58 techniques of radial nerve plasty described until then and contributed a new standard technique using the FDS 4 tendon as donor [47]. Despite this enormous variety, a muscular distribution pattern can be observed in the most frequently used techniques, which, however, show differences in the international comparison of the various "surgical schools". Wrist extension is usually restored by transferring the median-innervated pronator teres muscle to the extensor carpi radialis brevis muscle (according to Jones 1916). In Germany, however, the Perthes wrist tenodesis lasted until after the Second World War before the advantages of active wrist mobility were appreciated. In Germany and France, the Merle d'Aubigné operation is still the most common basic technique which restores finger extension by transfer of the flexor carpi ulnaris tendon. According to Brand's advice to keep the FCU as a wrist stabilizer, the flexor carpi radialis muscle is more frequently used for this purpose in the USA.

Due to medical progress (e.g., vaccinations since 1962) poliomyelitis disappeared, but the indications for muscle transfer surgery are extended to other patient groups with irreparable functional losses, for example, due to brachial plexus lesions, spinal cord injuries (tetraplegia), spastic paralysis, rheumatoid arthritis or nerve diseases such as leprosy. Here, again, the use of

innovatively thinking individuals was crucial, who are considered by their contemporaries often with scepticism or even resistance. Two examples illustrate this impressively.

The Swedish surgeon **Erik Moberg** (1905–1993) (Fig. 2.5) devoted himself entirely to the functional reconstruction of the arms and hands of tetraplegic individuals after his retirement, for which he had previously not had sufficient time. Through worldwide contacts and untiring pioneering work, he managed to reopen this "forbidden field" internationally after failed attempts from the 1950s to the 1960s. The international classification and meaningful guidelines conceived by Moberg and others stand at

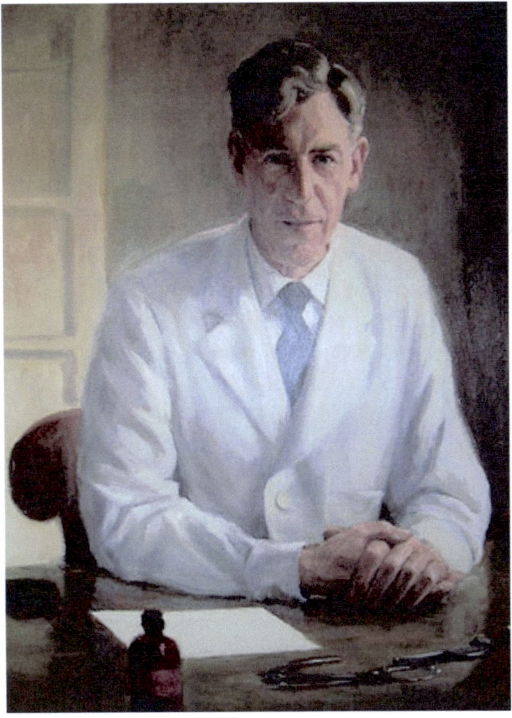

Fig. 2.5 Erik Moberg (1905–1993) became head of the first independent department for hand and extremity surgery in Europe in Gothenburg, Sweden in 1958. After his retirement in 1970, he devoted himself primarily to the surgical reconstruction of arm and hand function in tetraplegic individuals and through his commitment achieved a worldwide exchange of experience, which led to a classification and recognized therapy principles in this field that is still valid today. An international meeting, founded by him for the first time in 1978, continues to take place every 3 years

the beginning of an ongoing development of specialized tetraplegia hand surgery ([48, 49, 50]), which still today gives many patients more self-determination, mobility, privacy and independence.

The British hand surgeon **Paul Brand** (1914–2003) showed that in Hansen's disease (leprosy), ulcers and loss of extremity parts result from a lack of protective sensitivity caused by bacterial neuropathy—and not, as previously assumed, as a direct consequence of the disease itself. He became famous for his tendon transfers on the hands and plastic surgical restoration of the face in leprosy. His experience was based on the surgical treatment of victims of the London bomb war and the treatment of polio patients during the Second World War. For research, rehabilitation and facilitated reintegration of leprosy patients, he founded the New Life Centre in 1950 in Vellore, India, with workshops and huts where patients lived and learnt new skills. Later he transferred his studies and therapy concepts for pain perception ("The Gift of Pain") to other neuropathies, for example, diabetic polyneuropathy. His research on the biomechanics of muscle function in the forearm and hand, particularly with regard to muscle transfer, became the basic knowledge of hand surgeons and physiotherapists [51, 52].

2.3.6 1970s Until Today

Increased motorization in the post-war period increased the number of brachial plexus injuries, particularly due to motorcycle accidents. With the establishment of microsurgery, however, muscle transfer operations were decreasing, even being partially forgotten. Patients with complex nerve injuries, where microsurgical reconstruction attempts failed, are often left without further treatment. However, the emerging awareness of the often remaining residual defects after microsurgical reconstruction—especially in proximal lesions—led to a return of muscle transfers in the 1980s. Patients with extremity preservation in malignant soft tissue tumours often also benefited from muscle trans-

fer surgery, which markedly improved the usability of an arm or leg, even after oncological resection of entire muscle groups [53]. Lieber and Fridén (2002) used experimental and clinical studies to clarify the important role played by the architecture and tension of the donor muscle in excursion and force development during muscle transfer. They measure the intraoperative length differences of the sarcomere, the smallest contractile muscle unit, by means of laser diffraction.

2.4 Historical Development of Peripheral Nerve Surgery and Nerve Transfer Surgery

2.4.1 Beginnings

Parallel to tendon transfers, peripheral nerve reconstruction and nerve transfer surgery developed (Table 2.4). A prerequisite for this evolution was an improved understanding of the anatomy, physiology and pathology of the peripheral nervous system. Since antiquity, the processes of nerve degeneration and regeneration were largely unknown until the works of Augustus Waller (1856–1922) and Santiago Ramon y Cajal (1852–1934) [54] at the end of the nineteenth century (Table 2.4). False ideas about nerve regeneration were often the reason for absurd treatment dogmata, erroneous techniques and poor clinical results. Examples are instruments for excessive nerve stretching or nerve flaps with the aim of bridging the defect [55, 56].

The orthopaedic surgeon **Adolf Stoffel** (1880–1937) (Fig. 2.6), who has fallen into oblivion today, recognized as early as 1909 that nerves are not "rope-like structures" like tendons, but that their "topography" consists of functionally different motor and sensory fibres. Based on nerve cross-section studies, he developed techniques for neurotomy and nerve transfers in the upper and lower extremities. Stoffel worked at the University Institute of Anatomy in Heidelberg before starting his orthopaedic surgical training with his mentor Vulpius who promoted his anatomical studies and later development of clinical

Table 2.4 Development of peripheral nerve reconstruction surgery and nerve transfer surgery

Year/period	Protagonist, country of origin	Event/description
Old Testament, Bible (ca. 1500 BC)	Jacob, Israel	First description of a nerve lesion—presumably sciatic nerve lesion during a fight with a renegade angel (Genesis 32: 25–33): "... and he limped at his hip"
Antiquity, ca. 400 B.C.	Hippocrates (460–377 BC), Greece	No treatment of nerve injuries, fear of complications (convulsion and death)
About 300 BC	Herophilus (325–255 BC), Greece	Greatest anatomist of antiquity, distinguishes between tendons and nerves (sensitive and motor parts)
1608	Ferrara, Italy	First suture after nerve transection
1828	Fluorens (Italy)	Nerve transfer from the flexor to extensor side of the chicken wing
1851	Waller, UK	Degeneration and regeneration of nerves after transection
1863/1870	Phillipeaux/Vulpian, France	Nerve interposition (hypoglossal nerve/lingual nerve)
1864	Nélaton, France	Secondary nerve suture
1871	Hueter, Germany	Primary epineural nerve suture
1873	Létiévant, France	Nerve plasty, e.g., end-to-end neurorrhaphy
1875	Albert, Austria	Clinical use of (xenogenic) nerve interposition grafts
1882	Vanlair, France	Successful nerve tubulation (bone) to bridge about 3 cm of sciatic nerve
Since 1890	Ramon y Cajal, Spain	Histology of peripheral nerves, detection of axonal sprouting after cutting nerves
1910, 1912	Stoffel, Germany	Nerve cross-section studies, topography of sensitive and motor fibres, selective neurectomy in spasticity (Stoffel operation, 1911)
1915	Hofmann, Germany Tinel, France	Tapping sign for nerve damage/regeneration
1914	Heineke, Erlacher, Germany [57, 58, 59]	Direct muscle neurotization (implantation of a nerve stump)
1914–1920	Foerster, Germany	Special symptomatology and therapy of more than 4000 gunshot wounds of peripheral nerves—Basis for modern techniques of nerve suture, reconstruction with interposition grafts and nerve transfers (summarized in 1929)
1939	Bunnell and Boyes, USA	"Cable grafting for nerve bridging"
1940	Young and Medawar, England	Fibrin glue for nerve coaptation (spinal accessory and ulnar nerve)
1943	Seddon, England	Classification of nerve injury into 1. Neuropraxia, 2. Axonotmesis and 3. Neurotmesis
1948	Lurje, Russia	Nerve transfers at shoulder and upper arm
1951	Sunderland, Australia [60]	Five degrees of nerve lesions (based on Seddon's classification)
1960	Jacobsen, USA	Surgery under the microscope for injuries to extremities
1962	Millesi, Austria [61]	Tension-free fascicular nerve suture and nerve graft interposition
1964	Smith, USA	Microsurgery of peripheral nerves
1965	Benassy, France	First nerve transfer in tetraplegia (Brachialis branch to median nerve)
1968, 1978	Sunderland, Australia	"Nerves and Nerve Injuries": mainly studies on nerve topography
1972	Seddon, UK	"Disorders of the Peripheral Nerves"
1976	Taylor and Ham, Australia	Free vascularized nerve transplants
1988	Mackinnon and Dellon, USA [62]	"Surgery of the Peripheral Nerve", summary of the state of knowledge, in particular microsurgery, nerve decompression, pain treatment (neuroma) and sensitivity measurement, subdivision of nerve injuries into 6 grades
1988	Lundborg, Sweden	"Nerve Injury and Repair" (nerve injury and regeneration)

(continued)

Table 2.4 (continued)

Year/period	Protagonist, country of origin	Event/description
1992	Millesi, Austria	"Surgery of the peripheral nerves"—anatomy and surgical techniques
1994	Oberlin, France, Leechavengvongs, Thailand etc.	Proximal nerve fascicle transfers for the reconstruction of biceps and shoulder function, especially in upper plexus lesion
2004	Kuiken, Dumanian, USA [63]	"Targeted muscle reinnervation" (targeted nerve transfer for intuitive control of bionic prostheses after arm and leg amputation)
2004	Lundborg, Sweden	"The Nerve and the Brain"—interaction of hand and brain—brain plasticity
2010 until today	Bertelli, Brazil, Mackinnon, USA and others.	Proximal and distal nerve transport transfers in injuries of the brachial plexus, distal trunk nerves and spinal cord injury (tetraplegia)
2011, 2017	Xu, China	Contralateral C7-reinnervation in spastic hemiplegia

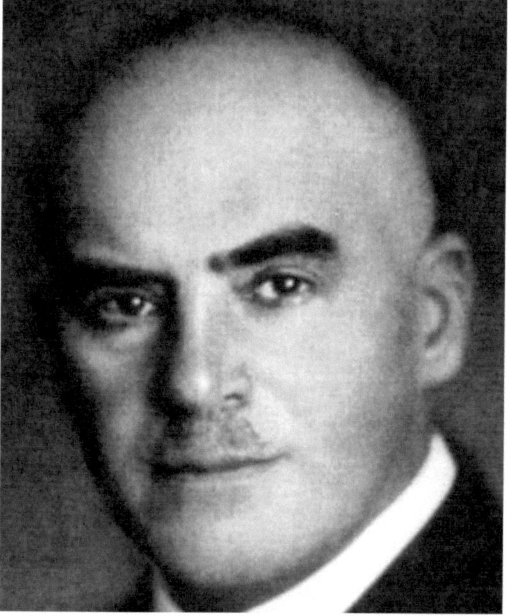

Fig. 2.6 Adolf Stoffel (1880–1937), a pioneer of fascicular nerve anatomy, selective neurectomy and nerve transposition, anticipated many ideas of proximal and distal nerve transfers that have been rediscovered in recent decades

Table 2.5 Adolf Stoffel's Techniques of (Fascicular) Nerve Transfers (1920)

Donor nerves	Recipient nerve
Upper extremity	
Fascicle to caput longum/ mediale of triceps muscle of the radial nerve	Axillary nerve
Fascicle of the radial nerve	Musculocutaneous/ median nerve
Subscapulary nerve (branch to M. teres major)	Axillary nerve
Fascicle of the median nerve	Ulnar nerve (intrinsic hand function)
Lower extremity	
Donor nerves	Recipient nerve
Fascicle of sciatic nerve	Nn. gluteales (gluteus maximus and medius muscles)
Obturatory nerve	Femoral nerve
Tibial nerve	Peroneal nerves (profundus et superficialis)

techniques to treat patients with peripheral nerve injuries [64].

In 1911, Stoffel developed an operation for selective neurotomy in spastic paralysis of the extremities, which still bears his name today. In recent, years it has experienced a renaissance as a "partial neurectomy" with spasticity on the arm and hand called "hyperselective neurectomy"

[65]. The textbook of "Orthopaedic Surgery" written with Vulpius contains a multitude of selective nerve transfers in the upper and lower extremities (Table 2.5). Some of those techniques were "newly" discovered 80 years later, for example, the restoration of axillary nerve paralysis by nerve fascicle transfer of the radial nerve (to the caput longum and medial) or the transfer of fibres of the peroneal nerve to the tibial nerve (Table 2.5) [66]. Stoffel used electrical nerve stimulation intraoperatively for these operations

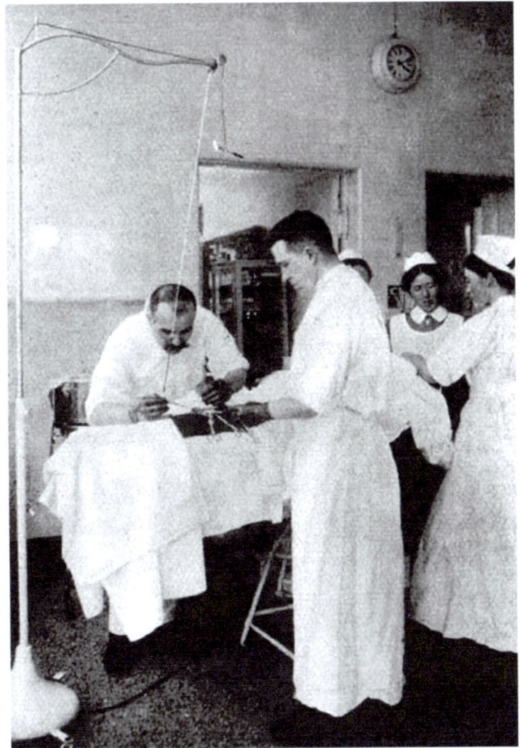

Fig. 2.7 Adolf Stoffel using intraoperative nerve stimulation during surgical exploration of the fibres of the sciatic nerve in the popliteal fossa of the knee

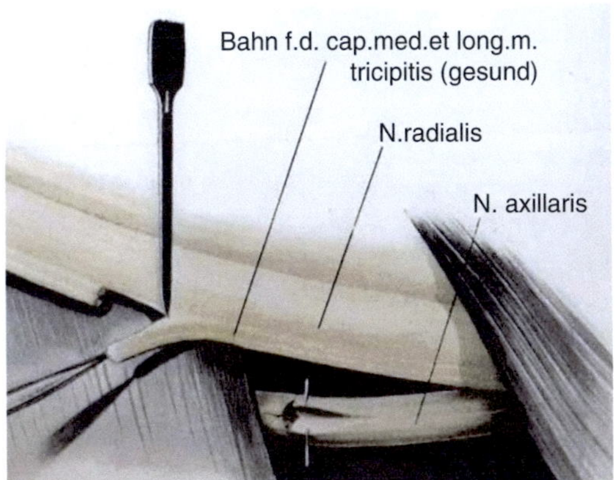

Fig. 2.8 Selective nerve transposition of motor axons of the radial nerve to the axillary nerve to restore shoulder abduction (deltoideus muscle function) according to Stoffel, illustrated in colour by his wife Edda [8]

in order to reliably identify and transfer motor donor fascicles at the level of the recipient (Figs. 2.7 and 2.8). Already in 1910 Vulpius prophesied: "If we compare the degree and safety of success today by means of tendon transplantation and nerve plasty surgery, the former is of course Goliath. But it can be guessed that a victorious David may rise in the nerve transfer" [8].

2.4.2　First World War

The treatment of peripheral nerve injuries changed dramatically due to the mass casualties of the First World War which flooded the military hospitals since 1914. The French Service de Santé alone is responsible for an estimated 30,000 nerve injuries, and by 1918 at least as many on the British side. It is estimated that 20% of all "seriously injured" also have nerve injuries. Research laboratories and a register for periph-

eral nerve injuries are set up in specialized military hospitals, headed in Great Britain by Sir Robert Jones (1857–1933) and in the USA by Gorgas and Frazier [67].

On the German side, the neurologist **Otfrid Foerster** (1867–1942) (Fig. 2.9) worked as a self-taught nerve surgeon and treated a total of 4787 gunshot wounds to peripheral nerves between 1914 and 1920 of which he himself operated 745 patients. Foerster meticulously recorded the symptomatology, therapy and course of his patients and thus created important foundations for modern reconstruction, transplantation and transfers of peripheral nerves. Confronted with thousands of gunshot wounds— and the disinterest and miserable results of his surgical colleagues—he decided in 1914 to operate as a neurologist himself, although he never received any formal surgical training. He explains this as follows: "I had to make the diagnosis, take the patient to the operating theatre, tell the surgeon where to operate, tell him what to do when he is inside. And then all the patients died—I decided that I couldn't make it worse" [68].

Foerster successfully performed neurolysis and nerve reconstruction by interposition of dispensable sensitive nerves (e.g., sural nerve from 1916), intraplexal neurotizations and numerous nerve transfers in the upper and lower limbs. For nerve sutures, he paid atten-

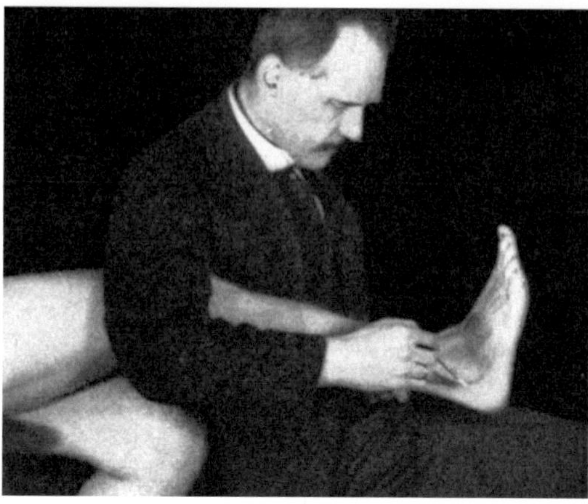

Fig. 2.9 Otfrid Foerster (1867–1942) investigating the sensory innervation area of the sural nerve which he probably first used since 1916 to bridge numerous motor nerve defects after gunshot wounds during the First World War

tion to the finest and tension-free technique. He attached great importance to postoperative rehabilitation with the help of electro-stimulation and physiotherapy in order to optimize the results after nerve regeneration through the plasticity of the brain. His long-time pupil, **Sir Ludwig Guttmann** (1899–1980), who after his emigration to England became the father of modern treatment for paraplegic individuals during the Second World War, saw this extremely careful and systematic aftercare as the main reason for Foerster's success, despite adverse conditions: "In other words, a better understanding of rehabilitation" [68].

Foerster's Principles and Techniques for Functional Restoration in Peripheral Nerve Lesions (1929)
- Complete removal of scar tissue to allow nerve coaptation
- Superfine suture material (thinnest silk threads or woman's hair)
- Suture of perineurium only
- Careful haemostasis
- Strict antisepsis
- Mobilization of the nerve stumps/relaxation through adapted (flexed) joint position
- Bridging of nerve defects with sensory nerve cables

- Direct nerve-muscle implantation if suture impossible (e.g., in musculocutaneous, radial, median, peroneal nerve)
- Nerve reconstruction ("nerve grafting") in brachial plexus lesions (donor nerves: pectoral, subscapular, thoracicus longus and thoracodorsal nerves)

2.4.3 1920s to 1930s

After the war, a careful follow-up examination in many centres was problematic because records are lost and patients are released from observation. The lack of a standardized assessment systems impaired the ability to document clinical changes and compare results [67]. In contrast, Foerster was able to personally track the progress of most of his patients. He also documented the postoperative development several years postoperatively with muscle and sensory tests, photographs and films, and even ink colourings of the sweat production to prove the return of sensory function. After Lenin's stroke, being his personal doctor Foerster spent almost 2 years in Siberia, where he condensed his experiences and documents into two volumes that were published in 1929 in German language. Unfortunately, these masterpieces have never been translated from German and have therefore not become generally known [68]. Research into nerve regeneration intensified in the 1930s in anticipation of an imminent global conflict. Bunnell and Boyes published the concept of "cable grafting" in 1939 to bridge nerve defects.

2.4.4 Second World War (1939–1945)

During the Second World War, neurosurgeons dominated the field of peripheral nerve surgery in the US Army and orthopaedic surgeons in the United Kingdom. Neurologists contribute very valuable innovations to the diagnosis and evaluation of nerve injuries and their treatment results, for example, renowned neurologists of the British Medical Research Council published an important brochure, which described a quantitative evaluation of muscle strength and showed in an atlas with diagrams how the key muscles with their innervation and the most important sensory dermatomes were clinically tested [69].

The surgical experience of the Second World War led to a new classification of nerve injuries and a refined timing for surgical procedures. The research group from Oxford led the way here, where **Herbert Seddon** (1903–1977), Professor of Orthopaedic Surgery, was supported by a team of outstanding young surgeons and neuroscientists. Seddon clarified important aspects of the pathology of peripheral nerve injury and defined three degrees of damage (neurapraxia, axonotmesis, neurotmesis) and suggested appropriate management [70, 71]. Since 1941, the Australian armed forces transferred all peripheral nerve injuries to the General Hospital in Heidelberg near Melbourne run by the Professor of Anatomy and Experimental Neurology, **Sidney Sunderland** (1910–1993). Until 1945, Sunderland studied the treatment results of hundreds of peripheral nerve injuries using clinical parameters and laboratory tests [16, 72].

2.4.5 Post-War Period

After 1945, follow-up data of more than 7000 nerve injuries from centres in Great Britain and the USA became available, but often poor results are found after peripheral nerve suture and nerve transfer, particularly discouraging were the results after brachial plexus injuries. Post-war research was therefore concerned with the goals of an improved technique for nerve transplantation, intraoperative diagnostic procedures and strategies for functional reconstruction after brachial plexus injuries. Sunderland's ability to combine clinical, anatomical and pathological findings gives him great authority over a long period of time. In 1968 he published his monumental book "Nerves and Nerve Injuries" (second edition 1978). He performed excellent research on the internal topography of the peripheral nerves, which was of particular rele-

vance when, in the 1960s, new microsurgical methods were used to optimize the results by fascicular nerve reconstruction [73].

2.4.6 Era of Microsurgery (Since 1960s)

Anticoagulation drugs and the surgical microscope are the technological prerequisites for the break-through of microsurgery of vessels less than 1 mm in diameter. Peripheral nerve surgery developed parallel to the establishment of microvascular surgery by replantation (e.g., of a completely separated thumb in 1965 by Komatsu and Tamai) and later tissue transplantation in the 1970s and 1980s. The "tension-free" technique for direct suturing or bridging with autologous interponates was mainly used by **Hanno Millesi** (*1927–2017) from Vienna establishing a recognized "gold standard".

His astonishingly good clinical results were often doubted initially. Millesi and his co-workers Meissl and Berger in Vienna publish several globally acclaimed series of tension-free nerve sutures on the upper nerves [74, 75]. Millesi proved that "total absence of tension at the suture site is a very important factor for successful nerve repair" and that interfascicular nerve reconstruction leads to better functional recovery. Despite initial enthusiasm, free vascularized nerve grafts [76] were not able to establish themselves in the clinical practice. The research of the following decades to the present concentrated on refinement of basic surgical techniques, a better understanding of nerve biology and anatomy (e.g., gliding tissue), and better sutures and biological implants for nerve transfer, including allografts [77, 78].

2.4.7 Twenty-First Century

A modern focus of research was targeted at influencing the central reorganization or "brain plasticity" after peripheral nerve injury in order to achieve functional improvements. The transfer of dispensable donor axons is also experiencing a renaissance in patients with cervical spinal cord injury (tetraplegia) and complements classical methods, such as tendon transfers. To restore an active hand opening, Bertelli recommends transferring the supinator branches to the interosseous posterior nerve (S-PIN operation) and axon transfers to restore elbow extension and flexor function of the hand. In some cases, nerve transposition is also combined with classical muscle transfers and joint stabilizations [50]. Bahm reconstructs important arm functions in arthrogryposis multiplex by means of nerve transfers [79]. For some years now, arm amputees have been controlling their bionic prostheses by means of targeted muscle reinnervation. Using the same technique, it is possible to amplify very weak nerve impulses with transplanted muscles and replace completely functionless hands after forearm amputation with thought-controlled prostheses [80]. In patients with hemiplegia, reinnervation from the contralateral C7 nerve root can reduce spasticity and improve limb function [81, 82].

2.5 Treatment of Brachial Plexus Injuries

2.5.1 Of World-Historical Importance?

The historical development of injuries of the plexus brachialis is to be presented separately (Table. 2.6)—not least because it is considered to be of world historical importance [83]. The most famous brachial plexus patient is the last German **Emperor William II** (1859–1941) (Fig. 2.10). Numerous contemporaries and later historians and psychologists see the key to understanding this unfortunate historical personality in his lifelong struggle against the weakness of his physical disability and the compensatory desire for dominance and strength. Wilhelm himself was convinced: "… an Englishman has crippled my arm" accusing the obstetrician sent by his grandmother Queen Victoria.

The therapy attempted by the most famous capacities at that time appears today like a "horrible child abuse" [90] (Table 2.7). In addition to constant cold baths, massages and movement exercises, the prince had to undergo "animal baths" twice a week from the age of 6 months, that is, the left arm was put into a warm, freshly slaughtered rabbit for half an hour each time. In order to stimulate the use of the paralysed arm, the healthy arm was tied to the back, which led to Wilhelm constantly falling painfully on the face when he was a toddler. In addition, the left arm was regularly treated with electric shocks, and since the age of eight he has had to put on an "arm stretching machine" three times a day.

Whether this is the cause of Wilhelm's hatred of England, which may have influenced the course of history [83], can only be assumed. It seems understandable that this extremely painful and completely unsuccessful treatment triggered a lasting disturbance of the Prince's (and later Emperor's) personality development [90]. The helplessness of his doctors becomes more understandable when one realizes how little knowledge there is about complex nerve injuries at that time.

2.5.2 First Medical Descriptions (1746–1861)

Almost 3000 years ago, Homer described in his "Iliad" flail arm paralysis due to spear stab injury and a stone falling on the shoulder area, and Albrecht Dürer (1471–1528) depicted around 1505 in his painting "Madonna with Child at the Window" baby Jesus with typical features of an upper brachial plexus paralysis (Fig. 2.11). It was not until 1768, however, that the first medical report of a Scottish obstetrician named Smellie (1697–1763) appeared, who in 1746 observed a bilateral brachial plexus lesion after forceps birth. The father of the famous French writer Gustave Flaubert (1821–1880), Achille-Chleophas Flaubert (1784–1846), documented two catastrophic traction injuries of the

Table 2.6 Development of the treatment of brachial plexus lesions

Year	Author, origin	Description/knowledge
Antiquity Around 700–800 BC	Homer, Ilias, Greece	First description of arm paralysis after brachial plexus injury (by spear stab and impact of stone in shoulder area)
Approx. 1505	Dürer, Germany	Picture "Madonna with child" shows typical signs of upper brachial plexus lesion
1768	Smellie, Scotland	First English language description of a brachial plexus lesion after forceps delivery (1746)
1827	Flaubert, France	Neurovascular traction injuries of the brachial plexus (with tear-out of C6-Th1 and axillary nerve) in reduction of delayed shoulder dislocations
1861	Duchenne, France	Concept of "obstetric brachial plexus lesion" on the basis of four newborns
1872	Mitchell, USA	Pain syndrome after brachial plexus lesions in the American Civil War ("causalgia")—only decompression, no suture performed
1875	Erb, Germany	Erb's point (Punctum nervosum), upper plexus lesion (C5–6, type Erb)
1877	Seeligenmüller, Germany	Complete (total) obstetric traumatic brachial plexus lesion
1885	Augusta Klumpke, USA, France [84, 85]	Lower brachialis plexus lesion (C7-Th1, Klumpke type) with Horner syndrome
1885	Sécretan, France	Study of 24 cases of brachial plexus lesion in German, French and English literature
1898 1899	Duval and Guillain, France Horsley, UK	Experimental studies have shown that in closed brachial plexus lesions either elongation (spontaneous improvement) or root rupture (therapy impossible) is present
1900	Thoburn, UK	First surgical treatment of the brachial plexus 7 months after severe traction damage (partial functional recovery)—clairvoyant analysis of the surgical problem
1903	Kennedy, Scotland	Surgical neuroma resection and direct suture of the nerve stumps after obstetric plexus lesion
1903	Harris and low, UK	Intraplexual neurotization ("cross-union") in cervical root tearing due to birth trauma
1913	Tuttle, UK [86]	Neurotization of cervical plexus and intraplexal roots in brachial plexus lesions
1913	Fairbanks, USA	Subluxation and internal rotation of the shoulder as a consequence of plexus paralysis
1914–1920	Foerster, Germany	Successful operation of 64 plexus injuries during and after the First World War (summarized in 1929)
1916, 1918	Sever, USA	36-page monograph on brachial plexus lesions, investigation of more than 1100 cases: scepticism towards nerve surgery, instead physiotherapy and muscle transfer recommended
1916, 1917	Sharpe and Wyeth, USA	Evaluation of 81 child plexus surgeries—intervention during the first year of life recommended
1920	Taylor, USA	Comparison of 70 operated and 130 non-operated cases of plexus paralysis—often astonishing improvement after surgery, only 1% spontaneous recovery
1934	Stevens, USA	Immediate revision recommended for plexus lesion, but surgery for traction injury with root rupture is "hopeless"
1936	Bonola, Italy	Report on increasing plexus injuries caused by motorcycle accidents
1934, 1939	L'Episcopo, USA [87]	Operations for secondary reconstruction, especially for external shoulder rotation

(continued)

Table 2.6 (continued)

Year	Author, origin	Description/knowledge
1942	Scaglietti, Italy	Several hundred cases of neurolysis and direct sutures in brachial plexus lesions
1961/1963	Seddon, UK	Intercostalis transfer to biceps replacement with interponate—only modest success
Since 1964	Millesi, Austria	Start of microsurgical brachial plexus operations, especially neurolysis and reconstructions with tension-free interfascicular suture and interposition
1966	SICOT (Societé Internationale de Chirurgie Orthopédique et Traumatologique)	International meeting in Paris with decision that the treatment of traction injuries of the brachial plexus is not useful: amputation and prosthesis treatment recommended
Since the mid-1960s	Narakas, Switzerland (Lithuania)	Establishment of microsurgical operations on the brachial plexus, classification, international meeting on plexus brachialis surgery
1972	Tsyuyama and Hara	Direct intercostalis transfer (without interposition grafts)—Improved results
1980	Wynn-Parry, UK	Series of 275 patients show pain syndromes especially in root avulsions
1981	Narakas, Switzerland (Lithuania)	Surgical therapy can significantly reduce the occurrence of pain
1977	Millesi, Austria	Microsurgical reconstruction in 56 patients, 70% with functional improvement
1984	Gilbert and Tassin, France	Convincing results after early microsurgical primary reconstruction of the child's brachial plexus in 180 cases
1987	Narakas, Switzerland (Lithuania) [88, 89]	Classification of paediatric brachial plexus palsy: Type II (C5–6), II (C5–7), III (C5-Th1), IV (C5-Th1) with Horner syndrome
1989	Narakas, Switzerland (Lithuania) [88, 89]	Worldwide surgical experience in more than 4000 cases of brachial plexus lesions
1989	Gu, China	Neurotization of the brachial plexus with contralateral C7 root
1994	Oberlin, France Mackinnon, USA and others	Proximal nerve (fascicular) transpositions in brachial plexus lesions
2010–today	Bertelli, Brazil Mackinnon, USA and others	Distal nerve transfers in trunk nerve lesions
2011	Xu, China	Contralateral C7 neurotization of the upper extremity in hemiplegia
2015	Aszmann, Austria	Forearm amputation and replacement of the functionless hand with a bionic prosthesis (controlled by selective nerve transfer)

brachial plexus in adults in Rouen 1827 in autopsy findings. The attempt to reposition a delayed shoulder dislocations by pulling of up to eight men ends fatally for both patients. The autopsy showed strong bleeding and root tears of C6-Th1 (C5 is intact), in one case the axillary artery was also torn.

The French physician Guillaume Benjamin Armand Duchenne (1806–1875) first coined the term "obstetric plexus lesion" in 1861—2 years after Kaiser Wilhelm's birth—based on the examination of four newborns and cites excessive traction forces on the arm during the birth process as the cause [91]. He tried to evaluate the severity of the paralysis by electrodiagnosis (similar to an electromyogram). He was already interested in prognostic and therapeutic aspects of the treatment [92].

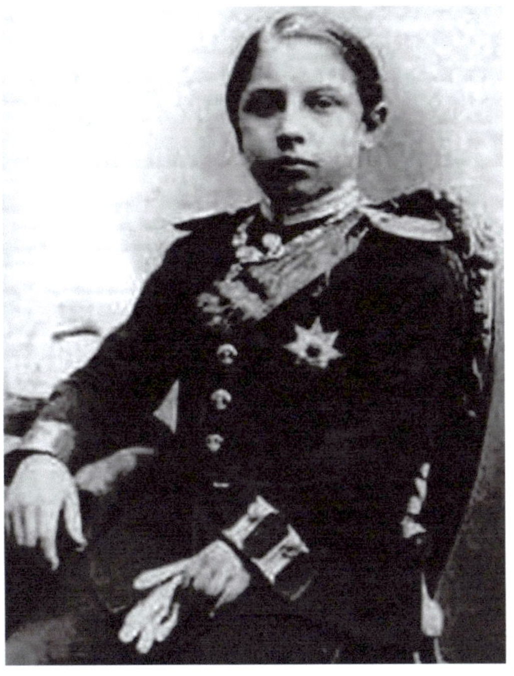

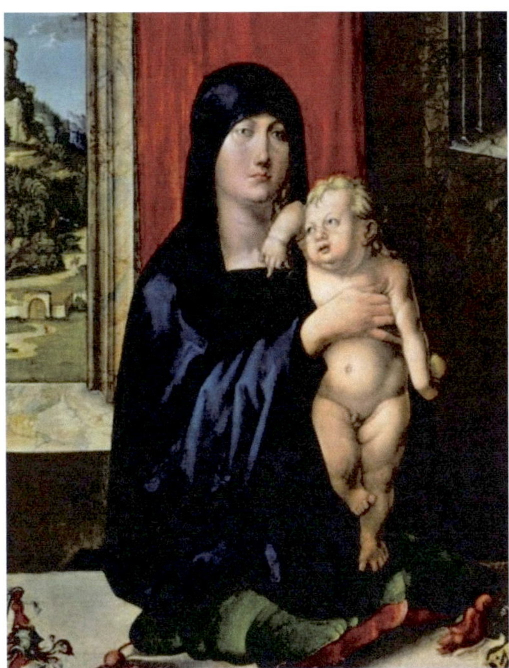

Fig. 2.10 The last German Emperor Wilhelm II (1859–1941) as a child. His left arm, probably paralysed by birth-related brachial plexus lesion and shortened (in adulthood by about 15 cm), is optically extended by a glove. (Courtesy of the Archive des Hauses Hessen)

Fig. 2.11 The painting "Madonna with Child at the Window" (1498) by the Nuremberg Renaissance painter Albrecht Dürer (1471–1528) shows little Jesus with typical features of an upper brachial plexus lesion on the left side: internal rotation and adduction of the shoulder, extension of the arm and flexion of the wrist—today called "waiter's tip" deformity

Table 2.7 Treatment methods for (suspected) brachial plexus paralysis by Emperor Wilhelm II (1859–1941) during his childhood

Inception	Forms of therapy
Since the first months of life	Cold baths in the first months, regular sea water showers
Since the fourth month of life	Passive movement exercises (three times daily)
Since the age of 1 year	Regular electrical stimulation (alternating current and galvanization)
Since the sixth month of life	Forced use of the paralysed left arm (healthy arm tied to the back for hours every day), thus frequently falling on the face as a toddler "Animalic baths": 2 times a week for 30 min, insertion of the left arm into a still warm, freshly slaughtered rabbit
From the age of 4 years	Torticollis treatment with painful stretching devices and multiple operations
From the age of 8 years	Regular clamping of the paralysed arm in a stretching machine

2.5.3 Classification into Different Lesion Types (1875–1885)

The German neurologist **Wilhelm Heinrich Erb** (1840–1921), founder of the Deutsche Zeitschrift für Neurologie (German journal of neurology) and the Deutsche Gesellschaft für Neurologie (German society of neurology), proved by anatomical observations and electro-stimulation in 1875 that brachial plexus damage occurs most frequently in the area of the roots C5 and C6, today known as Erb's point. The upper brachial plexus paralysis until today bears his name [93].

Two years later, Seeligenmüller documented a complete (total) obstetric plexus lesion (C5-Th1) before Augusta Klumpke (1859–1927) examined the lower brachial plexus lesion (C7-Th1, type Klumpke) in 1885 [84, 85]. She was the first woman to receive a full training position at the Sorbonne Medical Faculty in Paris. Together with her professor and later husband, the neurologist Joseph Jules Dejerine (1849–1917), she discovered that damage to the lower plexus not only damages the function and sensation of the forearm, wrist and hand but also causes pupil constriction (miosis) and drooping eyelid (ptosis), as already observed in 1869 by the Swiss ophthalmologist Georg Johann Friedrich Horner (1831–1886), thus called "Horner syndrome [94]".

2.5.4　Surgical Treatment Firsts (Around 1900)

It was not until 15 years later that the first surgical therapy for nerve suture in a closed plexus lesion became known, performed by **William Thoburn,** assistant surgeon at the Royal Infirmary in Manchester on 13 April 1896 [95]. Seven months after a severe traction damage, he exposed the brachial plexus transclavicularly in a 16-year-old mill worker and performed a direct suture of the nerves with finest silk, supposedly free of tension. At the follow-up 4 years later, the patient showed only little shoulder control and almost no elbow extension and hand function, yet useful elbow and wrist flexion. Thoburn honestly admitted his limited success and concluded with astonishing clairvoyance: "With the experience gained here, there can be no doubt that delayed injuries of the brachial plexus, when they are accessible, will be surgically treated and not condemned as hopeless—an attitude that has even led to amputation to remove a useless strain. Only in cases where the plexus is avulsed from the spinal cord surgery is impossible." Kennedy in Scotland also succeeds in 1903 utilizing neuromuscular resection and primary direct suture of the nerve stumps after obstetric plexus lesion. In the same year, the British neurologists Harris and Low performed intraplexual neurotization ("cross-union") for the first time to bypass a root avulsion due to birth trauma. In 1913, Tuttle performed neurotization of the cervical plexus and intraplexal roots.

2.5.5　Conservative Primary and Operative Secondary Reconstruction (Until 1970s)

In spite of these surgical glimmers of hope, the treatment of brachial plexus lesions for many decades usually consisted only of physiotherapy—in anticipation of spontaneous regeneration or permanent complete loss of function. Surgery was only performed in exceptional cases, the results achieved were modest and larger patient series rare. Even later, only unsatisfactory results were usually obtained, especially in traction injuries despite nerve interposition graftings, so that only conservative measures were usually applied in birth-associated lesions. In 1925, James W. Sever (1878–1964) compiled a 36-page monograph on brachial plexus lesions including more than 1100 cases. He primarily recommended physiotherapy and secondary muscle transfers and confirmed the scepticism towards nerve operations, due to mostly poor results. Joseph B. L'Episcopo (1890–1947) published in 1934 and 1939, based on Sever, classical surgical techniques to restore muscle balance at the shoulder. The aim was to increase abduction and external rotation through muscle transfer and release (Sever-L'Episcopo operation).

In the time between the two world wars, operations on the brachial plexus seemed to be almost forgotten. Rare exceptions included the work of Otfrid Foerster, who reconstructed 64 lesions in the German city of Breslau (today Wroclaw, Poland) during the First World War, sometimes with admirable results [96]. Taylor presented in 1920 an interesting comparison between 70 operated and 130 non-operated cases of plexus paralysis. Surgery often brought amazing improvements, a comparable spontaneous recovery with conservative therapy occurred only in 1%.

During the Second World War, the Italian orthopaedic surgeon, Oscar Scaglietti (1906–1993), treated several hundred cases of gunshot wounds to the brachial plexus, mainly through neurolysis and direct suturing.

The attitude towards surgical primary care remained pessimistic for a long time, although new diagnostic methods made it possible to investigate, grade and plan therapy more precisely: cervical myelography was introduced in 1947, electromyography in 1948, the recording of nerve action potentials in 1949 and the histamine test (to distinguish between pre- and post-ganglionic nerve damage) in 1954. Seddon had been investigating peripheral nerve injuries in soldiers and civilians on behalf of the British government since 1943 and was developing numerous strategies for autologous reconstruction together with his colleagues. In 1963, he presented the intercostal nerve transfer to the musculocutaneous nerve to restore biceps function [97].

However, the results were often disappointing and in 1966 Seddon and Robert Merle d'Aubigné, at an international SICOT conference in Paris, claimed that despite surgical treatment for complete paralysis a satisfactory result was practically impossible. The treatment of traction injuries would be pointless, surgical exploration of the brachial plexus, especially of infraclavicular lesions, had no diagnostic benefit, surgical repair was often impossible and even after surgery no useful effect could be guaranteed. As a result, several authors recommended amputating the patients' paralysed arms at upper arm level and having prostheses fitted [98]. Few surgeons opposed this therapeutic nihilism.

2.5.6 Era of Microsurgery (1960 to Present)

However, the perspective changed fundamentally in the late 1960s and early 1970s due to the emergence of microsurgical techniques. Through preparation under the microscope, external and interfascial neurolyses could be successfully performed and nerve regeneration could be initiated or accelerated. Microsurgical nerve transplantation permitted tension-free bridging of defects and precise suturing in the event of nerve displacement.

The leading pioneer was **Hanno Millesi** (1927–2017) from Vienna who had been working intensively with peripheral nerve sutures since 1958, and with the aid of a borrowed Zeiss microscope since 1964 on nerve reconstruction and plexus surgery using microsurgery. He designed multi-stage treatment algorithms. These initially aimed at microsurgical neurolysis or nerve transplantation and then at partly traditional, partly new methods of muscle transfer in order to achieve optimum results even with extensive paralysis patterns. For example, even with root lesions that were previously considered hopeless, he achieved satisfactory results for elbow flexion in over 80% of the cases [78, 99].

A second pioneer was particularly prepared for his tasks as a plexus surgeon through his life. **Algimantas Otonas Narakas** (1927–1993) from Lithuania, aged 11, suffered a deep hip wound while playing with ammunition, which developed into bone infection and hip arthrosis. In 1938, he left his homeland for a cure in Switzerland, to which he could not return even after the Second World War. Until antibiotics healed his osteomyelitis shortly after 1945, he spent most of his years in bed, learning languages, reading and working on fine motor activities such as model making. A stateless person, he completed his medical studies in 1957 but was unable to work as a physician, so he continued his education in a variety of surgical fields, including neurosurgery, orthopaedics and limb surgery. This work familiarized him with all the important aspects of brachial plexus injuries, which he treated—after obtaining Swiss citizenship—in operations lasting up to 19 h from 1966 onwards. His operation drawings prove to be a valuable tool for understanding complex injury patterns. He drafted a classification on the basis of which four categories with corresponding therapy and probable prognosis were formed and set up a meeting (Narakas Club) at which people interested in plexus surgery exchanged their experiences every 2 years until today [100].

With the obstetric plexus lesions—today more objectively "birth-associated"—the perspective also changed at the beginning of the 1980s. Gilbert and Tassin [101] presented convincing results after primarily microsurgical treatment on 180 patients and others as authors confirmed this approach. In 1989, the working group around Gu from Shanghai devised a neurotization using the contralateral C7 root. In 1993, Oberlin expanded the treatment spectrum for C5–7 lesions. By means of a single or double transfer of fascicles from the ulnar nerve and median nerve directly transferred to the biceps or brachialis motor branch of the musculocutaneous nerve, good elbow flexion could be restored [102]. About 100 years after Adolf Stoffel's pioneering work, authors such as Jayme Bertelli (Florianopolis, Brazil) or Susan Mackinnon (St. Louis, USA) subsequently developed a large number of innovative proximal and later distal fascicular transfer operations. These accelerated and improved the return of function both in the shoulder and upper arm area as well as on the forearm and hand considerably [103, 104].

2.6 Conclusions

The review of the development of muscle and nerve transfer surgery gives us a fascinating insight into the beginnings of orthopaedic and surgical specialties and the pioneering achievements of our predecessors, who founded the principles of these operations that are still valid today. The resulting findings can be summarized as follows:

- Anatomical studies are a prerequisite for clinical knowledge progress and thus improved surgical treatment methods, since structure and function cannot be separated from each other.
- Technical developments are significantly influenced by social changes and contemporary events, especially the polio epidemics since about 1880, the introduction of insurance systems and the care for the countless shot-gun injuries of the First and Second World Wars.
- The decisive factor, however, is often the tireless commitment of individuals who think far ahead of their time, even if their contemporaries often treat them with scepticism or even resistance.
- The significance of many innovations is not adequately recognized at the time of their initial description, they are forgotten and some only rediscovered much later. A careful examination of the old thoughts of our predecessors not only confirms our actions today, but also offers the opportunity to "re-evaluate" some of these ideas in our time and technological context and to apply them profitably.
- The historical analysis of the beginnings of motor and nerve replacement surgery shows us, against the background of an extremely eventful period, the exemplary inventiveness, endurance and accuracy of our predecessors, who can serve us as inspiration and role models in our daily work and in looking to the future of functional reconstructive surgery.

References

1. Ackerknecht E. Kurze Geschichte der Medizin. Stuttgart: Thieme; 1967.
2. Smith RJ. History of tendon transfers. In: Smith RJ, editor. Tendon transfers of the hand and forearm. Boston: Little, Brown; 1987.
3. Bismarck O. Gesammelte Werke (Friedrichsruher Ausgabe). Bandolier. 1924/1935;9:S195/196.
4. Lange F. Lehrbuch der Orthopädie. 3rd ed. Stuttgart: Gustav Fischer; 1928.
5. Osten P. Über den Aufbau einer "modernen Krüppelfürsorge" 1905–1933. Frankfurt/Main: Mabuse; 2004.
6. Thomann KD. Geschichte der Reichskrüppelzählung von 1906. Orthopade. 2000;29:1055–66.
7. Thomann KD, Rauschmann M, Heine MC. Die Deutsche Orthopädische Gesellschaft von 1918–1932. Entwicklungen und Strömungen. Orthopade. 2001;30:685–711.
8. Vulpius O, Stoffel A. Orthopädische Therapie. In: Lewandowsky M, Hrsg. Handbuch der Neurologie, Bd. I, Teil. 1910; 2. p. S1299–S1321.
9. Perthes O. Die Funktionellen Ergebnisse der Sehnenoperationen bei irreparabler Radialislähmung. Klein Wochenschr. 1922;3:127–9.
10. Vulpius O. Die Sehnenüberppflanzung und ihre Verwertung in der Behandlung der Lähmungen. Leipzig: Veit & Comp; 1902.
11. Vulpius O. Die Behandlung der spinalen Kinderlähmung. Leipzig: Thieme; 1910.

12. Vulpius O, Stoffel A. Orthopädische Operationslehre, Enke, Stuttgart; 1913, 1920, 1924.
13. Mayer L. The physiological method of tendon transplantation. Surg Gynecol Obstet. 1916;22:182–97.
14. Steindler A. Orthopaedic reconstruction work on hand and forearm. New York Med J. 1918;108:1117–9.
15. Huber E. Hilfsoperationen bei Medianuslähmung. Dtsche Zeitschr Chir. 1921;162:271–5.
16. Sudeck P. Gedanken zur Radialislähmung. Chirurg. 1943;15:665.
17. Bunnell S. Surgery of the hand. 2nd ed. Philadelphia: Lippincott; 1948.
18. Merle d'Aubigné R, Lange P. Transplantations tendineuses dans le traite-ment des paralysies radiales posttraumatiques. Sem Hôpitaux Paris. 1946;22:1666–80.
19. Littler JW. Tendon transfers and arthrodeses in combined median and ulnar nerve paralysis. J Bone Joint Surg. 1949;31A:225–34.
20. Pulvertaft RG. Tendon grafts for flexor tendon injuries in the fingers and thumb: a study of technique and results. J Bone Joint Surg. 1956;38B:175–94.
21. Boyes JH. Tendon transfer for radial palsy. Bull Hosp Jt Dis. 1960;21:97–105.
22. Boyes JH. Selection of a donor muscle for tendon transfer. Bull Hosp Jt Dis. 1962;23:1–4.
23. Zancolli EA. Claw-hand caused by paralysis of the intrinsic muscles: a simple surgical procedure for its correction. J Bone Joint Surg Am. 1957;39:1076–80.
24. Zancolli E. Structural and dynamic bases of hand surgery. Philadelphia: Lippincott; 1968.
25. Tamai S, Komatsu S, Sakamoto H, Sano S, Sasauchi N. Free muscle transplants in dogs with microsurgical neurovascular anastomoses. Plast Reconstr Surg. 1970;46:219–25.
26. Lieber RL, Jacobson MD, Fazeli BM, Abrams RA, Botte MJ. Architecture of selected muscles of the arm and forearm: anatomy and implications for tendon transfer. J Hand Surg. 1992;17A:787–98.
27. Ninković M, Sućur D, Starović B, Marković S. A new approach to persistent traumatic peroneal nerve palsy. Br J Plast Surg. 1994;47:185–9.
28. Fridén J, Lieber RL. Mechanical considerations in the design of surgical reconstructive procedures. J Biomech. 2002;35:1039–45.
29. Hoffa A. Lehrbuch der orthopädischen Chirurgie. Stuttgart: Enke; 1891.
30. Wirth CJ, Rühmann O. Historische Entwicklung der Ersatzoperationen bei Armplexuslähmung. Orthopade. 1997;26:626–9.
31. Nicoladoni C. Nachtrag zum Pes calcaneus und zur Transplantation der Peronealsehnen. Arch Klin Chir Berlin. 1881;27:660.
32. Lexer E. Die Gesamte Wiederherstellungschirurgie. Leipzig: Barth; 1931.
33. Drobnik T. Über die Behandlung der Kinderlähmung mit Funktionsteilung und Funktionsübertragung der Muskeln. Dtsch Z Chir. 1896;43:473.
34. Franke F. Ueber operative Behandlung der Radialislähmung nebst Anmerkungen über die Sehnenüberpflanzung bei spastischen Lähmungen. Arch Klin Chir. 1898;57:763.
35. Codavilla A. Sui trapienti ttendinei nella practica orthopedia. Archivo Orth. 1899;16:225.
36. Codivilla A (1903) Meine Erfahrungen über Sehnenverpflanzungen. Verh Deutsch Orthop Ges 2: 221–251.
37. Braun A. Oscar Vulpius—Leben und Werk. Heidelberg: Verlag Brigitte Gunderjahn; 1997.
38. Hahn P, Braun AC, Unglaub F. Oscar Vulpius und die Sehnentranspositionen an der Hand. Handchir Mikrochir Plast Chir. 2012;44:187–8.
39. Mayer L. Transplantation of the trapezius for paralysis of abductors of the arm. J Bone Joint Surg. 1929;11:80–8.
40. Biesalski K, Mayer L. Die physiologische Sehnenverpflanzung. Berlin, Heidelberg/New York: Springer; 1916.
41. Stoffel A. Muskel- und Sehnenoperationen nach Kriegsverletzungen. Stuttgart: Enke; 1921.
42. Borchardt F. Nervenverletzungen. In: Schjerning, editor. Handbuch der ärztlichen Erfahrungen im Weltkrieg. Leipzig: Barth; 1922.
43. Jones R. Tendon transplantation in cases of musculospinal injuries not amendable to suture. Am J Surg. 1921;35:333–5.
44. Dellon AL. History of peripheral nerve surgery. In: Winn HR, editor. Youman's neurological surgery. 5th ed. Philadelphia: WB Saunders; 2004. p. 3798–808.
45. Perthes O. Über Sehnenoperationen bei irreparabler Radialislähmung. Beitr Klin Chir. 1918;113:289–96.
46. Boyes JH. On the shoulders of giants. Notable names in hand surgery. Philadelphia: Lippincott; 1976.
47. Boyes JH. Tendon transfer for radial palsy. Bull Hosp Jt Dis. 1960;21:97–105.
48. Moberg E (1979) The upper limb in tetraplegia. A new approach in surgical rehabilitation. Thieme, Stuttgart.
49. Fridén J. Tendon transfers in reconstructive hand surgery. London: Taylor & Francis; 2005.
50. Fridén J, Gohritz A. Update on tetraplegia management. J Hand Surg. 2015;40:2489–500.
51. Brand PW. The reconstruction of the hand in leprosy. The reconstruction of the hand in leprosy. Ann R Coll Surg Engl. 1952;11:350–61.
52. Brand P. Biomechanics of tendon transfer. Orthop Clin North Am. 1974;5:205–30.
53. Steinau HU, Biemer E. Plastisch-chirurgische Rekonstruktionsmöglichkeiten bei gliedmaßenerhaltender Resektion maligner Weichteiltumoren der Extremitäten. Chirurg. 1985;56:741–5.
54. Cajal RS. Degeneration and regeneration of the nervous system. London: Oxford University Press; 1928.
55. Lanska D. Historical perspective: neurological advances from studies of war injuries and illnesses. Ann Neurol. 2009;66:444–59.

56. Naff NJ, Ecklund JM. History of peripheral nerve surgery techniques. Neurosurg Clin N Am. 2001;12:197–209.
57. Erlacher P. Ueber die motorischen Nervendigungen. Z Orthop Chir. 1914;34:561.
58. Erlacher P. Hyperneurotisation; muskuläre Neurotisation; freie Muskeltransplanttion. Zentr Mbl f Chirurg Bd. 1914;15.
59. Heineke D. Die direkte Einflanzung des Nervs in den Muskel. Zentralbl Chir. 1914;41:465.
60. Sunderland S. A classification of peripheral nerve injuries producing loss of function. Brain. 1951;74:491–516.
61. Millesi H. Klinische und experimentelle Untersuchungen bei der Wiederherstellung peripherer Nervenläsionen. Langenbecks Arch Chir. 1962;301:893–7.
62. Mackinnon SE, Dellon AL. Surgery of the peripheral nerve. New York: Thieme; 1988.
63. Kuiken TA, Dumanian GA, Lipschutz RD, Miller LA, Stubblefield KA. The use of targeted muscle reinnervation for improved myoelectric prosthesis control in a bilateral shoulder disarticulation amputee. Prosthetics Orthot Int. 2004;28:245–53.
64. Stoffel A. Zum Bau und zur Chirurgie der peripheren Nerven. Verh Dtsch Orthop Ges. 1912;11(177–189):50.
65. Leclercq C. Selective neurectomy for the spastic upper extremity. Hand Clin. 2018;34:537–45.
66. Leechavengvongs S, Witoonchart K, Uerpairojkit C, Thuvasethakul P, Ketmalarisi W. Nerve transfer to biceps muscle using a part of the ulnar nerve in brachial plexus injury (upper type): a report of 32 cases. J Hand Surg. 1998;23A:711–6.
67. Hanigan W. The development of military medical care of peripheral nerve injuries during World War I. Neurosurg Focus. 2010;28:E24.
68. Gohritz A, Dellon AL, Guggenheim M, Spies M, Steiert A, Vogt PM. Otfrid Foerster—self-taught neurosurgeon and innovator of peripheral nerve surgery. J Reconstr Microsurg. 2013;29: m33–43.
69. Medical Research Council. Methods of investigating nerve injuries. In: Seddon HJ, editor. Peripheral nerve injuries, part 1. London: Her Majesty's Stationery Office; 1954.
70. Seddon HJ. Three types of nerve injury. Brain. 1943;66:237–88.
71. Seddon HJ. Surgical disorders of the peripheral nerves. Edinburgh: Churchill Livingstone; 1972.
72. Sunderland S. Nerve injuries and their repair. A critical appraisal. Melbourne: Churchill Livingstone; 1991.
73. Simpson D. From Lanfranc to Sunderland: the surgery of peripheral nerve. ANZ J Surg. 2009;79: 930–5.
74. Mackinnon SE. Nerve surgery. New York: Thieme; 2015.
75. Millesi H. Persönliche Mitteilung. 2016.
76. Taylor IG, Ham FJ. The free vascularized nerve graft. Plast Reconstr Surg. 1976;57:413–26.
77. Millesi H. Progress in peripheral nerve surgery. World J Surg. 1990;14:733–47.
78. Millesi H. Chirurgie traumatischer Plexus brachialis-Läsionen. Handchir Mikrochir Plast Chir. 2004;36:29–36.
79. Bahm J. Arguments for a neuroorthopaedic strategy in upper limb arthrogryposis. J Brachial Plex Peripher Nerve Inj. 2013;8:9.
80. Aszmann OC, Roche AD, Salminger S, Paternostro-Sluga T, Herceg M, Sturma A, Hofer C, Farina D. Bionic reconstruction to restore hand function after brachial plexus injury: a case series of three patients. Lancet. 2015;385(9983):2183–9.
81. Xu WD, Hua XY, Zheng MX, Xu JG, Gu YD. Contralateral C7 nerve root transfer in treatment of cerebral palsy in a child: case report. Microsurgery. 2011;31:404–8.
82. Hua XY, Qiu YQ, Li T, Zheng MX, Shen YD, Jiang S, Xu JG, Gu YD, Xu WD. Contralateral peripheral neurotization for hemiplegic upper extremity after central neurologic injury. Neurosurgery. 2015;76:187–95.
83. Ober WB. Obstetrical events that shaped Western European history. Yale J Biol Med. 1992;65:201–10.
84. Hohmann G. Ersatz des gelähmten Bizeps brachii durch den Pectoralis major. Münch Med Wochenschr. 1918;45:1132–3.
85. Klumpke A. Paralysies radiculaires de plexus brachiale: Paralysies radiculaires totales. Paralysies radicullaires inferiores. De la participation des filets sympathiques oculo-pupillaires dans ces paralysies. Rev Med Paris. 1885;5:739.
86. Tuttle H. Exposure of the brachial plexus with nerve transplantation. JAMA. 1913;61:15.
87. L'Episcopo JB. Tendon transplantation in obstetrical paralysis. Am J Surg. 1934;25:122.
88. Narakas AO. Traumatic brachial plexus injuries. In: Lamb D, editor. The paralyzed hand. Edinburgh: Churchill Livingstone; 1979. p. 100–115.
89. Narakas AO. Obstetrical brachial plexus injuries. In: Lamb D, editor. The paralyzed hand. Edinburgh: Churchill Livingstone; 1979. p. 116–35.
90. Röhl JCG, Wilhelm II. Die Jugend des Kaisers, 3. Aufl. 1859–1888. München: Beck; 2008.
91. Duchenne GB. Du l'électrisation localisée et de son application á la pathologie et á la thérapeutique par courants induits et par courants galvaniques interrompus et continus. Paris: Bailliére et fils; 1872.
92. Robotti E, Longhi P, Verna G, Bocchiotti E. Brachial plexus surgery—an historical perspective. Hand Clin. 1995;11:517–53.
93. Erb WH. Über eine eigenthümliche Lokalisation von Lähmungen des Plexus brachialis. Verhdl naturhistmed Vereins zu Heidelberg. 1874;2:130–6.
94. Horner JF. Über eine Form von Ptosis. Klin Monatsbl Augenheilkd. 1869;7:193–8.

95. Thoburn W. Secondary suture of brachial plexus. Br Med J. 1900;1:1073–5.

96. Foerster O. Die Therapie der Schussverletzungen der peripheren Nerven. Bumke Foersters Handb Neurol (Lewandowsky). 1929;3:1509–720.

97. Seddon HJ. Peripheral nerve injuries. Medical Research Council Special Report Series No. 282. London: Her Majesty's Stationary Office; 1954.

98. Fletcher I. Traction lesions of the brachial plexus. Hand. 1969;1:129.

99. Millesi H. Surgical management of brachial plexus injuries. J. Hand Surg. 1977;25:367–79.

100. Narakas AO, Hentz VR. Neurotization in brachial plexus injuries. Clin Orthop Relat Res. 1988;237:43–56.

101. Gilbert A, Tassin JL. Réeparation chirurgical du plexus brachial dans la paralysie obstétricale. Chirality. 1984;110:70–5.

102. Oberlin C, Beal D, Leechavengvongs S, Salon A, Dauge MC, Sarcy JJ. Nerve transfer to biceps muscle using a part of ulnar nerve for C5–C6 avulsion of the brachial plexus: anatomical study and report of four cases. J Hand Surg. 1993;19A:232–7.

103. Ray WZ, Chang J, Hawasli A, Wilson TJ, Yang L. Motor nerve transfer: a comprehensive review. Neurosurgery. 2016;78:1–26.

104. Wood MB, Murray PM. Heterotopic nerve transfers: recent trends with expanding indication. J Hand Surg [Am]. 2007;32:397–408.

T. Schwenzer

3.1 Shoulder Dystocia

3.1.1 Definitions and Frequency

In most cases of shoulder dystocia, this is the typical high shoulder straight line with the front shoulder trapped above the symphysis. It is much less common for a birth arrest to occur with the shoulders pinched already after the entry of the shoulders into the maternal pelvis. This is typically a shallow (platypelloid) basin. Even rarer is the bilateral shoulder dystocia with pinching of both the anterior and posterior shoulder.

However, there is no uniform definition for the shoulder dystocia [1]. The lack of a general definition of shoulder dystocia is one reason why the number of actually occurring shoulder dystocia is not fully recorded because, for example, lighter forms are not documented [2–8].

For birth weights between 2500 and 4000 g, the incidence is 0.6–1.4% [9] and for birth weights between 4000 and 4500 g, 5–9%. In children with a birth weight above 4500 g, the frequency of shoulder dystocia is reported to be more than 15% [10] (Fig. 3.1). In maternal diabetes mellitus, the frequency of shoulder dystocia is significantly higher even in comparison with non-diabetic pregnant women in the respective weight classes (Table 3.1).

The incidence of shoulder dystocia—at least in relation to vaginal births—is clearly increasing. This is confirmed by data from individual institutions that have consistently recorded the frequency of shoulder dystocia over long time intervals. Øverland et al. [10] report an incidence of 0.25% for the 10-year period 1967–1976 and in the following 10-year periods significant increases up to 1.21% in the last period 1997–2006. Dandolu et al. [11] report from the state of Maryland an increase of the shoulder dystocia incidence from 0.2% in 1979 to 2.11% in 2003 with nearly 280,000 vaginal births, which would correspond to a tenfold increase of the cases.

Data from other authors also underline an increase in cases of shoulder dystocia in vaginal births [12–17]. Nocon et al. [18] state 185 registered shoulder dystocia in 12,532 vaginal births, which corresponds to a rate of 1.4%. In these 185 cases, 14 clavicle fractures and 28 plexus pareses were found. In addition, they identified 19 patients in their patient population in whom no shoulder dystocia was coded, but in whom 5 plexus pareses and 14 clavicle fractures were nevertheless found.

These data underline the problem of under-recording the shoulder dystocia. If these 19 cases are added to the 185 originally recorded shoulder dystocia cases, the incidence is 1.6%. In a recent study by Grobman [19], the frequency of shoulder

T. Schwenzer (✉)
Direktor der Frauenklinik, Klinikum Dortmund gGmbH, Dortmund, Germany
e-mail: thomas.schwenzer@klinikumdo.de,
thomas@schwenzerdo.de

© Springer Nature Switzerland AG 2021
J. Bahm (ed.), *Movement Disorders of the Upper Extremities in Children*,
https://doi.org/10.1007/978-3-030-53622-0_3

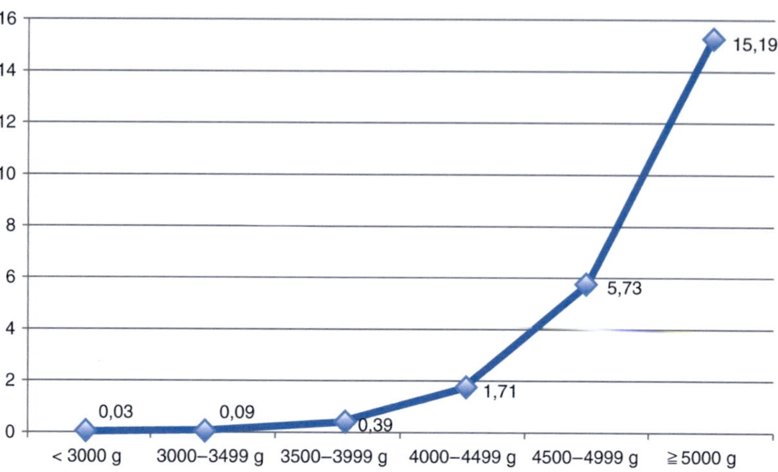

Fig. 3.1 Frequency of shoulder dystocia as a function of birth weight [10]

Table 3.1 Frequency of shoulder dystocia as a function of birth weight and the presence of diabetes mellitus

Birth weight (g)	Frequency of shoulder dystocia without diabetes mellitus (%)	Frequency of shoulder dystocia with diabetes mellitus (%)
<4000	0.1–1.1	0.6–3.7
4000–4499	1.1–10.0	4.9–23.1
≥4500	4.1–22.6	20.0–50.0

Modified after [2]

dystocia is even reported to be up to 3% of all vaginal deliveries.

> In a European or North American population, the incidence of shoulder dystocia must be assumed to be above 1% but well below 2%, taking into account the available literature.

The plexus paresis of the shoulder girdle is the most frequent complication of shoulder dystocia. Here you will find frequencies between 1.5‰ and 2‰ [20]. From this it can be estimated that about 10–15% of shoulder dystocia are associated with plexus paresis or that paresis may also occur without recorded shoulder dystocia.

Spong et al. [8] define the presence of a shoulder dystocia during an extended time between the birth of the head and the birth of the trunk and/or the need to take additional obstetric measures for the birth of the trunk. They gave an interval of 60 s, because in their collective the 60-s limit was about twice the standard deviation for the normal interval between head and torso birth.

Another definition diagnoses shoulder dystocia as a delayed birth of the shoulder or the inability of the shoulder to deliver spontaneously [21, 22]. The diagnosis of a shoulder dystocia is often made when the shoulder does not follow the child's head despite "normal," "usual," or "gentle" traction [21, 23].

The problem with applying this definition is that, according to many authors, any traction on the child's head is superfluous in the case of an unproblematic birth and, in the case of a shoulder dystocia, can even trigger plexus damage [22], and even if there is no blockage caused by a shoulder dystocia, a strong traction can possibly cause trauma to the plexus. In many maternity hospitals it is common for the midwife to wait for rotation after the birth of the head. If the torso does not follow in the same contraction, the midwife often grabs the head biparietally and tries to develop first the anterior and then the posterior shoulder. During this maneuver, a shoulder dystocia can be diagnosed if there is either a direct clear **"turtle sign"** exists if the fuselage does not follow with careful (!) pull at the head or at the latest with the next woe the fuselage is not born.

3.1.1.1 Definition of Shoulder Dystocia

One of the following situations exists:

- After the birth of the head, the head is firmly pressed onto the vulva—"turtle sign."
- With a careful (!) pull on the child's head, the torso does not follow.

– The hull will not be born without train with the next contraction or after 1 min at the latest.

If there is a corresponding finding, however, the diagnosis of a shoulder dystocia should always be made, regardless of how easy or difficult and with which measures the dystocia can be overcome. Other terms such as "difficult shoulder development," etc., are out of place and confusing only when plexus damage results.

These definitions of a shoulder dystocia are always based on the finding of a developmental disability of one of the two child shoulders. However, there may also be temporary blockages of one or even both shoulders during the passage through the mother's pelvis, which are not noticed at all, but which dissolve independently through a change of position of the mother and/or the force of the contractions and can nevertheless cause temporary plexus damage. This form of shoulder dystocia is given special consideration in a statement by the American College of Obstetricians and Gynecologists [24].

3.1.2 Risk Factors

Leading for the shoulder dystocia risk is the **fetal macrosomy** from 4000 g birth weight and especially from 4500 g. However, 41% of all shoulder dystocia occur in normal-weight fetuses under 4000 g [25].

In individual cases, it is difficult to differentiate to what the macrosomy is due. It is certainly a multifactorial event and consists of an increased risk of gestational diabetes, an increased incidence of maternal obesity, and an increased incidence of excessive intrapartum weight gain [26]. In a multivariate analysis, Stotland et al. [27] identified the following significant risk factors for a macrosomy >4500 g the male sex, multiparity, maternal age between 30 and 40 years, diabetes mellitus, and gestation >41 weeks of pregnancy.

The estimation of the actual birth weight is still associated with an estimation error, which is certainly influenced by the experience of the examiner and the examination conditions. This estimation error only allows a very limited risk stratification according to the expected birth weight. Particularly, the weight class from 4500 g, which is particularly affected by shoulder dystocia, is difficult to access for a meaningful risk assessment using ultrasound [28].

The **diabetes mellitus** both in the form of pre-existent diabetes and gestational diabetes definitely represents a risk factor for shoulder dystocia, which is relevant independently of the macrosomia frequently associated with the metabolic disorder and must be taken into account in clinical decisions. In all weight categories, diabetics have a significantly higher risk of shoulder dystocia than non-diabetic pregnant women. For diabetics, over 30% of the cases of shoulder dystocia in the weight group of 4000 g or more must be expected. This has also found its way into the guidelines of scientific societies in both the USA and Europe [29–32]. However, as the metabolic control of diabetic pregnant women improves, this factor becomes less important and non-diabetic fetal macrosomy dominates shoulder dystocia in macrosomal children.

The frequency of macrosomies is also associated with the weight of the mother, the maternal weight gain during pregnancy, the age of the mother and parity, without multivariate analyses being able to determine an independent risk. In terms of thought theory, the weight of the mother at the time of birth most likely represents an independent risk, because in the case of severe obesity, the birth ducts are also affected by the increase in fat deposits.

The weight gain of the fetus does not end at the estimated date of delivery. Rather, even after 40 completed weeks of pregnancy, there is still further fetal growth. The probability that the birth weight exceeds 4000 g is twice as high for 42 completed weeks of pregnancy as for 40 weeks of pregnancy. In a study with 519 pregnancies and one **gestation** of more than 41 weeks, 23% of newborns had a birth weight above 4000 g and 4% had a birth weight above 4500 g [33]. Boyd et al. [34] also found a 21% incidence of macrosomia at 42 completed weeks of pregnancy, as opposed to only 12% at 40 completed weeks.

The **parity** is also a risk factor associated with the incidence of macrosomia, because with increasing age of the pregnant woman the probability of a higher BMI increases. The male sex probably not only has a higher shoulder dystocia risk than girls due to the higher birth weight, but there are also constitutionally typical characteristics that favor the risk of shoulder dystocia at least in higher weight classes from 4500 g irrespective of the birth weight.

The **protracted opening and expulsion period** is found frequently in macrosome children, so that it is not certain whether the protracted course represents an independent risk for a shoulder dystocia. A protracted expulsion period can also be expected disproportionately often in the case of shoulder dystocia of children of normal weight, because in these cases a relatively narrowed (platypelloid) pelvis often triggers first the protracted course and then the shoulder dystocia.

The **vaginal-operative delivery** is undoubtedly an independent risk for shoulder dystocia. Here, too, the standstill during the expulsion period often determines the indication for forceps or vacuum delivery due to so-called relative disproportion and this indication is ultimately based either on a child that is (too) large for the specific situation or on a pelvis that is (too) narrow for the size of the child. The use of surgical delivery in this situation, however, creates an additional independent risk for shoulder dystocia. It is quite obvious that the forced lowering of the child's head blocks the physiological entry of the shoulders into the pelvic entrance and the lowering through the pelvis. The increased risk of shoulder dystocia after vaginal surgery is associated with both vacuum extraction and forceps delivery. Benedetti and Gabbe [35] have pointed out that macrosome children are more likely to use vacuum delivery. Anyone who performs a vaginal-

operative birth during the expulsion period with a protracted course of birth must be aware of this increased risk for shoulder dystocia, especially if the child's head is still in the middle of the pelvis. This is especially true for expectably large children.

The **condition after shoulder dystocia** is to be considered differentiated: The risk of macrosomia is often just as high or even higher than in the previous pregnancy with shoulder dystocia. In this case, a relatively high risk of shoulder dystocia will have to be assumed for a renewed vaginal delivery. If one can safely assume that, for example, with an improved metabolic control, a normal-weight child can now be expected, then the risk of recurrence for this complication is also low. In the case of a shoulder dystocia with a normal-weight or even rather light-weight child, there is a disproportionately high incidence of **constricted (platypelloid) pelvis** in front of you. In this situation there is a high risk that the same complication will occur as in the previous pregnancy.

3.1.3 Pathomechanisms

In American literature, **risk factors** of a shoulder dystocia with the **"3 P"** [26]:

- **P**assenger—birth object—child
- **P**assage—birth canals
- **P**ower—force

This characterization reflects well which factors influence the development of shoulder dystocia.

The child's shoulder normally enters the pelvis transversely or obliquely with its width. In this phase of birth, the child's head is typically located almost on the pelvic floor with the control center. The arrow seam is almost completely or already completely rotated. After the birth of the child's head, the shoulder girdle also rotates through the pelvis, recognizable by the backward rotation of the head. The front shoulder is then born under the symphysis without the support of traction on the head. It remains there because the contractions first push the torso with the rear shoulder cross-legward. Here there is normally room for unfolding. The symphysis acts as a hypomochlion for the anterior shoulder, which has already been partially born.

In typical shoulder dystocia, the shoulder girdle does not enter the pelvis transversely or obliquely due to the macrosomy of the child or the disproportion between child and pelvis (birth object and birth canal). Even before the head with the arrow seam in the straight diameter has been rotated out, the shoulder girdle, which is in the sagittal plane or slightly oblique, does not rotate with it (Fig. 3.2). It remains above the pelvic entrance level while the head completes its rotation in the birth canal under the pressure of the contractions and is finally born. This birth of the head becomes possible because the posterior shoulder usually goes deeper over the promontory and so the trunk covers the longer distance along the sacral cavity. The trunk rotates around the symphysis and the front shoulder is more and more fixed by the pressure of the contractions. This high shoulder straight line represents the most common form of shoulder dystocia and is clinically immediately detectable for the obstetrician. Clinically, this form of shoulder dystocia impresses with its **"turtle sign"** (Fig. 3.3) with the head firmly pressed onto the vulva and the face to the side or diagonally dorsally at most.

If the shoulders are very wide in relation to the straight pelvic diameter, a blockage of the posterior shoulder above the promontory very rarely occurs. In this situation, the head is normally not born, or at least not completely born, by the contractions. In this situation, the head is sometimes developed surgically by means of forceps or vacuum. This double shoulder dystocia is a particularly severe progressive form.

Plexus damage in newborns is rarely observed on the posterior shoulder and also in cases where there may be no external forces on the child in the form of manual traction or vacuum or forceps [36]. In a position paper of the American College, this form of shoulder dystocia is particularly thematized and seen as an explanation for the fact that birth-associated plexus paresis also occurs without previous, at least without documented, shoulder dystocia.

A shoulder dystocia can rarely develop without blocking the anterior shoulder behind the symphysis or the posterior shoulder by the promontory. For pelvic deformities, in particular for a flat pelvis (**platypelloid cymbal**), the shoulder girdle can enter the pelvis with both shoulders and then a birth arrest occurs because the shoulders are virtually pressed into the pelvic canal

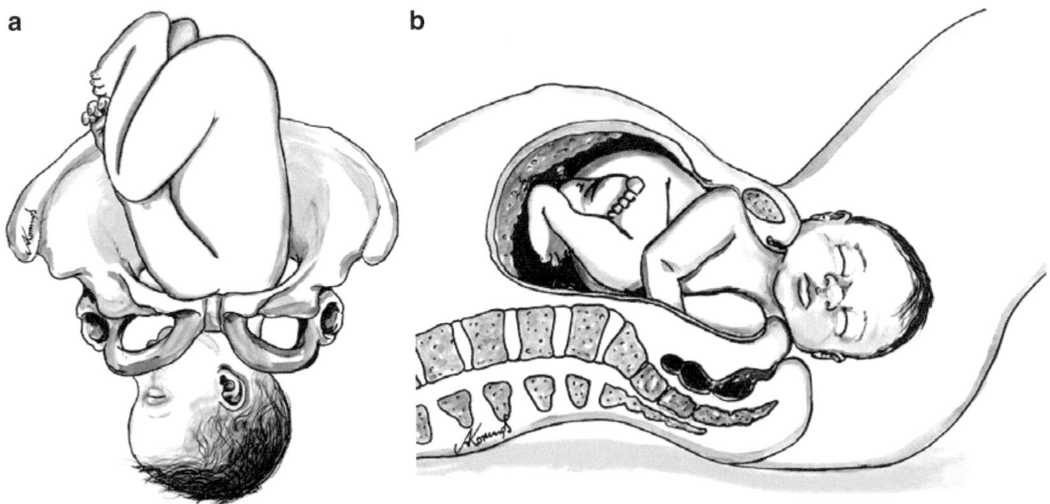

Fig. 3.2 (**a**, **b**) Typical high shoulder straightness with front shoulder trapped behind symphysis

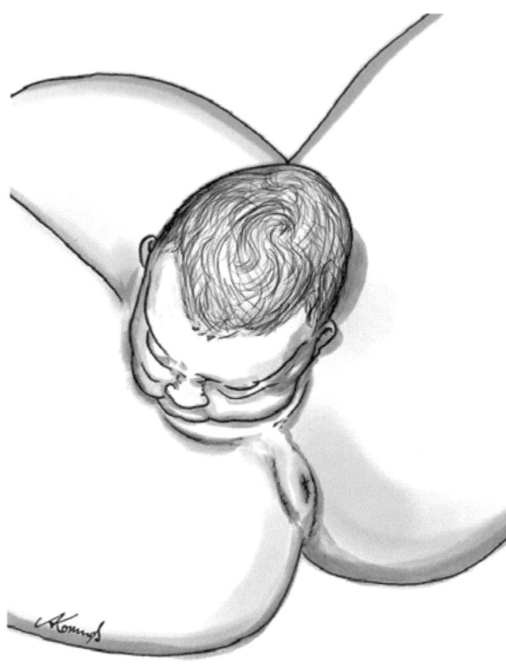

Fig. 3.3 Turtle phenomenon in shoulder dystocia with front shoulder pinching

[21]. This form of shoulder dystocia can also be observed in children of normal weight. The frequency of a shoulder dystocia in the shallow pelvis is 8–10 times higher than in the normally configured pelvis [21].

The fact that in many works about **plexus pareses** which occur without shoulder dystocia, at least without documented shoulder dystocia, and which in part also represent permanent damage, has led to considerations on the pathomechanism of these pareses. This work is further reinforced by the fact that these pareses frequently affect the posterior shoulder, which is averted from the symphysis [36]. The child as a birth object is driven through the birth canal by internal and occasionally additional external forces. Internal forces are built up by the contractions and in the expulsion period additionally by the active pressing of the pregnant women. External forces are generated by pulling on the child's head with the obstetrician's hands or during a vaginal-operative delivery by means of forceps or vacuum extraction. These forces can press the posterior shoulder against the promon-

tory and thus lead to a strain on the brachial plexus. The statement of the American College [24] deals with the possible development of a paresis of the brachial plexus without shoulder dystocia, at least without documented dystocia. These cases do not appear to the clinician sub partu but are only relevant for the development of postpartal plexus paresis without clinical shoulder dystocia.

3.2 Plexus Damage

It is important for the obstetrician to minimize the risk of developing plexus paresis. Two main strategies must be pursued to this end.

First strategy: risk stratification at the end of pregnancy whether there is a significantly increased shoulder dystocia risk in the specific pregnancy and whether the alternative of a caesarean section should therefore be discussed with the pregnant woman. According to the established case law of the Federal Court of Justice, an explanation of the alternative of a caesarean section to vaginal birth is necessary if the risk of vaginal birth is significantly increased [37–39]. In a conversation about birth planning, the obstetrician must draw up a corresponding risk profile based on his experience and advise the pregnant woman on this basis. The indication of an increased risk for shoulder dystocia does not mean that the pregnant woman must always be delivered by a caesarean section. The pregnant woman only has to be able to make a self-determined decision on the basis of comprehensive risk information. Every obstetrician must be aware that he or she is in the clarification trap if, when a foreseeable complication occurs, he or she has not fully clarified the delivery alternatives in an open-ended manner.

The second component for reducing the risk of obstetric plexus paresis is to control the measures that can be taken in the event of shoulder dystocia to develop the unborn child without damage. Even the most experienced obstetrician does not always succeed. He may also be surprised by a severe shoulder dystocia in a woman under childbirth who never imagined giving birth before and who carried a severely macrosome child of over 4500 g or even 5000 g in her own massive overweight. Thus, a defect in the plexus alone should not be interpreted as an error on the part of the obstetrician. However, if the obstetrician is able to take the necessary external and internal measures to correct the shoulder dystocia [28], the risk of plexus damage can be minimized. This also includes regular **training of doctors and midwives** on the phantom and a structured emergency plan to implement all necessary steps in the event of shoulder dystocia.

References

1. Gottlieb AG, Galan HL. Shoulder dystocia: an update. Obstet Gynecol Clin N Am. 2007;34(3):501–31, xii. https://doi.org/10.1016/j.ogc.2007.07.002.
2. ACOG Practice Patterns. Shoulder dystocia. Number 7, October 1997. American College of Obstetricians and Gynecologists. Int J Gynaecol Obstet. 1998;60(3):306–13. http://www.ncbi.nlm.nih.gov/pubmed/9544722.
3. ACOG Technical Bulletin. Number 159—September 1991. Fetal Macrosomia. Int J Gynaecol Obstet. 1992;39(4):341–5. http://www.ncbi.nlm.nih.gov/pubmed/1361472.
4. Gherman RB, Ouzounian JG, Miller DA, et al. Spontaneous vaginal delivery: a risk factor for Erb's palsy? Am J Obstet Gynecol. 1998;178(3):423–7. http://www.ncbi.nlm.nih.gov/pubmed/9539501.
5. Gonik B, Hollyer VL, Allen R. Shoulder dystocia recognition: differences in neonatal risks for injury. Am J Perinatol. 1991;8(1):31–4. https://doi.org/10.1055/s-2007-999334.
6. Romoff A. Shoulder dystocia: lessons from the past and emerging concepts. Clin Obstet Gynecol. 2000;43(2):226–35. http://www.ncbi.nlm.nih.gov/pubmed/10863622.
7. Rouse DJ, Owen J, Goldenberg RL, Cliver SP. The effectiveness and costs of elective cesarean delivery for fetal macrosomia diagnosed by ultrasound. JAMA. 1996;276(18):1480–6. http://www.ncbi.nlm.nih.gov/pubmed/8903259.
8. Spong CY, Beall M, Rodrigues D, Ross MG. An objective definition of shoulder dystocia: prolonged head-to-body delivery intervals and/or the use of ancillary obstetric maneuvers. Obstet Gynecol. 1995;86(3):433–6. https://doi.org/10.1016/0029-7844(95)00188-W.
9. Baxley EG, Gobbo RW. Shoulder dystocia. Am Fam Physician. 2004;69(7):1707–14. http://www.ncbi.nlm.nih.gov/pubmed/15086043.
10. Øverland EA, Vatten LJ, Eskild A. Risk of shoulder dystocia: associations with parity and offspring birthweight. A population study of 1 914 544 deliveries. Acta Obstet Gynecol Scand. 2012;91(4):483–8. https://doi.org/10.1111/j.1600-0412.2011.01354.x.
11. Dandolu V, Lawrence L, Gaughan JP, et al. Trends in the rate of shoulder dystocia over two decades. J Matern Fetal Neonatal Med. 2005;18(5):305–10. https://doi.org/10.1080/14767050500312730.
12. Acker DB, Sachs BP, Friedman EA. Risk factors for shoulder dystocia. Obstet Gynecol. 1985;66(6):762–8. http://www.ncbi.nlm.nih.gov/pubmed/4069477.
13. Dodd JM, Catcheside B, Scheil W. Can shoulder dystocia be reliably predicted? Aust N Z J Obstet Gynaecol. 2012;52(3):248–52. https://doi.org/10.1111/j.1479-828X.2012.01425.x.
14. Gherman RB, Chauhan S, Ouzounian JG, et al. Shoulder dystocia: the unpreventable obstetric emergency with empiric management guidelines. Am J Obstet Gynecol. 2006;195(3):657–72. https://doi.org/10.1016/j.ajog.2005.09.007.
15. Hamilton E, Ciampi A, Dyachenko A, et al. Is shoulder dystocia with brachial plexus injury breventable? Fetal Matern Med Rev. 2008;19:293–310.
16. Hedegaard M, Lidegaard Ø, Skovlund C, Mørch L. Perinatal outcomes following an earlier post-term labour induction policy: a historical cohort study. BJOG. 2015;122:1377. https://doi.org/10.1111/1471-0528.13299.
17. Nesbitt T, Gilbert W, Herrchen B. Shoulder dystocia and associated risk factors with macrosomic infants born in California. Am J Obstet Gynecol. 1998;179:476–80.
18. Nocon JJ, McKenzie DK, Thomas LJ, Hansell RS. Shoulder dystocia: an analysis of risks and obstetric maneuvers. Am J Obstet Gynecol. 1993;168(6 Pt 1):1732–7; discussion 1737–9. http://www.ncbi.nlm.nih.gov/pubmed/8317515.
19. Grobman W. Shoulder dystocia. Obstet Gynecol Clin N Am. 2013;40(1):59–67. https://doi.org/10.1016/j.ogc.2012.11.006.
20. Okby R, Sheiner E. Risk factors for neonatal brachial plexus paralysis. Arch Gynecol Obstet. 2012;286(2):333–6. https://doi.org/10.1007/s00404-012-2272-z.
21. Kreitzer MS. Recognition, classification, and management of shoulder dystocia: the relationship to causation of brachial plexus injury. In: O'Leary J, editor. Shoulder dystocia and birth injury. 3rd ed. Totowa, NJ: Humana Press; 2009. p. 179–208.
22. Smeltzer JS. Prevention and management of shoulder dystocia. Clin Obstet Gynecol. 1986;29(2):299–308. Retrieved from http://www.ncbi.nlm.nih.gov/pubmed/3720062.
23. Revicky V, Mukhopadhyay S, Morris EP, Nieto JJ. Can we predict shoulder dystocia? Arch Gynecol Obstet. 2012;285(2):291–5. https://doi.org/10.1007/s00404-011-1953-3.
24. American College of Obstetricians and Gynecologists' Task Force on Neonatal Brachial Plexus Palsy. Executive summary: neonatal brachial plexus palsy. Obstet Gynecol. 2014;123(4):902–4. https://doi.org/10.1097/01.AOG.0000445582.43112.9a.
25. Gupta M, Hockley C, Quigley MA, Yeh P, Impey L. Antenatal and intrapartum prediction of shoulder

dystocia. Eur J Obstet Gynecol Reprod Biol. 2010;151(2):134–9. https://doi.org/10.1016/j.ejogrb.2010.03.025.

26. O'Leary J. Shoulder dystocia and birth injury. 3rd ed. Totowa, NJ: Humana Press; 2009.

27. Stotland NE, Caughey AB, Breed EM, Escobar GJ. Risk factors and obstetric complications associated with macrosomia. Int J Gynaecol Obstet. 2004;87(3):220–6. https://doi.org/10.1016/j.ijgo.2004.08.010.

28. Schwenzer T, Bahm J. Schulterdystokie und geburtsassoziierte Plexusparese. Berlin, Heidelberg/New York: Springer; 2016.

29. ACOG Practice Bulletin. Clinical management guidelines for obstetrician-gynecologists. Number 40, November 2002. Obstet Gynecol. 2002;100(5 Pt 1):1045–50. http://www.ncbi.nlm.nih.gov/pubmed/12434783.

30. Arbeitsgemeinschaft Medizinrecht der Deutschen Gesellschaft für Gynäkologie und Geburtshilfe. Empfehlungen zur Schulterdystokie Erkennung, Prävention und Management. 2010. http://www.awmf.org/uploads/tx_szleitlinien/015-024_S1_Empfehlungen_zur_Schulterdystokie_05-2008_05-2013.pdf.

31. Chauhan SP, Gherman R, Hendrix NW, Bingham JM, Hayes E. Shoulder dystocia: comparison of the ACOG practice bulletin with another national guide-line. Am J Perinatol. 2010;27(2):129–36. https://doi.org/10.1055/s-0029-1224864.

32. Royal College of Obstetricians and Gynaecologists. Shoulder dystocia green-top guideline No 42. 2012. www.rcog.org.uk/files/rcog-corp/GTG42_150713.pdf.

33. Carpenter MW. Rationale and performance of tests for gestational diabetes. Clin Obstet Gynecol. 1991;34(3):544–57. http://www.ncbi.nlm.nih.gov/pubmed/1934706.

34. Boyd ME, Usher RH, McLean FH. Fetal macrosomia: prediction, risks, proposed management. Obstet Gynecol. 1983;61(6):715–22. http://www.ncbi.nlm.nih.gov/pubmed/6843930.

35. Benedetti TJ, Gabbe SG. Shoulder dystocia. A complication of fetal macrosomia and prolonged second stage of labor with midpelvic delivery. Obstet Gynecol. 1978;52(5):526–9. http://www.ncbi.nlm.nih.gov/pubmed/724169.

36. Gherman RB, Ouzounian JG, Goodwin TM. Brachial plexus palsy: an in utero injury? Am J Obstet Gynecol. 1999;180(5):1303–7. http://www.ncbi.nlm.nih.gov/pubmed/10329894.

37. BGH. VI ZR 300/91 Urteil v. 16.2.1993. NJW. 1993;2372.

38. BGH. VI ZR 186/03 Urteil v. 14.9.2004. NJW. 2004;3703.

39. BGH. VI ZR 69/10 Urteil v. 17.5.2011. 2011.

Part II
Diagnostics

Diagnostics and Therapy Planning from the Perspective of the Neuropaediatrician

T. Becher and C. Bußmann

4.1 What Is the Goal of Diagnostics?

The majority of focal movement disorders are chronic and not life-threatening. Only a small proportion of these occur acutely and make it necessary to go to an emergency clinic or to get an appointment in a special neuropaediatric clinic at short notice. The acute occurrence of a focal neurological disorder requires immediate diagnostic clarification in order to (as far as possible) immediately initiate therapeutic measures. The first step in diagnostics should therefore always be the primary subdivision of acute, subacute and chronic disorders. In addition, this classification is an indispensable prerequisite for the etiological classification of the movement disorder. It should be noted that movement disorders that can be classified as subacute can develop either slowly, progressively or rapidly. Only in the course of the disorder can it be assessed whether it is transient or permanent.

The primary goal of neuropaediatric diagnostics is the **etiological classification** of the movement disorder. In the second step, the diagnosis of the **extent of functional disorder** and its **impact in the everyday life** of the child is at least just as important. The purely functional testing of the neuropaediatric examination should be supplemented here by questionnaires on hand/arm function (e.g., Children's Hand-use Experience Questionnaire, CHEQ) and function-oriented classification systems (e.g., Manual Ability Classification System, MACS). On this basis, the possible therapy options for the individual child must be weighed up. In addition, they offer good measuring instruments for assessing the course of therapy.

As experts, we often think we know what the right and necessary therapy for our patients is. In the case of somatic acute diseases, this is indeed usually correct; the therapy goals result from the disease because healing is the goal. With regard to movement disorders, this applies to all acutely occurring forms as well as to reconstructive procedures that take place at an early stage, for example, microsurgical nerve reconstruction. In the case of chronic illnesses, especially movement disorders for which no cure is possible, we need a different orientation because the interests and environmental conditions of the patient determine the relevance of activities in everyday life. With increasing age, preferred activities become more and more differentiated.

On the basis of many findings from rehabilitation research, we cannot assume that an intervention in the domain of structure and function

T. Becher (✉)
Kinderneurologisches Zentrum Gerresheim,
SANA Kliniken Düsseldorf, Duesseldorf, Germany
e-mail: thomas.becher@sana.de

C. Bußmann
Praxis for Kinderneurologie, Heidelberg, Germany
e-mail: bussmann@atos.de

automatically leads to an improvement in the domain of activities. A very well studied example is the treatment with botulinum toxin (BoNT) on the upper extremity.

In a Cochrane review [1] of upper extremity therapy for unilateral spastic cerebral palsy, it was clearly stated that botulinum toxin should not be used alone, but in combination with planned occupational therapy. A combination of botulinum toxin and ergotherapy is more effective than ergotherapy alone in reducing impairment, improving activity levels and achieving goals, but not in improving quality of life or self-efficacy. This systematic review found strong evidence for the use of BoNT as an additional therapy for upper extremity management in children with spastic CP.

The emphasis on individual therapy goals and the demand that BoNT should not be used alone, but only in combination with planned occupational therapy ("BoNT-A should not be used in isolation but should be accompanied by planned occupational therapy"), are decisive. Similarly, this requirement must also be applied to all operational measures.

In order to arrive at common therapy goals in an interdisciplinary manner together with the patient, individual diagnostics are used here to define the goal of the therapeutic activity. Precisely because no cure is possible, reasonable therapy plans result from the analysis of everyday activities and the patient's difficulties.

Traditional diagnostics aim at "objective parameters", measurable structural deficits such as strength reduction, active range of motion, contractures and innervation. Modern diagnostics also focuses on performance—so what the patient does with his or her reduced possibilities in everyday life—and the limitations that inhibit him or her in everyday life.

4.2 The International Classification of Functioning as a Guide

The International Classification of Functioning (ICF) is a WHO classification that was initially established and published in 2001 to describe the functional health status, disability, social impairment and relevant environmental factors of human beings. The ICF encompasses the objectively comprehensible dimensions of human life; the subjective dimension of functionality and disability (subjective well-being) is not included. A German version of the ICF for children and adolescents was published in 2011 by Olaf Kraus de Camargo and Judith Hollenweger [2]; a presentation of the application in practice was published in 2013 by Olaf Kraus de Camargo and Liane Simon [3].

The ICF distinguishes between **five domains** to describe a health problem and associated factors. The different domains are briefly explained in Fig. 4.1 and in the following tables.

4.2.1 Participation and Activities (Table 4.1)

This domain describes the activities that are important for participation in age-appropriate fields of activity, which differ from child to child according to his or her personal preferences and environment. From primary school age onwards, all activities related to self-sufficiency (washing, braiding hair, dressing, zippers and buttons, being able to eat alone, preparing food), school (using a ruler) and sports (catching and throwing a ball) are frequently mentioned. Very often, however, very individual problem areas are named as well.

> When talking with the child, it is important to develop an interest in the child's everyday life, to ask what he or she enjoys, to talk about the daily routine together, to identify successful and difficult activities, and to identify beneficial and inhibiting influencing factors.

4.2.2 Structure and Function (Table 4.2)

In these domains, the physical impairments are described in the narrower sense, and they reflect the neurological disorder and its immediate consequences for the function.

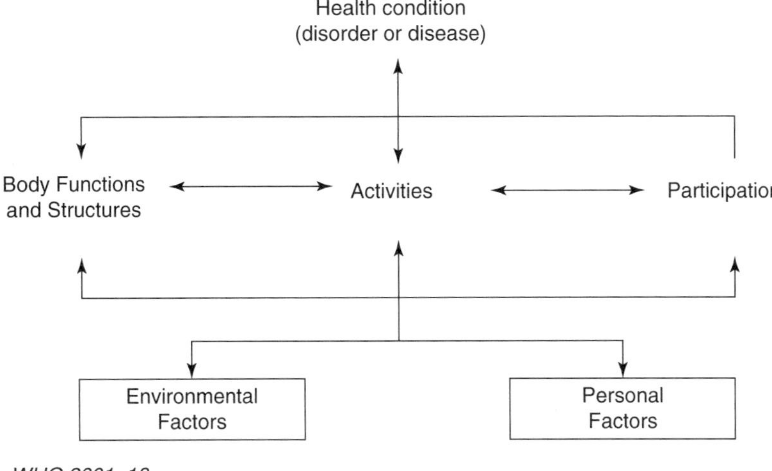

Fig. 4.1 The biopsychosocial model of ICF. World Health Organization. How to use the ICF: A practical manual for using the International Classification of Functioning, Disability and Health (ICF). Exposure draft for comment. October 2013. Geneva: WHO

Table 4.1 Classification of activities and participation [4]

Activities and participation	Examples
Learning and knowledge application	Conscious sensual perceptions; elementary learning; application of knowledge
General tasks and challenges	Taking on tasks; performing a daily routine; dealing with stress and other mental challenges
Communication	Communicating as receiver; communicating as sender; conversation and use of communication devices and techniques
Mobility	Changing and maintaining body position; carrying, moving and handling objects; walking and moving; moving by means of transport
Self-sufficiency	Washing; body care; dressing and undressing; using the toilet; eating, drinking; taking care of one's health
Domestic life	Procurement of the necessities of life; household tasks; cleaning and maintaining household items; helping others
Interpersonal interactions and relationships	General interpersonal interactions; special interpersonal relationships
Important spheres of life	Education/training; work and employment; economic life
Community life, social and civic life	Community life; recreation and leisure; religion and spirituality

Plexus paresis as an example:

- Structures of the nervous system: C5+C6 (Erb's paralysis)
- Structures related to movement: deltoid m. + infraspinatus m. (C5) and biceps m (C6)
- Movement-related functions: upper arm adducted, internally rotated; lower arm stretched; free hand and finger mobility

4.2.3 Environment and Personal Factors (Table 4.3)

Classification of Personal Context Factors [4]

- Age
- Gender
- Character
- Lifestyle
- Fitness

Table 4.2 Classification of bodily functions and structures [4]

Classification of bodily functions	Classification of bodily structures
Mental functions	Structures of the nervous system
Sensory functions and pain	The eye, the ear and related structures
Voice and speech function	Structures involved in voice and speech
Functions of the cardiovascular, haematological, immune and respiratory systems	Structures of the cardiovascular, immune and respiratory systems
Functions of the digestive, metabolic and endocrine systems	Structures related to the digestive, metabolic and endocrine systems
Functions of the urogenital and reproductive system	Structures related to the urogenital and reproductive system
Neuromusculoskeletal and motion-related functions	Structures related to movement
Functions of the skin and the skin appendages	Structures of the skin and the skin appendages

Table 4.3 Classification of environmental factors [4]

Environmental factors	Examples
Products and technologies	Food, medication, aids, assets
Natural and man-made environment	Demographic change, plants, animals, climate, sounds, noises, air quality
Support and relationships	Family, friends, superiors, helpers and caregivers, strangers
Settings	Individual attitudes of family and friends; social attitudes
Services, systems, operational principles	Housing, utilities, transportation, health care, economy, justice, politics

- Social background
- Upbringing
- Education/training
- Occupation
- Experience
- Coping strategies
- Genetic predisposition

The description of these domains encompasses the world in which the child and his or her family live; the resources, the inhibitory factors, motivation and willingness to undergo therapy are all reflected here. These domains are of utmost importance for the formulation of interdisciplinary and consensual therapy goals. Failure to consider the conditions of child and family in view of intensive therapy or surgery can

Table 4.4 Documentation of the recorded ICF domains

Component	Participation	Activities	Structures Functions
Techniques	Training in a sports club	Strength training Climbing wall Specific workout	BoNT Silicone hand orthosis
Therapy goals	Better goalkeeper Keep up with the others	Catching a ball on the right side of the body with both hands	Shoulder mobility Supination Wrist strength Orientation in the room

Environmental factors: Stabilising family, sustainable relationships with friends, football club

Personal factors: High motivation, good intellect, willingness to work hard

lead to significant complications, disappointment and unsatisfactory results.

4.2.4 Integration of the Levels

In our interdisciplinary work, we have developed a simple questionnaire (Table 4.4) with which we can present a documentation of the recorded domains to the various disciplines as well in talks with children and parents.

Showing the different dimensions of everyday, therapy-relevant problems this way has proven to be effective in the planning of operations, treatments with botulinum toxin, intensive therapy measures (such as rehabilitation stays) and in long-term therapy planning.

Objectives at Different Levels

- **Participation goals:** Arise from the occupational needs and problems, the hobbies and the living environment.
- **Activity targets:** Analysis of the child's everyday life. What troubles the child particularly? In what situations does is the child annoyed about missing skills? Formulate this as concretely as possible. Select verifiable criteria.
- **Functional goals:** Which motor requirements must be developed in order to achieve the occupational goal?
- **Structural targets:** Which structural conditions need to be changed or created?
- **Environmental factors/consulting:** What can be added, adapted or changed, for example, adapted products and technology for playing (e.g., remote-controlled cars) or auxiliary products for personal daily use, for example, orthoses.
- **What action is to be taken:** Which therapy is suitable taking into account the neurological findings, individual interests and resources?

4.3 Clinical Examination

First impressions of the extent of the child's movement disorder can already be gained at the beginning of the first consultation. Particular attention should be paid to the **spontaneous posture** of the affected arm, both when walking (e.g., when entering the examination room) and in the spontaneous motor activity of the upper extremity (e.g., taking off the jacket, climbing on a chair, passing objects to a parent) as well as when at rest.

> During the anamnesis following the welcoming of the child and its parents, it is strongly recommended to keep an eye on the child's motor skills and behaviour. Even this "relatively unobserved" situation allows important conclusions to be drawn about the motor deficit.

4.3.1 Cognition

The neurological examination of a movement disorder in childhood and adolescence always includes an assessment of the cognitive developmental status. This is largely done via the anamnesis. In the examination situation, particular attention must be paid to language comprehension and behavioural problems in addition to expressive language. Additional information is provided by tasks of drawing simple shapes and figures and, depending on the stage of development, in writing and reading. If there are indications of a mental developmental disorder, supplementary standardised psychological diagnostics should be sought if this has not yet been done already.

The neurological diagnosis of the upper extremity described below represents the ideal case of an examination of a child who is able and also willing to cooperate, approximately from primary school age. However, the neuropaediatrician is often confronted with examination situations that do not correspond to this ideal. In these cases, the power of observation is needed. Try to play with the child, but if this is not tolerated, try to create a play situation for parents and the child. This is also a way to obtain important examination results:

- Spontaneous posture of the upper extremity?
- Use of both hands? Transfer? Fine and gross motor skills of both hands approximately the same on both sides? The second hand is only the auxiliary hand? Complete neglect of the second hand?
- Range of movement of the arm? (Toys are held at different heights)
- Posture of arm and hand during walking and fast running?

4.3.2 Motor Skills

The motor diagnostics of the upper extremity begin with the **comparison** of both arms and both hands. The following points must be observed:

- Spontaneous posture: Position of the joints (e.g., flexion of the elbow, pronation of the forearm in case of pyramidal tract disorder)? Wrist and finger position?
- Muscle contour: focal or global atrophy signs? Difference in length?
- Pathological movements (tremor, choreoathetosis, dystonia)?

An assessment of the **muscle tone** (isolated and in side comparison) follows. The child should be encouraged to say immediately if any movement is painful. Muscle tone is best assessed by passive flexion and extension of the elbow, pronation and supination of the forearm, as well as flexion, extension and rotation of the wrist. Here, it is evaluated whether a normal muscle tone, hypertonus or hypotonus is present. An increased muscle tone is usually found in a lesion of the first motor neuron; a reduced muscle tone indicates a lesion of the second motor neuron, a cerebellar lesion, a peripheral nerve lesion or a neuromuscular disease.

For hypertonus due to spasticity (pyramidal tract damage), a catch phenomenon is typical: rapid movement, for example, of the elbow joint, results in sudden resistance (catch). This does not occur with an increased muscle tone due to an extrapyramidal disturbance (rigor); here, a cogwheel phenomenon may be present.

The **muscle power** is evaluated according to the **MRC scale**. The paresis scale of the Medical Research Council (MRC) is divided into 6 levels (0–5) (Table 4.5).

As this division is too inaccurate for cases of lighter pareses, there are various modifications of this scale. A more differentiated classification is offered by the **scaling of Luc Noreau** from [5] (Table 4.6).

Table 4.5 MRC scale

0	No contraction visible or perceptible
1	Visible or perceptible contraction
2	Movement possible without the influence of gravity
3	Movement possible against gravity
4	Movement possible against gravity and resistance
5	Normal muscle power

Table 4.6 MRC scale (Luc Noreau)

0	No muscle contraction
1	Visible or perceptible muscle contraction
1.5	Movement without influence of gravity with partial range of movement
2	Movement without influence of gravity with full range of movement
2.5	Movement against gravity with partial range of movement
3	Movement against gravity with full range of movement
3.5	Movement against slight resistance with full range of movement
4	Movement against moderate resistance possible
4.5	Muscle works against strong resistance, but not yet entirely normal
5	Normal muscle power

It makes sense to examine the movements listed in Tables 4.7 and 4.8 in the shoulder and arm musculature area. Table 4.9 lists the examinations of extension and finger flexion.

The following questions should be considered when assessing muscle weakness:

- Is there a proximal, distal or generalised weakness?
- Does the weakness correspond to the supply area of a nerve or of a myotome?

4.3.3 Reflexes

The proprioceptive reflexes of the upper extremity, like all reflexes, are subject to great interindividual variability. A valid statement on increased or reduced reflexes is only possible by side comparison (provided it is not a bilateral disorder).

Table 4.7 Movements to be examined in the shoulder and arm musculature area

Motion	Muscle
Shoulder abduction	First 90°: M. supraspinatus (C5); Second 90°: M. deltoid (C5)
Shoulder adduction	M. latissimus dorsi, M. pectoralis major (C7)
External shoulder rotation	M. infraspinatus (C5)
Internal shoulder rotation	M. subscapularis, M. teres minor (C5)
Elbow flexion (in supination)	M. biceps (C5–6)
Elbow flexion (in middle position)	M. brachioradialis (C5–6)
Elbow extension	M. triceps (C7)

Table 4.8 Standard values for active and passive shoulder movement (Neutral 0 method)

Adduction/abduction	20–40/0/180°
Anteversion/retroversion	150/170/0–40°
Horizontal extension/flexion	135/0/40–50°
Internal/external rotation in adduction	95/0/40–60°
Internal/external rotation in 90° abduction	70/0/70°

Table 4.9 Examination of the hand/finger musculature

Wrist extension	M. extensor carpi ulnar (C7–8)
Finger extension	M. extensor digitorum (C7–8)
Abduction of the thumb	M. abductor pollicis brevis (C8-Th1)
Finger abduction	Mm. interossei (C8-Th1)

- Biceps tendon reflex (BTR) tests C5,6 and the musculocutaneous nerve
- Brachioradial reflex (BRR) tests C5,6 and the radial nerve
- Triceps tendon reflex (TTR) tests C7,8 and radial nerve

If the reflexes cannot be triggered spontaneously, an attempt can be made to trigger them by means of the **Jendrasik manoeuvre**. Here, the examiner counts up to three, and at three the patient clenches his or her teeth and the examiner simultaneously triggers the reflex.

4.3.3.1 Coordination

The main tests of the coordination test are carried out with the **finger-nose test** to assess intention tremor or dysmetry and rapidly alternating pronation and supination movements of the palms of the hands (dysdiadochokinesis).

4.3.3.2 Mirror Movements

To check the innervation of the affected extremity in central lesions, it is advisable to check the mirror movements of the **affected** hand. For this purpose, testing of unilateral pronation/supination in alternation, alternating fist closing and opening, and finger-thumb opposition is carried out. If mirror movements (not only an increase in tonus) occur in the affected hand, this indicates ipsilateral innervation.

4.3.4 Sensitivity

More than any other examination, the sensitivity test is dependent on the understanding and willingness of the child to cooperate and be examined.

Proprioception, sharp/blunt differentiation and the sense of vibration are to be tested.

Depending on the clinical picture, the sensitivity test must also be carried out along the C5-Th1 dermatomes.

If a peripheral nerve lesion is suspected, the sensitivity test is carried out specifically in the sensitive supply areas of the peripheral arm nerves:

- N. radialis, C5-Th1 (radial back of the hand, first spatium interosseum).
- N. medianus, C5-Th1 (radial edge of the index finger).
- N. ulnaris C8-Th1 (ulnar margin of the little finger).
- N. musculocutaneous, C5–C7 (radial side of forearm).
- N. axillaris, C5–C6 (dorsolateral shoulder arch).

The following questions must be clarified on the basis of the neurological examination findings:

- Is there a central lesion (pyramidal or extrapyramidal)?
- Is there a lesion of the nerve root?
- Is there a lesion of a peripheral nerve?

4.3.5 Specific Lesion Patterns

4.3.5.1 Root Syndromes

Knowledge of specific lesion patterns facilitates classification (Table 4.10).

4.3.5.2 Plexus Paresis

Table 4.11 gives an overview of the different forms of obstetric brachial plexus palsy.

4.3.5.3 Lesions of Peripheral Nerves

These include radial, median and ulnar paresis (Table 4.12).

4.4 Techniques

4.4.1 Neurophysiological Diagnostics

The result of neurophysiological diagnostics depends on the child's willingness to cooperate. In

Table 4.10 Special root syndromes

	Dermatome	Identifying muscle
C5	Centre of lateral upper arm	M. deltoid
C6	Radial side of forearm, ball of thumb, thumb and radial side of index finger	M. biceps brachii M. brachioradialis
C7	Ventral and dorsal middle hand with middle finger and adjacent finger halves	M. triceps brachii Thenar M. pronator teres
C8	Ulnar hand side and ulnar side of the ring finger, little finger	Hypothenar muscles To a lesser extent also Mm. interossei
Th1	Centre medial forearm	M. abductor pollicis brevis

Table 4.11 Obstetric brachial plexus palsy

Height of the lesion	Frequency	Clinical symptoms
C5+C6 (Erb's palsy) M. deltoid + M. infraspinatus (C5) and M. biceps (C6)	50% of all cases	Upper arm is adducted, internal rotation, forearm stretched, hand and finger movement is free
C5–C7 (Erb's palsy plus)	35% of all cases	Upper arm is adducted, internal rotation, forearm extended + pronated, ulnar abduction, flexion of the wrists and finger joints = "waiter's tip"
C5-Th1		Paresis of the entire arm
C5-Th1 with severe root injury		Paresis of the entire arm with additional Horner syndrome ipsilateral
C8-Th1 (Klumpke's palsy)	Extremely rare (!)	Insolated palsy of the hand ("claw hand") with additional Horner syndrome
Upper plexus paresis (Erb)+C4 (N. phrenicus)		Additional unilateral diaphragm paralysis

children below primary school age, diagnosis is often only possible when the child is under sedation, although there are exceptions. The examination can also be successful with young children in a quiet, trusting atmosphere where a parent is present. Distraction with a small DVD player or tablet has proven to be extremely helpful.

- **Nerve compression syndromes:**
  - **Carpal tunnel syndrome: Nerve conduction studies (median n.): distal motor latency (DML) and distal sensory latency (DSL).**
  - **Cubital tunnel syndrome: Nerve conduction studies (ulnar n.): motor conduction velocity across the elbow and that below the elbow.**
  - **Ulnar tunnel syndrome: Nerve conduction studies (ulnar n.)** to abductor digiti minimi m. and interosseous dorsalis m.

Table 4.12 Lesions of peripheral nerves

Lesion site	Motor signs	Sensory failure
Radial nerve palsy		
Upper arm	"Wrist drop" (paresis of hand and finger extensors)	1. Spatium interosseum dorsal back of the hand
Proximal forearm	Paralysis of the finger extensors in the metacarpophalangeal joint and thumb abduction, no wrist drop – hand with radial extension	Intact
(Axilla)	Wrist drop + stretch failure elbow	1. Spatium interosseum dorsal back of the hand
Median nerve palsy		
Proximal	"Hand of benediction" (flexion weakness of thumb, index and middle finger), positive "bottle sign" (abduction weakness of thumb)	Radial palm +3½ radial fingers
Carpal tunnel	Abduction weakness and opposition weakness of thumbs	3½ radial fingers
Ulnar nerve palsy		
Upper arm/ elbow	"Claw hand" (failure of Mm. interossei), positive "Froment sign" (adduction weakness of the thumb)	Ulnar palm and back of the hand +1½ ulnar fingers
Forearm/ wrist	Claw hand, positive Froment sign	Depending on level of lesion only ulnar palm + 1½ ulnar fingers or only fingers

- **Traumatic nerve lesions:** Motor and sensitive neurography of the affected nerves, F-wave, EMG.
- **Plexus lesions:**
  - The value of neurophysiological examinations in the diagnostics of childhood plexus paresis continues to be controversially discussed [6].
  - Some authors use electromyography (EMG) and nerve conduction studies to distinguish between neuropraxia and axonotmesis or neurotmesis within a few days [7].
  - The electromyography of the back muscles is certainly most conclusive for the differential diagnosis of a root rupture, but is difficult to carry out in practice with an infant. Prognostically, the compound muscle action potential (CMAP) is regarded as valuable. According to one study, a reduction of the CMAP to below 10% of the opposite side after the first 2 weeks of life already correlates with a significant weakness at 6 months of age [8]. Reinnervation can also be proved with the help of the EMG, but the prognosis often seems to be too positive. In older children, the EMG can be used for specific questions on the function of individual nerves.

All neurophysiological findings can only be interpreted in conjunction with the clinical course. A standard for their use in childhood brachial plexus palsy has not yet been established.

- **Root lesions:**
  - EMG examinations in the characteristic muscles of the cervical nerve roots have the highest significance.
  - Polyneuropathy: Motor and sensitive nerve conduction velocities (on both sides) of two arm nerves and at least one leg nerve including F-wave.
  - EMG (distal, if possible).

4.5 Classifications

To describe motor skills, the "Gross Motor Function Classification System" (GMFCS) and the "Manual Ability Classification System" (MACS) are available [9], as well as the "Bimanual Fine Motor Function (BFMF) Classification" [10].

4.5.1 Gross Monitor Function Classification System (GMFCS)

The Canadian working group around Peter Rosenbaum has developed the instruments gross motor function measurement (GMFM) and GMFCS for measuring gross motor abilities in cerebral palsy. The GMFCS is a classification tool that allows an international age-based classification (from <2 years to 18 years) of cerebral palsy by severity level.

The GMFCS classifies the severity of functional impairment into 5 levels and takes into account the need for aids, including walking aids. Levels 1–5 are described for different age groups and serve as a guideline. Until their second year of life, the age of premature babies should be corrected accordingly.

The classification takes place according to the best everyday—not the best possible –motor ability that can be independently initiated at that time. The distance between the individual steps corresponds to an ordinal scale.

4.5.2 Bimanual Fine Motor Function (BFMF) Classification

The BFMF was developed in 2002 by Beckung and Hagberg analogous to the GMFCS, it divides the abilities of the hands separately into 5 levels (Table 4.12; [11, 12]).

The classification is used to describe unilateral and bilateral pareses, but in our experience, it does not adequately reflect the different levels of restriction. The ability to "transport" is completely missing, the gap between restrictions for "more complex fine motor tasks" and "only grasping and holding" is quite large.

4.5.3 Manual Ability Classification System (MACS)

The MACS describes the bimanual performance abilities of children aged 4–18 years in 5 levels (Fig. 4.2). A mini-MACS has been available for younger children since 2016 but is not yet available in German. The child's ability to deal with objects that are important for the activities of daily life (e.g., playing, leisure activities, eating, getting dressed) is recorded. In which situations is the child independent? To what extent does he or she need support and relief? The differentiation between the individual levels is made easier by descriptions in the available material. For example, "Children in level 2 can deal with most items, but in a slower and clumsy manner. Due to their limited ability to grasp or use objects, children in level 3, usually need help preparing the activity and/or adapting the environment" (www.macs.nu).

What is examined is the child's usual performance at home, in school and in community life. The classification should not be based on a special test procedure, but on interviews with people who know the child well. The interpretation must be adapted to the age of the child, and the different manual skills at different ages should be taken into account. The MACS is useful for communication with parents, among professionals, with politicians and social services, as well as for evaluation, the definition of goals and for establishing groups in research. The classification follows an ordinal scale.

A comparison between MACS and BFMF was published by Elvrum et al. [10] (Table 4.13).

4.6 Questionnaires

4.6.1 Children's Hand-Use Experience Questionnaire

The CHEQ is an online questionnaire for children from 6 years of age and adolescents with reduced hand function that covers 29 activities which are typically performed with two hands. The questionnaire can be completed by the children themselves (recommendation: from 13 years) or with their parents. A mini-CHEQ version has been developed for children aged 3–8. The questions refer to activities that are carried out independently and not independently, the use of hands during the activity, the effectiveness of grasping/stabilising, the speed

What do you need to know to use MACS?
The child's ability to handle objects in important daily activities, for example during play and leisure, eating and dressing. In which situation is the child independent and to what extent do they need support and adaptation?

I. **Handles objects easily and successfully.** At most, limitations in the ease of performing manual tasks requiring speed and accuracy. However, any limitations in manual abilities do not restrict independence in daily activities.

Distinctions between Levels I and II
Children in Level I may have limitations in handling very small, heavy or fragile objects which demand detailed fine motor control, or efficient coordination between hands. Limitations may also involve performance in new and unfamiliar situations. Children in Level II perform almost the same activities as children in Level I but the quality of performance is decreased, or the performance is slower. Functional differences between hands can limit effectiveness of performance. Children in Level II commonly try to simplify handling of objects, for example by using a surface for support instead of handling objects with both hands.

II. **Handles most objects but with somewhat reduced quality and/or speed of achievement.** Certain activities may be avoided or be achieved with some difficulty; alternative ways of performance might be used but manual abilities do not usually restrict independence in daily activities.

Distinctions between Levels II and III
Children in Level II handle most objects, although slowly or with reduced quality of performance. Children in Level III commonly need help to prepare the activity and/or require adjustments to be made to the environment since their ability to reach or handle objects is limited. They cannot perform certain activities and their degree of independence is related to the supportiveness of the environmental context.

III. **Handles objects with difficulty; needs help to prepare and/or modify activities.** The performance is slow and achieved with limited success regarding quality and quantity. Activities are performed independently if they have been set up or adapted.

Distinctions between Levels III and IV
Children in Level III can perform selected activities if the situation is prearranged and if they get supervision and plenty of time. Children in Level IV need continuous help during the activity and can at best participate meaningfully in only parts of an activity.

IV. **Handles a limited selection of easily managed objects in adapted situations.** Performs parts of activities with effort and with limited success. Requires continuous support and assistance and/or adapted equipment, for even partial achievement of the activity.

Distinctions between Levels IV and V
Children in Level IV perform part of an activity, however, they need help continuously. Children in Level V might at best participate with a simple movement in special situations, e.g. by pushing a button or occasionally hold undemanding objects.

V. **Does not handle objects and has severely limited ability to perform even simple actions.** Requires total assistance.

Fig. 4.2 Manual ability classification system (MACS) (https://www.macs.nu/files/MACS_English_2010.pdf)

compared to peers and the perceived load. The questionnaire is very suitable for defining therapy goals together with the child and the parents that are relevant to everyday life, and for measuring the effectiveness of a therapy. The evaluation with the questionnaire nicely shows the results of multimodal therapy (botulinum toxin, orthotics, physiotherapy and occupational therapy) (www.cheq.se).

4.7   Assessment

4.7.1   Assisting Hand Assessment

The Assisting Hand Assessment (AHA, [13]) was developed for children with an impairment of the hand function of an extremity (e.g., unilateral cerebral palsy or plexus palsy). It measures the performance of the affected hand in

Table 4.13 Comparison between MACS and BFMF [10]

BFMF	MACS
Level I One hand manipulates without restrictions. The other hand manipulates without restrictions or has limitations in more advance fine motor skills	*Level I* Handles objects easily and successfully. At most limitations in the ease of performing manual tasks requiring speed and accuracy. However, any limitations in manual abilities do not restrict independence in daily activities
Level II (a) One hand manipulates without restrictions. The other hand has only ability to grasp or hold. (b) Both hands have limitations in more advanced fine motor skills	*Level II* Handles most objects, but with somewhat reduced quality or speed of achievement Certain activities may be avoided or achieved with some difficulty; alternative ways of performing might be used, but manual abilities do not usually restrict independence in daily activities
Level III (a) One hand manipulates without restrictions. The other hand has no functional ability (b) One hand has limitations in more advanced fine motor skills. The other hand has only ability to grasp or worse. *The child needs help with tasks*	*Level III* Handles objects with difficulty; needs help to prepare and/or modify activities. The performance is slow and achieved with limited success regarding quality and quantity. Activities are performed independently if they have been set up or adapted
Level IV (a) Both hands have only ability to grasp (b) One hand has only ability to grasp. The other hand has only ability to hold or worse *The child needs support and/or adapted equipment*	*Level IV* Handles a limited selection of easily managed objects in adapted situations. Performs part of activities with effort and limited success. Requires continous support and assistance and/or adapted equipment for even partial achievement of the activity
Level V Both hands have only ability to hold or worse. *The child requires total assistance, even with adaptations*	*Level V* Does not handle objects and has severely limited ability to perform even simple actions. Requires total assistance

its function as an assisting hand. Assuming that "the hand fulfils its role as a supporting, holding and stabilising hand, it is referred to in the AHA concept as an "assisting hand" (not as a "non-dominant hand")." The test thus clearly differentiates between the roles of a dominant hand, a non-dominant hand and an assistant hand, which has considerable effects on the formulation of therapy goals and the selection of therapy methods for children with unilateral impairments. Thus, therapy does not focus on functions that are based on a healthy dominant hand or a non-dominant hand, but on functions that are important for an assisting hand.

There are two versions for infants and young children (6–18 months, mini-AHA) and for children (from 18 months to 12 years). In a videographed game situation, 20 items are each evaluated in six categories: general use, use of the arm, grasping/letting go, fine motor adjustment, coordination and speed. The quality of the most frequently observed execution is evaluated. This evaluation results in a total score that can be converted to an ordinal scale ("equal interval unit logits"). The AHA is standardised and valid, measures the child's performance in the use of the assisting hand and provides a good basis for planning and evaluating an activity-oriented therapy. A certification course is also required for this assessment (http://www.ahanetwork.se).

4.8 Definition and Review of the Therapeutic Objective

For the definition of therapy goals, various instruments are available that make a qualitative and quantitative assessment of the achievement of goals possible. In addition to the procedures mentioned here, the **Canadian Occupational Performance Measurement** (COPM), which is described in Chap. 10, should, in particular, be mentioned for the area of the upper extremity and the activities related to everyday life.

4.8.1 SMART Targets

The formulation of therapy goals is easier if it takes into account the criteria recorded in the SMART acronym:

- **S**pecific
- **M**easurable
- **A**ttractive, accepted
- **R**ealistic
- **T**imed

Therapeutic goals should be specific to the patient, measurable, accepted by child and environment, realistic in terms of the desired effect, and timed in terms of a temporal dimension of the assessment of success. Bovend'Eerdt and colleagues point out that each goal should consist of four parts: target activity, support needs, quantitative measurement of performance, and time to achieve the desired status. The quantity of performance can be measured by the time required to perform, the quantity achieved by continuous activity (e.g., distance travelled in a defined time) or by the frequency at which an activity can be performed in a defined time [14].

4.8.2 Goal Attainment Scale

The Goal Attainment Scale can be used to operationalise specific goals (Table 4.14; [15]). The

Table 4.14 Bimanual Fine Motor Function (BFMF) Classification—version 2.0[a]

BFMF version 2.0	
Level I One hand: manipulates without restrictions. The other hand: manipulates without restrictions or limitations in more advanced fine motor skills	
Level II (a) One hand: manipulates without restrictions. The other hand: only ability to grasp or hold (b) Both hands: limitations in more advanced fine motor skills	(a) (b)
Level III (a) One hand: manipulates without restrictions. The other hand no functional ability (b) One hand: limitations in more advanced fine motor skills. The other hand: only ability to grasp or worse	(a) (b) (b)
Level IV (a) Both hands: only ability to grasp (b) One hand: only ability to grasp. The other hand: only ability to hold or worse	(a) (b)
Level V Both hands: only ability to hold or worse	

[a]https://www.siv.no/seksjon/CP-registeret_/Documents/Klassifikasjonsverktoy/Bimanual%20Fine%20Motor%20Function%202.0.pdf

Table 4.15 Goal attainment scale

Points	Description	Occupational goal
+2	Goal achieved well above the expected level	Florian writes fluently with both hands on the keyboard
+1	Goal achieved slightly above the expected level	Florian tries to write with the other fingers as well
0	Goal achieved, expected outcome	Florian writes with his right hand (index and middle finger) on the right half of the keyboard
−1	Goal partially achieved	Florian uses the right index finger to press individual right-sided keys
−2	Current stage of development	Florian mainly writes with his left hand on the laptop

meaningfulness and stability of goals of children was investigated in a multicentre study with children from 7 to 11 years of age, according to which goals of children are just as achievable as those stated by parents. Children can therefore be trusted to define their own goals—and thus influence their participation in the intervention programme [16] (Table 4.15).

A common definition of the subgoals has proved to be particularly effective for children who can adhere to agreements, as this increases motivation and the achievement of subgoals can be assessed positively as a joint success.

4.9 Planning and Verification

Together with the child and/or its parents, goals are described and defined. In our experience, children of primary school age and older can provide information about their everyday life, their difficulties and their goals when the appropriate questions and examples are used (also using semi-structured interviews such as COPM, Chap. 10). At a defined point in time, progress and convergence towards the goal are recorded in a manner that is as qualitative and quantitative as possible.

In ambulatory settings, the Goal Attainment Scale and the CHEQ are particularly suitable instruments, as they can be applied quickly and effectively.

References

1. Hoare B J, Wallen M A, Imms C, et al. Botulinum toxin a as an adjunct to treatment in the management of the upper limb in children with spastic cerebral palsy (Cochrane update). Cochrane Database of Systematic Reviews. 2010.
2. Kraus de Camargo O, Hollenweger J. ICF-CY: Internationale Klassifikation der Funktionsfähigkeit, Behinderung und Gesundheit bei Kindern und Jugendlichen, Bern. 2011.
3. Kraus de Camargo O, Simon L. Die ICF-CY in der Praxis. Bern. 2013.
4. BAR—Bundesarbeitsgemeinschaft für Rehabilitation. ICF Praxisleitfaden 2—medizinische Rehabilitationseinrichtungen. Frankfurt. 2008.
5. Noreau L, Vachon J. Comparison of three methods to assess muscular strength in individuals with spinal cord injury. Spinal Cord. 1998;36:716–23.
6. Russmann B. Neonatal brachial plexus palsy. In: Post TW, editor. UpTo-Date. 2015. http://www.uptodate.com/contents/neonatal-brachial-plexus-palsy. Accessed 20 Apr 2020.
7. Giunta RE, et al. Geburtstraumatische Armplexusparesen. Monatsschr Kinderheilkd. 2010;158:262–72.
8. Heise CO, et al. Motor conduction studies for prognostic assessment of obstetrical plexopathy. Muscle Nerve. 2004;30:451–5.
9. Becher T, Horn A. GMFCS, MACS, AHA und andere Akronyme. Kann man wirklich damit arbeiten? Neuropädiatrie in Klinik und Praxis. 2016;15:11–8.
10. Elvrum A-KG, et al. Bimanual fine motor function (BFMF) classification in children with cerebral palsy: aspects of construct and content validity. Phys Occup Ther Pediatr. 2016;36:1–16.
11. Beckung E, Hagberg G. Neuroimpairments, activity limitations, and participation restrictions in children with cerebral palsy. Dev Med Child Neurol. 2002;44:309–16.
12. Elvrum A-KG, Beckung E, Sæther R, et al. Bimanual capacity of children with cerebral palsy: intra- and interrater reliability of a revised edition of the bimanual fine motor function classification. Phys Occup Ther Pediatr. 2017;37:239–51.

13. AHA Network. Assisting hand assessment web site. 2016. http://www.ahanetwork.se. Accessed 20 Apr 2020.
14. Bovend'Eerdt TJ, Botell RE, Wade DT. Writing SMART rehabilitation goals and achieving goal attainment scaling: a practical guide. Clin Rehabil. 2009;23:352–61.
15. Maloney FP, Mirrett P, Brooks C, Johannes K. Use of the goal attainment scale in the treatment and ongoing evaluation of neurologically handicapped children. Am J Occup Ther. 1978;32:505–10.
16. Vroland-Nordstrand K, Eliasson A-C, Jacobsson H, Johansson U, Krumlinde-Sundholm L. Can children identify and achieve goals for intervention? A randomized trial comparing two goal-setting approaches. Dev Med Child Neurol. 2016;58:589–96. https://doi.org/10.1111/dmcn.12925.

Surgical Diagnostic and Measurement Procedures

5

Jörg Bahm

5.1 Clinical Characteristics

The first knowledge base is given by the observation of the children and their disability, appropriate examination, and the recording of those findings that are important for developmental description and decision-making.

5.1.1 Extent of Active/Passive Movement

Each joint is examined passively and actively in all degrees of freedom (in the infant lying down—thus eliminating gravity, then sitting and standing: against gravity); the relevant restrictions compared to the healthy opposite side are noted. Active range of motion is strongly dependent on patient compliance and must be tested in a motivating manner and repeated if necessary.

Joint ankyloses are rare in infants and indicate either unrecognized subluxation or dislocation or arthrogryposis.

5.1.2 Muscle Weakness and Scoring

As early as [1], the British Medical Research Council (BMRC) drew up a muscle strength score that is still generally accepted today; Gilbert modified it for the examination of supine infants [2, 3].

This type of grading remains debated, as the functional correlation may vary. There is a dividing line at force grade M3 (movement against gravity, i.e., visible and applicable for upright patients is, therefore, a meaningful functional threshold). For shoulder movements and wrist extension, grade 4 and more are mandatory for function. Conversely, an M2 strength of intrinsic hand muscles may correct a paralytic deformity. So it is important to understand that the BMRC grade is relevant for the different muscles and functional movements being tested.

BMRC Muscle Strength Score
- 0: no muscle contraction
- 1: visible or palpable muscle contraction without movement
- 2: movement under conditions eliminating gravity
- 3: movement against gravity (dead weight of the arm)
- 4: movement against resistance
- 5: normal development of strength.

J. Bahm (✉)
Department of Plastic, Hand and Burn Surgery,
Section for Plexus Surgery, University Hospital,
Aachen, Germany
e-mail: jbahm@ukaachen.de,
jorg.bahm@belgacom.net

© Springer Nature Switzerland AG 2021
J. Bahm (ed.), *Movement Disorders of the Upper Extremities in Children*,
https://doi.org/10.1007/978-3-030-53622-0_5

5.1.3 Cutaneous Sensation

Although very good examination methods are available for adults, these are only rarely applied, recorded, or included in a plan of therapy (Chap. 9), especially for small children, due to a lack of compliance and feedback, but unfortunately sometimes also out of disinterest—the affected dermatomes are maybe difficult to delimit or determine. Obviously, we must try harder in this field to improve our knowledge in the future.

5.1.3.1 Cocontractions

As already mentioned in Chap. 1, the observation of cocontraction movement patterns and their objective determination by parallel surface electromyography is very important.

Treatment with botulinum toxin is discussed in Chap. 11.

5.1.4 Avoidance Movement or Adaptation Posture (Compensations)

Some compensation patterns are very typical, such as the throwback or lateral displacement of the upper body or the trumpet sign (Fig. 5.1).

5.1.5 Growth Disorder

One may find differences in the length of the long bones. When analyzing various joint contractures, joint dysplasia may be observed in ultrasound imaging due to the hypotrophic development of joint partners (Fig. 5.1), axial deviations, or an incongruent articulation (subluxation). These are usually triggered by long-lasting muscle imbalances between antagonists, which must first be corrected in order to have a lasting effect on the forces influencing the joint [4].

We have little influence on the hypoplasia of the epiphyses and the slower growth of the long bone. Angle corrections, for example, concerning the neck of the humeral head or glenoid, are carried out only hesitantly, since they sometimes correct the radiological image, but do not significantly improve the function in the sense of increasing the passive range of motion [5].

In older children, the existing joint status is therefore maintained and a rotational osteotomy is performed in the distal diaphysis to correct the positioning.

5.2 Surgical Decision Criteria

In the case of severe traumatic nerve damage without the likelihood of spontaneous recovery,

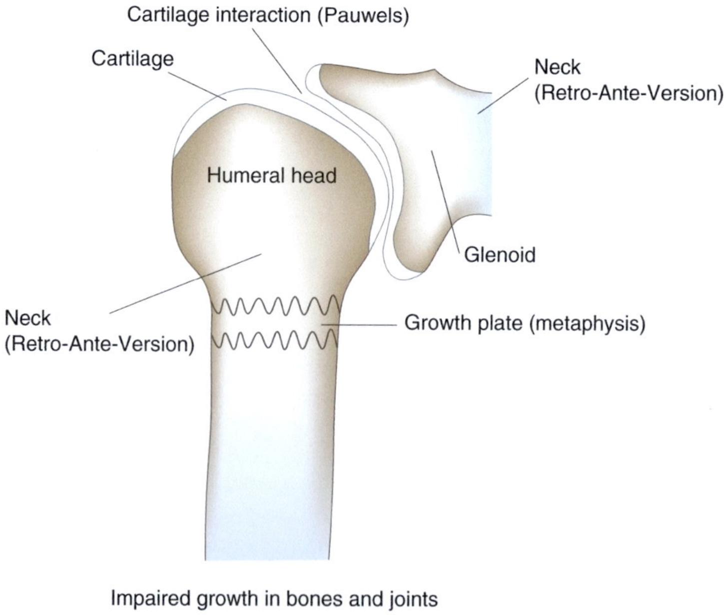

Fig. 5.1 Growth disorders in joints and bones

the decision to undergo surgery is made in the first 3 months after the trauma, mainly to overcome the progressive reduction of the motor target organs (progressive denervation amyotrophy).

This applies as much to the complete plexus palsy involving all roots (experience frequently has shown preganglionic lesions of the lower nerve roots supplying the hand) as it does to the injury or loss of individual nerves.

Surgical exploration is first and foremost the safest form of *diagnostic assessment, prior to* the actual reconstruction, performed in the same operative session [6, 7].

Partial lesions, as well as upper plexus damages, can be followed, according to the reinnervation period of 6–9 months at a rate of 1–2 mm/day, from the level of injury; only in the absence of one or more significant reinnervation targets will the operation be indicated.

Exceptions include preganglionic lesions seen on CT or MRI imaging or similar lesions with no or only little chance for reinnervation. Those must, therefore, be explored soon and reconstructed appropriately by nerve transfers.

Electrodiagnostic evidence of severe spinal nerve lesions with poor prognosis also may add valuable arguments for surgery, but this technique is only established in multidisciplinary centers with high expertise in this type of investigation in little children [8].

5.3 Accompanying Symptoms

Various of the following signs indicate an increased severity of injury and may strengthen an indication:

- The *Claude Bernard-Horner sign* suggests a preganglionic avulsion of spinal nerve Th1 and, in the case of complete plexus paresis, means a clear, urgent indication for surgery, which is then postponed only with regard to the infant's general condition (weight, concomitant diseases, relative immaturity of the lungs, etc.).
- The *paralysis of the ipsilateral hemidiaphragm* signs a serious lesion of the spinal nerve C4 or of the phrenic nerve in its course

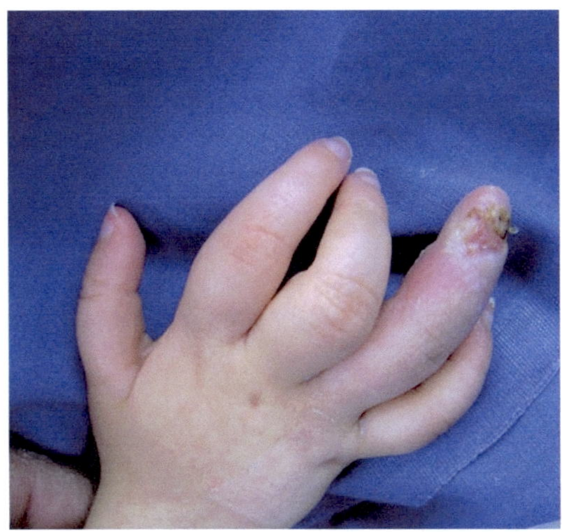

Fig. 5.2 Nail dystrophy as an expression of severe damage to the spinal nerves C8 and Th1

on the scalenus anterior muscle, where it can be embedded in a neuroma or other scarring.
- *Nail dystrophy:* torn or chewed nails are until further notice a sign of a severe loss of cutaneous sensation in the area of C8 and Th1 spinal nerves and are usually associated with severe proximal nerve damage, a proximal rupture, or true preganglionic lesion) (Fig. 5.2).

5.4 Measuring Methods

These include

- *Clinical examination:* passive and active range of motion (ROM), strength (BMRC M0-5), sensibility, daily activities: see Chap. 4.3.
- Objective methods of *motion analysis* (Chap. 6).
- *Imaging:* X-rays, ultrasound, MRI [9].

The use of imaging techniques in (young) children is rather limited for the following reasons:

- No precise direct insight into the nerve injury is provided nowadays by any imaging procedure. Only spinal nerve root tears can be seen in myelo-CT and MRI both directly (absence of radicles in the spinal canal) and indirectly (existence of meningomyeloceles); however, these investigations require sedation of the child and are naturally burdened by false-positive and negative results (Fig. 5.3).

- Radiation-intensive examinations without clear and powerful reasons should be avoided in children for reasons of radiation protection (especially shoulder CT), as other investigations like ultrasound may suffice.
- In addition to imaging, it is also a matter of skillful interpretation of the findings in uncommon disorders.

5.4.1 Standard Radiographs

Radiographs are helpful in the assessment of long bones (exclusion of fractures, postoperative documentation after osteotomy, subluxation of the radius head, joint assessment in arthrogryposis). Examples are shown in Fig. 5.4.

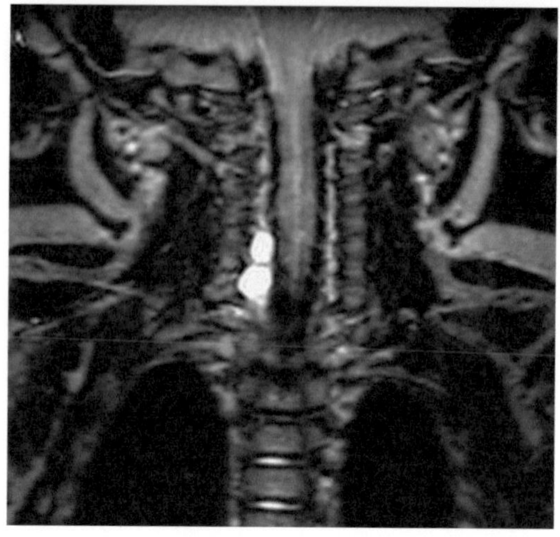

Fig. 5.3 Root avulsion in MRI: The light fluid pockets (so-called pseudo-meningocele) surrounding the injured rootlet attachment area onto the spinal cord are clearly visible, compared to the opposite unaffected side

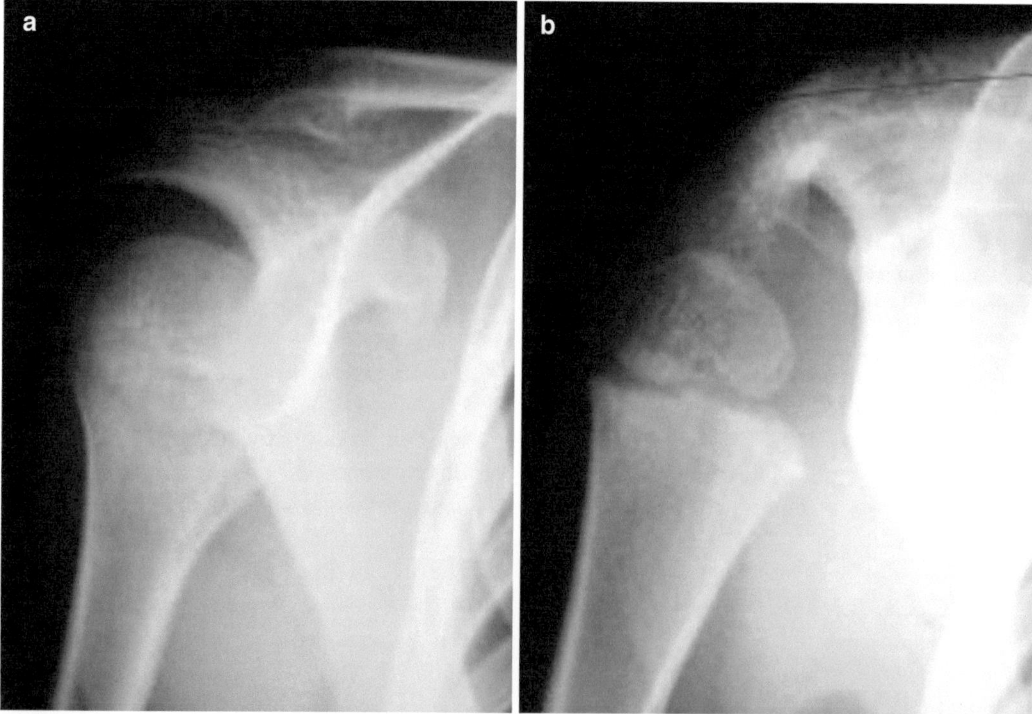

Fig. 5.4 (**a**, **b**) Radiological findings of the glenohumeral joint on the healthy side (**a**) in comparison with the shoulder altered by an internal rotation malposition in child-hood plexus palsy (**b**). The deformed, less ossified humeral head, which develops with delay due to the misalignment, is clearly visible in a side comparison

Fig. 5.5 Ultrasound findings of the same clinical situation as in Fig. 5.4 for internal rotation misalignment of the shoulder: *Left: Normal; right:* glenohumeral dysplasia. The ultrasound image also shows the comparative morphology of the subscapular and infraspinatus muscles

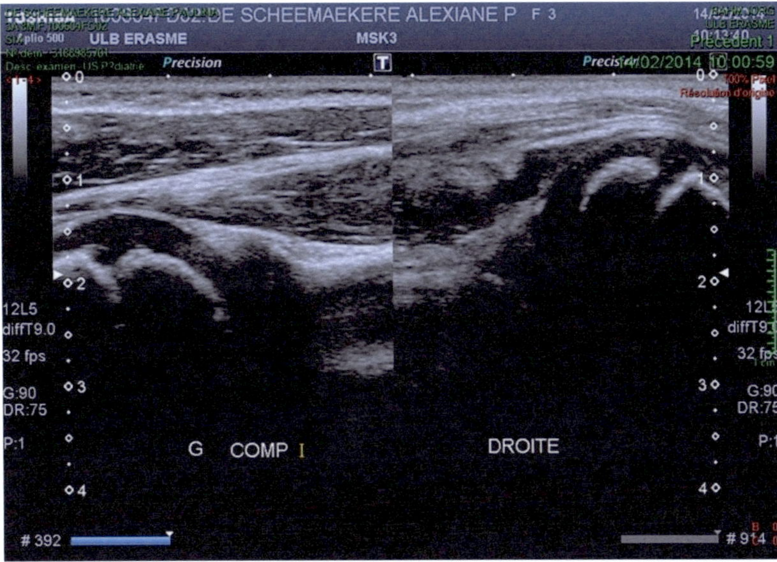

5.4.2 Ultrasound

Ultrasonography allows on the one hand a good and noninvasive assessment of the congruence of the shoulder joints in an experienced hand, but has also been increasingly used for structural diagnosis of peripheral nerves in recent years. We may anticipate more extensive application of this innocuous technique in lesions of spinal and peripheral nerves in the adult and child, mainly in the case of a structural lesion to larger nerves like a neuroma in continuity.

Ultrasound may also be used for morphological examinations and the measurement of questionable denervated muscles: fatty degeneration or atrophy during denervation (Fig. 5.5).

5.4.3 Magnetic Resonance Imaging (MRI): Cervical Spinal Cord and Meninges Lesions

MRI is currently the most important instrument to enable good morphological imaging in the central and peripheral nervous system, but it requires the sedation of the child under inpatient conditions and therefore a hospital stay. Figure 5.6 shows some examples.

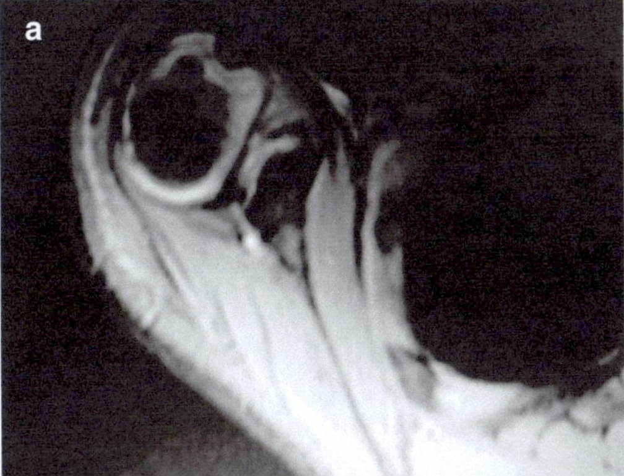

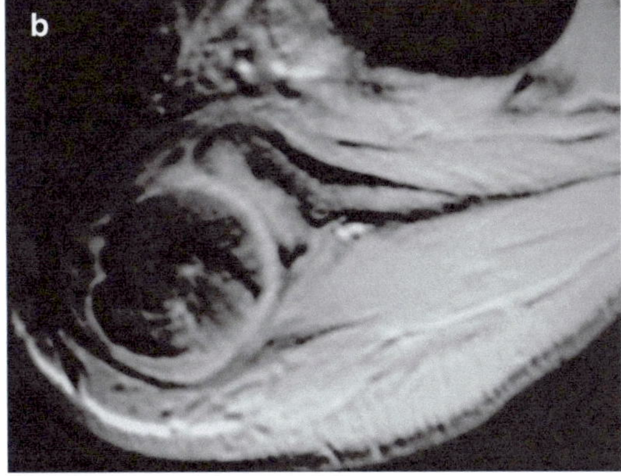

Fig. 5.6 (**a, b**) Two examples of the dorsally subluxated position of the humeral head in the transversal image section in MRI

References

1. British Medical Research Council. Aids to the investigation of peripheral nerve injuries. London: His Majesty's Stationery Office; 1943.
2. Gilbert A, Hentz VR, Tassin FL. Brachial plexus reconstruction in obstetric palsy: operative indications and postoperative results. In: Urbaniak JR, editor. Microsurgery for major limb reconstruction. St Louis: Mosby; 1987.
3. Gilbert A, Pivato G, Kheiralla T. Long-term results of primary repair of brachial plexus lesions in children. Microsurgery. 2006;26(4):334–42.
4. Döderlein L. Bedeutung der muskulatur für die entwicklung neuromuskulärer deformitäten–neue diagnostische und therapeutische aspekte. Orthopade. 2010;39:7–14.
5. Graichen H, Koydl P, Zichner L. Der Stellenwert der Glenoidosteotomie in der Behandlung der posterioren Schulterinstabilität. Z Orthop. 1998;136: 238–42.
6. Bahm J. Die kindliche armplexusparese–übersicht zur klinik, pathophysiologie und chirurgischen behandlungsstrategie. Handchir Mikrochir Plast Chir. 2003;35(2):83–97.
7. Blaauw G, Muhlig RS, Vredeveld JW. Management of brachial plexus injuries. In: Advances and technical standards in neurosurgery, vol. 33. Wien New York: Springer; 2008. p. 201–31.
8. Bisinella GL, Birch R, Smith SJM. Neurophysiological prediction of outcome in obstetric lesions of the brachial plexus. J Hand Surg. 2003;28B(2):148–52.
9. Gasparotti R, Garozzo D, Ferraresi S. Radiographic assessment of adult brachial plexus injuries. In: Chung KC, Yang LJS, Mc Gillicuddy JE, editors. Practical management of pediatric and adult brachial plexus palsies. Amsterdam: Elsevier; 2012.

6

C. Disselhorst-Klug

6.1   Introduction

To move independently is the basis for the human being's ability to act. Movement disorders and functional movement restrictions cause pain and hinder. If the upper extremities are affected, the performance of everyday activities is often hardly possible or impaired. Therefore, in addition to diagnosis, the restoration of the patient's mobility through suitable individually adapted measures plays an important role. This is a prerequisite for a quicker restoration of mobility and an independent lifestyle.

The main problem associated with movement disorders is the objective evaluation of the patient's movement performance. In addition to the clinical examination, the physician has so far primarily relied on the visual observation of the movements, a qualitative approach that is essentially based on the **subjective impression** of the investigator.

Semi-objective methods are scores and questionnaires. However, they do not describe the actual motion sequence and thus do not take malposition or coping movements into account. Imaging procedures are mostly not dynamic and therefore do not provide any information about the execution of the movement.

However, an objective analysis of the cause, extent and severity of the movement restriction improves diagnostics and is a prerequisite for an individual adaptation of the therapy measures and for control of the therapy success. For this reason, movement analysis methods which provide quantitative information on individual deficits are becoming increasingly important. The aim is to support the physician in his decision making on the therapy of patients by using objective measures. This allows optimizing the therapy and its better adaption to the individual needs of the patient.

Two aspects are fundamentally essential when it comes to describing human motion quantitatively (Fig. 6.1) [1]. One aspect is the purely phenomenological description of the actual movement, mostly according to the laws of mechanics. This includes, for example, the consideration of joint positions, movement speeds or symmetries (kinematics) as well as the acting forces and torque (kinetics) [2]. In the pathological context in particular, the muscular component must also be taken into consideration as an essential cause of movement. About the so-called **muscular coordination patterns**, the circle between the control of movement by the central nervous system and the resulting execution of movement closes. Most functional limitations

C. Disselhorst-Klug (✉)
Department of Rehabilitation and Prevention
Engineering, Institute of Applied Medical
Engineering, RWTH Aachen University,
Aachen, Germany
e-mail: disselhorst-klug@ame.rwth-aachen.de

© Springer Nature Switzerland AG 2021
J. Bahm (ed.), *Movement Disorders of the Upper Extremities in Children*,
https://doi.org/10.1007/978-3-030-53622-0_6

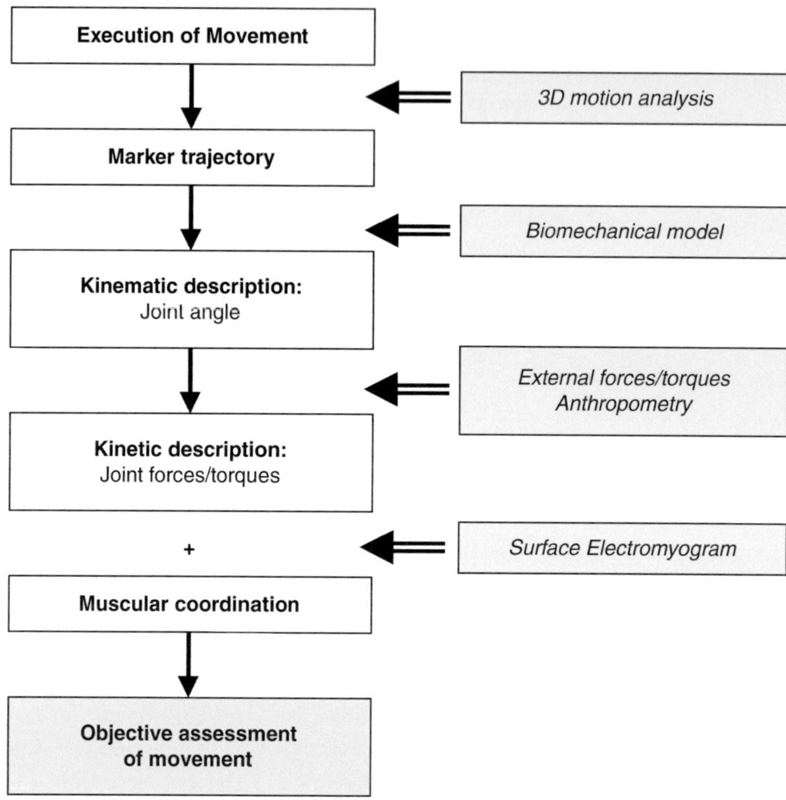

Fig. 6.1 Necessary steps leading to a quantitative and objective description of human motion. The gain in information through the addition of further measured variables and biomechanical models leads to an increasingly detailed description of the movement. (Modified according to [1])

lead to deviations in the muscular coordination pattern. Three alternatives tend to be possible:

– Due to neuromuscular diseases, individual muscles can no longer or only with reduced strength contribute to the execution of movement.
– Cerebral damage means that individual muscles or muscle groups can no longer be controlled in isolation.
– Painful changes in the musculoskeletal system cause malposition and coping movements with altered muscular coordination patterns.

Changes in the muscular coordination pattern have a long-term effect on the entire musculoskeletal system and often lead to **consequential damages**, which in turn restrict the functionality. Information about changes in the muscular coordination pattern is therefore not only important for the evaluation of movement performance; from them, conclusions can often be drawn about consequential damages and their prevention.

6.2 Objective Detection of Upper Limb Movements

6.2.1 Motion Analysis Methods

All methods and procedures used to record human motion are referred to as motion analysis procedures. In recent years, motion analysis methods have become increasingly important, especially in clinical gait analysis. Many of the motion analysis techniques used in clinical gait analysis either looked at the symmetry of the gait or determined path-time parameters. This approach is based on the periodic repetition of the gait cycle, which in the physiological case is performed symmetrically by both body halves.

In contrast to gait, movements of the upper extremities are neither symmetrical nor periodic. Therefore, motion analysis methods for the quantitative assessment of movements of the upper extremities aim at the determination of joint angles, joint angle velocities and joint angle accelerations. This form of description, known as kinematics, is often supplemented by kinetics, in which the forces and torques acting on the joints are included in addition to the kinematics [1, 2].

Many simple motion analysis techniques, such as **goniometer**, already provide diagnostically valuable quantitative and objective information, for example, on the maximum range of motion of a patient. However, this information is only static and thus represents only a snapshot of the motion. In addition, usually only one angle can be measured at a time, while the joints of the upper extremity have at least two degrees of freedom of rotation, most of them three.

Video analyses allow the evaluation of the movement performance and document the status quo of the patient, but do not provide quantitative information and are therefore dependent on the subjective impression of the observer. In addition, the image they provide is two-dimensional, while the movements of the upper extremities usually take place in three planes. Three-dimensional motion analysis methods (**3D motion analysis**) combine the advantages of video analysis with a quantitative description of the movement and thus allow an objective recording of dynamic movements in three dimensions.

Significant technical progress was made with the introduction of the **photometric measuring method** in the last 30 years, so that today reliable 3D motion analysis systems with sufficient accuracy are available. With the photometric measurement method, the movement of passive infrared light-reflecting markers (Fig. 6.2b), which are glued to the test object, is detected with at least two cameras. The movement of the markers in space is then reconstructed three-dimensionally from the image data. Fig. 6.2a shows a typical infrared camera used for motion analysis. Since the cameras film the movement of the marker with a high temporal resolution, the position of the marker in space results as a function of time (trajectory) (Fig. 6.2c).

Compared to gait, the movements of the upper extremities are more complex and less reproducible. Therefore, a high number of infrared cameras is necessary to ensure that at any time of movement a marker attached to the arm is seen by at least two cameras. Modern motion analysis laboratories often have ten or more cameras arranged in a circle. This ensures that even with complex movements, the markers are captured by at least two cameras. If the marker positions are linked to a biomechanical model of the human body, joint positions and their changes in time can be determined (Fig. 6.1). In this way, conclusions can be drawn about the actual movement performed by the patient. Today, marker-based

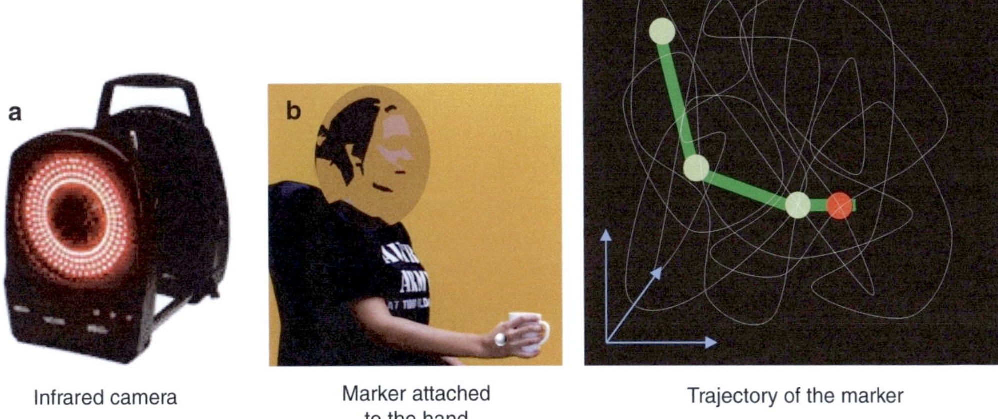

Fig. 6.2 (a–c) Photometric motion analysis. (a) Infrared camera. (b) Markers on the hand. (c) Three-dimensional trajectory of the marker during a 1-min movement of the hand

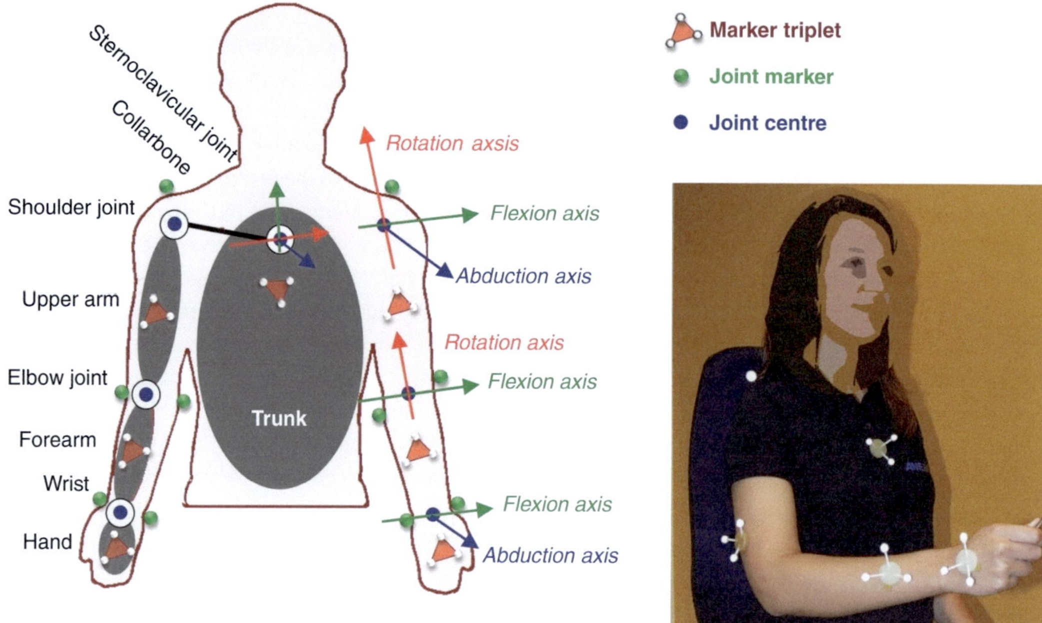

Fig. 6.3 Structure of the biomechanical model of the upper limb and the resulting marker arrangement. The movement of each segment is determined by a marker triplet (*red*). To define the joint centres and anatomical joint axes, additional markers (*green*) are required

3D motion analysis systems are a reliable, fast and extremely accurate tools for analysing motion in all degrees of freedom [3, 4].

6.2.2 3D Motion Analysis of the Upper Extremity (Kinematics)

6.2.2.1 Objective Determination of the Joint Position and Joint Angle

A biomechanical model is necessary to link the three-dimensional marker movements with the rotational movements around anatomical joint axes established in everyday clinical practice (Fig. 6.1) [2]. Like most biomechanical models, the biomechanical model of the upper extremity assumes of rigid segments connected by ideal ball joints [1, 5]. The hand, forearm, upper arm, collarbone and trunk are each regarded as a rigid segment connected by the wrist, the elbow, the shoulder joint and the sternoclavicular joint (Fig. 6.3) [1, 5, 6].

The movement of each individual segment in space can be detected in all degrees of freedom by three noncollinear markers per segment, which must not move relative to each other. Such a marker arrangement is usually represented by **marker triplets** (Fig. 6.3). The collarbone is an exception, as this segment is not accessible through markers attached to the skin. The collarbone is therefore assumed to be the rigid connecting line between the sternum and the humeral head [5].

With the help of the marker triplets, the movement and orientation of the individual segments in space is defined. However, the orientation of the individual segments relative to each other is important for the clinical evaluation of a movement, since this describes the actual joint position. To ensure that the calculated joint position corresponds with the anatomical joint position, the centre of rotation must correspond to the anatomical joint centre and the axes of rotation to the anatomical axes of the joint connecting two rigid segments. The joint centres are determined by a static calibration measurement in which joint markers are attached to anatomically defined positions (Fig. 6.3—green markers). With the aid of additional anthropometric information such as height, weight and joint width, the position of the anatomical joint centres (Fig. 6.3—blue dots) relative to the marker triplets can be estimated from the position of the joint markers [5].

Because of the strong skin movement at the joints, the joint markers are only used during the static calibration measurement and are removed later. After calibration, the rotation around the individual anatomical joint axes can be calculated from the trajectories of the triplet markers [5, 6]. As in clinical gait analysis, Euler/Kardan angles are used for this resulting in:

- Flexion/extension angles
- Abduction/adduction angles
- Rotation angles performed around the longitudinal axis of a segment

It should be noted that anatomically no abduction/adduction axis is defined in the elbow joint and no rotation axis in the wrist (Fig. 6.3). By definition, all joint angles are zero in the neutral zero position.

In comparison to the gait, different movement strategies are chosen by different persons to solve a movement task of the upper extremity. This usually leads to a large variability between the individual measurements [1]. It is therefore urgently necessary to give the patient or test person the most precisely defined movement task possible. This can be, for example, defined goal-oriented everyday movements in which the start and the desired end position are known. Examples of this are the so-called "cookie tests" in which the hand moves from the knee to the mouth or the movement task "parking ticket" which is described below. An alternative procedure is the method of the so-called **3D tracking** [7], in which a robot specifies a defined three-dimensional trajectory which the subject should follow with his finger. By this procedure the position of the hand is given at any time of the movement and thereby limits the possibilities of variation in joint positions and movement speed. Compared to freely executed, targeted movements, a higher reproducibility of the movement can be achieved by the method of 3D tracking [7].

6.2.2.2 Pathological Changes in Movement Patterns

Figure 6.4 shows the typical movement pattern for the everyday movement **"Parking ticket"**. Here, healthy test persons were asked to perform a movement that is necessary to pull from a seated position (car) a parking ticket from a machine at the entrance of a parking garage. The magnitudes of the movements around the anatomical axes of the shoulder, elbow and sternoclavicular joints calculated based on the biomechanical model from the positions of the markers of the triplets are plotted. The example of the complex everyday movement "Parking ticket" shows that with the method of the 3D motion analysis a quantitative detection of the movements of upper extremities becomes possible. In addition, it is shown that movement sequences between individual subjects are reproducible and that, like clinical gait analysis, a base-line of healthy movement patterns can be created [5].

Pathological movements can now be evaluated on a patient-specific basis against the baseline of healthy subjects. Figure 6.4 shows the example of a patient with frozen shoulder. A pathologically reduced abduction as well as a slightly reduced rotation of the shoulder joint is clearly visible. This special patient compensates for the limited movement of the shoulder by an increased flexion of the shoulder and a lowering of the shoulder in the sternoclavicular joint. Furthermore, the temporal interaction of the different joints has changed significantly. Thus, the extension of the elbow during the holding phase takes considerably longer [5]. It has also been shown in patients with shoulder stiffness that it is possible to achieve quality control in the rehabilitation of upper extremities with this procedure [8, 9].

Bahm and colleagues have been the first who used 3D motion analysis information for therapy planning in children with obstetric plexus brachialis lesions [10, 11]. The individual movement

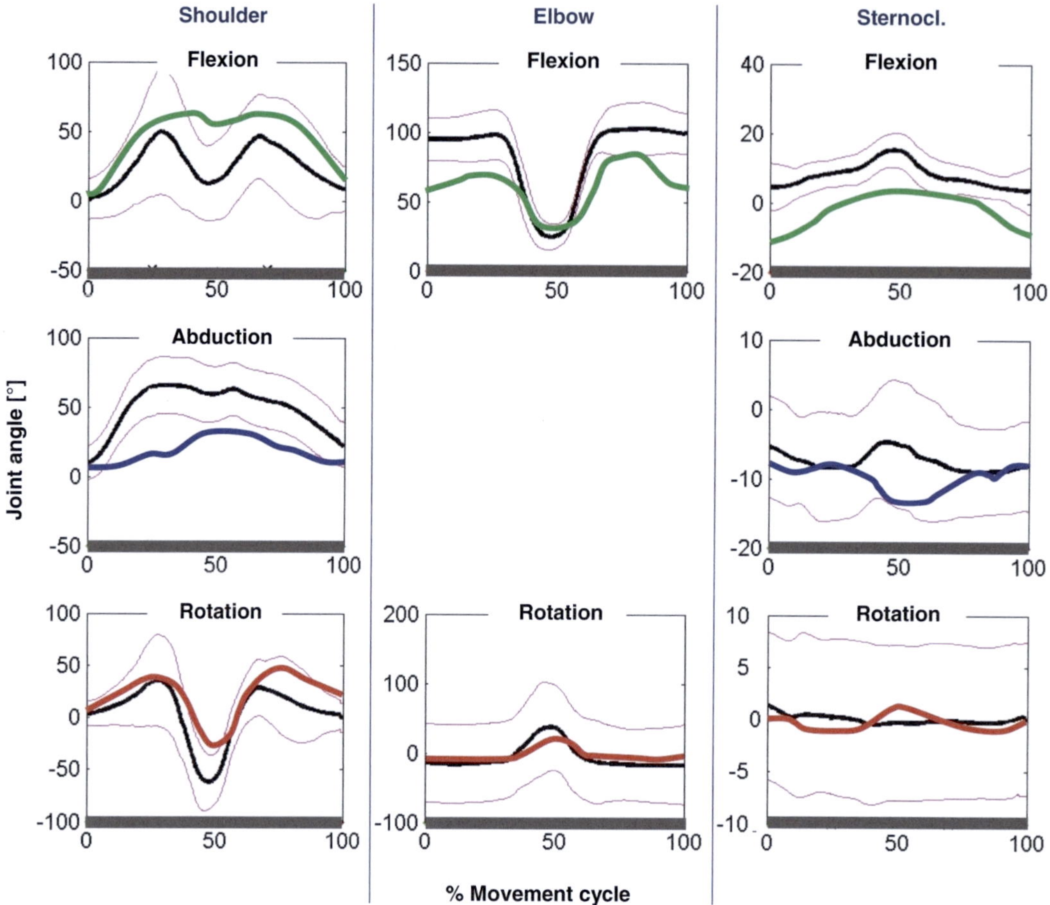

Fig. 6.4 Movement pattern of the movement task "Parking ticket" for healthy subjects (base line) and a patient with shoulder stiffness. *Black:* Average motion of healthy subjects. *Magenta:* Standard deviation of the motion of healthy subjects. *Green:* Flexion movement of the patient in shoulder, elbow and sternoclavicular joint. *Blue:* Abduction movement of the patient in shoulder and sternoclavicular joint. *Red:* Rotational movement of the patient in shoulder, elbow and sternoclavicular joint. In the elbow joint, anatomically the abduction/adduction is not defined. (Modified after [5])

patterns of the children were analysed during different everyday tasks and the degree of movement restriction was determined by comparing the affected side with the non-affected side.

Many patients suffering from a obstetric plexus-brachialis lesion experience a pathological internal rotation malposition of the shoulder. Figure 6.5a shows that the degree of pathological misalignment during movement can be quantified using 3D motion analysis of the upper extremities. In the example shown, during the execution of a flexion/extension movement of the shoulder compared to the unaffected side, a rotational malposition of an average of 60° can be seen in the shoulder joint, while the movements about the other joint axes are unchanged (Fig. 6.5a).

Figure 6.5b shows the example of a more complex everyday movement in which the patient's hand moves from the knee to the mouth in a seated position. While the patient was able to successfully perform the movement task with the unaffected side, the hand did not reach the mouth on the affected side. The reason for this is a significant restriction of the active range of motion in the elbow joint (Fig. 6.5b), which prevents

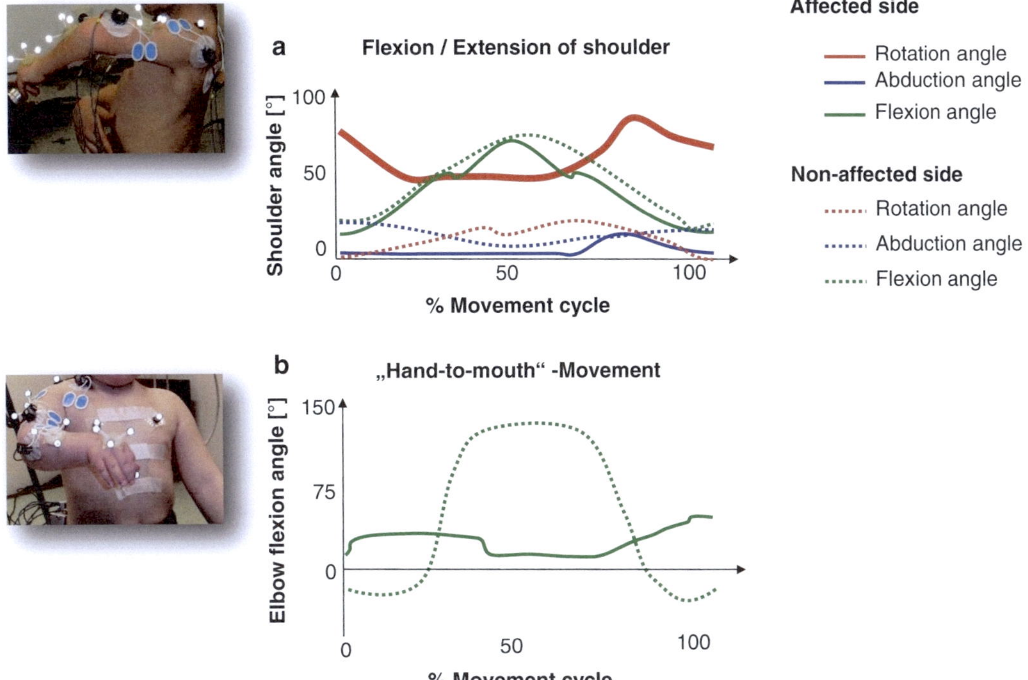

Fig. 6.5 (**a**, **b**) Typical changes in the movement pattern of patients with obstetric plexus lesions. (**a**) Pathologically changed movement pattern of a shoulder flexion/extension movement (0–90°) with pathological internal rotation of the shoulder. (**b**) Active limitation of elbow joint movement during "hand-to-mouth movement" (cookie test).

flexion of the elbow during the movement. It is typical for these patients that the limitation of movement occurs only during the active execution of movement, while passive elbow flexion is possible.

6.2.3 Forces and Torques Acting on the Joints During Movements of the Upper Extremity (Kinetics)

The 3D motion analysis of the upper extremity provides objective information about pathological deviations in the patient's movement patterns. The degree of movement restriction and coping movements performed by patients to execute successfully a movement task can be quantified.

However, motion analysis alone does not provide any information on the harmfulness of pathological motion patterns for joints and surrounding structures (Fig. 6.1). The forces and torques acting on the joints during movement are decisive for the stress on the joints. Since bony structures can adapt functionally to the acting forces [12, 13], this adaptation manifests itself macroscopically in the shape and size of bones and the points of attack of tendons, ligaments and muscles. This was systematically described by Pauwels [14], who was able to show that unphysiological stress leads to a strain on the bone, which increases the risk of joint deformations and joint wear. In fact, movement disorders of the upper extremities also lead to changes in the joint shape, which are very likely attributable to pathological forces acting on the joints during pathological movement executions [15, 16]. For this reason, in addition to kinematics, it makes sense to also consider the kinetics of the movement performed, which includes the forces and torques acting (Fig. 6.1).

6.2.3.1 Determination of Joint Forces and Torques

The forces and torques acting on the joints of the extremities during movement can be divided into internal forces generated by the body itself and external forces due to the interaction of the body with its environment [2]. The **internal forces** include the active muscle forces as well as passive forces of tendons, ligaments or bony structures. In the kinetic description of the movement, the forces and torques are calculated which arise in the individual joint either through the movement itself or through the external forces. They are usually in equilibrium with the internal forces. The kinetic description of the movement therefore ignores the internal forces, the active muscle forces. The muscular coordination pattern (see below) provides an estimate of the share of the musculature in the joint forces and torques.

A prerequisite for the kinetic description of the movement of the upper extremities is the acquisition of the kinematics of the wrist, the elbow, the shoulder and the sternoclavicular joint according to the anatomical axes as described above. During movement, the individual body segments (hand, forearm and upper arm) are affected by gravity and inertia forces [17]. These can be calculated from the anthropometric data of the subject and the joint positions of each individual joint [18]. According to Zatsiorsky, the masses of the individual body segments, their moments of inertia and the distance between the centres of gravity of the body segments from the centre of rotation of the adjacent joints can be calculated using easily measurable quantities such as body weight, body height and segment lengths [19]. If only one's own body is moved, anthropometric and kinematic data are enough to calculate the forces acting on the joints (Fig. 6.6).

If additional external forces are applied during movement by the subject, they must be known and added to gravity and inertial forces (Figs. 6.1 and 6.6) [18]. These additional external forces can be given, for example, by a dumbbell or an isokinetic device. Innovative new processes use robotics to specify and control external forces. In this procedure, the robot guides the hand of the subject. At the same time, the acting forces and torques are measured using a force-torque sensor located between the robot and the hand. The advantage of this approach is a high reproducibility of both the movement and the applied forces [7].

If the anthropometric data, the kinematics of the movement and the external forces are known, it is possible to use the **inverse dynamics** to estimate the forces acting in the individual joints (Fig. 6.6). In the case of the upper extremity, inverse dynamics means that first the joint forces and torques in the wrist are calculated regarding the external forces as well as inertia and weight of the hand. The joint forces and torques in the elbow joint are the sum of the inertia and weight of the lower arm and the joint forces acting in the wrist. The forces and torques in the shoulder joint

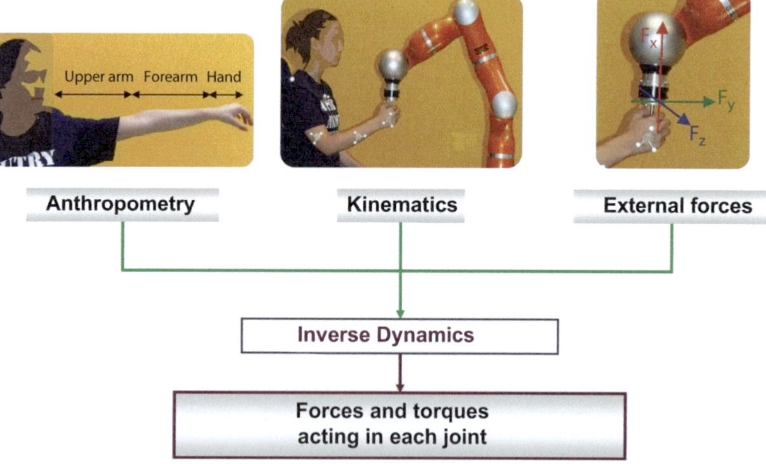

Fig. 6.6 Procedure for the kinetic description of the movement. The forces and moments acting in the individual joints can be calculated from anthropometric data, kinematic motion description and measured external forces

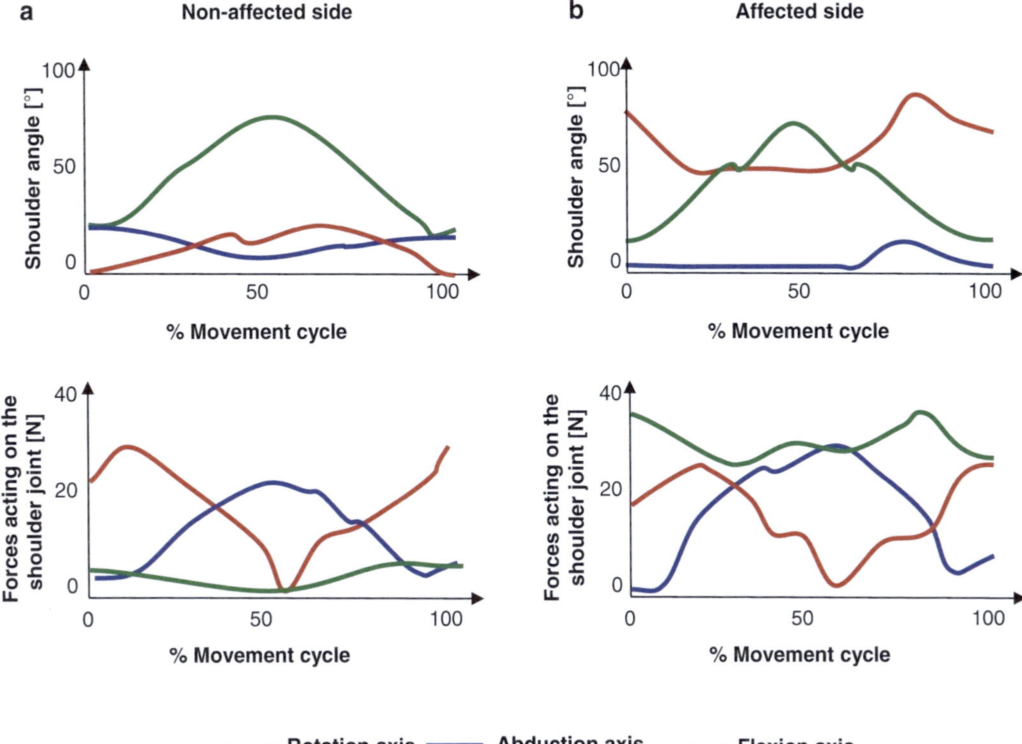

Fig. 6.7 Forces acting on the shoulder joint during a flexion/extension movement (0°–90°) of the shoulder when the elbow has a flexion angle of 120° during the movement and the hand has been held in pronated position. (**a**) Physiological movement. (**b**) Pathological movement with an average of 60° internally rotated shoulder. (Modified according to [18])

correspond to the sum of the weight and inertia of the upper arm and the joint forces acting in the elbow joint [2, 18].

Figure 6.7a shows the typical forces that act in the shoulder joint during a flexion/extension movement from 0° to approx. 90° shoulder flexion. Since the forces acting on the joints are added up from distal to proximal by means of inverse dynamics, the forces acting on the shoulder joint can only be interpreted correctly if the joint positions of the distal joints are known. In the movement underlying Fig. 6.7a, the flexion angle of the elbow was approximately 120°. In addition, the hand was in pronated position [18].

At the beginning of the movement, while the arm is hanging downwards, the weight of the hand, forearm and upper arm acts along the humerus and thus in the direction of the rotation axis of the shoulder joint. During the execution of the movement, the direction of action of the force changes in relation to the position of the anatomical joint axes. With a flexion position of 90° of the shoulder, the weight forces act exclusively along the anatomical abduction/adduction axis of the shoulder joint, which is directed towards the ground during this phase of movement. At no time during the physiologically performed movement did forces act along the flexion/extension axis of the shoulder.

6.2.3.2 Pathological Joint Damaging Forces

Kleiber et al. have dealt extensively with the question of how pathological **coping movements** (trick movements) affect the joint forces in the upper extremities [18]. His calculations were based on investigations of coping movements of patients with obstetric plexus-brachialis lesions.

Figure 6.7b shows an example of the forces acting on the shoulder joint of the same patient shown in Fig. 6.5a, who suffered from a malposition of the shoulder joint of average 60° internal rotation. Apart from the rotational malposition of the shoulder, the execution of the movement corresponded to that shown in Fig. 6.7a (shoulder flexion 0° to approx. 90°; elbow flexed by 120°; hand pronated). It can clearly be seen that an additional force acts along the flexion/extension axis over the entire range of motion.

Kleiber et al. were also able to show, through simulations, that with increasing internal rotation of the shoulder there is an additional increase in the force along the abduction/adduction axis of the shoulder. The resulting force vector shows medial-posterior. The body reacts to these unphysiological forces with a bony growth that is opposite to the direction of force. Corresponding morphological changes of the shoulder joint in connection with a obstetric plexus-brachialis lesion is described in the literature and confirmed by imaging procedures [15, 16].

6.3 Objective Assessment of Muscular Coordination

Although kinematics and kinetics provide quantitative measures of the execution of movement tasks that enable an objective description of the subject's condition and a follow-up check, they do not provide any information about the cause of the restriction of movement. However, information about possible causes can be found in the **muscular coordination patterns** that reflect motion control by the central nervous system.

The temporal coordination of individual muscles or muscle groups leads to the targeted and highly precise execution of a movement. Agonistic, synergistic and antagonistic muscles always work hand in hand as active driving power sources to control the movement [20]. The aim is to achieve the most precise, targeted movement possible while at the same time keeping energy consumption low. The neuro-musculoskeletal system uses passive forces, such as gravity, mass inertia or passive forces of muscles, tendons and ligaments, in addition to active force develop-

ment through the musculature. Movement and muscular coordination always go hand in hand. Accordingly, the interpretation of a movement execution always requires information about the underlying muscular coordination pattern. On the other hand, an interpretation of the muscular coordination pattern is not possible if there is no information about the movement performed.

6.3.1 Surface Electromyography (sEMG)

When the muscles are excited by the central nervous system, an electric field develops on the skin surface. Its strength reflects the degree of activation of the muscles and it can be measured by means of surface electrodes. This procedure, called surface-electromyography (sEMG), is an established method for studying muscle function [21].

Compared to needle electromyography, which is widely used in neurology and in which the signals are derived directly from the muscle fibre, the sEMG has a much lower spatial resolution and thus provides only a statement about the global activity of individual muscles or muscle groups [22]. Due to its non-invasive character, it is particularly suitable for investigations of the muscular coordination pattern during movements. For this purpose, the sEMG signals of several muscles or muscle groups are simultaneously derived using surface electrodes and recorded synchronously with the movement [2].

Figure 6.8 shows the typical electrode arrangement for recording the muscular coordination pattern of the upper extremity, which generates the coordinated movement of the elbow and shoulder during a hand-to-mouth movement (Cookie test). The sEMG signals are derived bipolar with relatively large electrodes (diameter 0.8 cm) and a wide electrode spacing (electrode spacing 2 cm). The EMG signals are amplified immediately behind the electrodes to ensure a sufficiently good signal quality. In order to be able to relate the muscular coordination pattern to the movement performed, the execution of the movement is simultaneously recorded by means of 3D movement analysis (Figs. 6.1 and 6.8). The muscular coordination pattern obtained in this

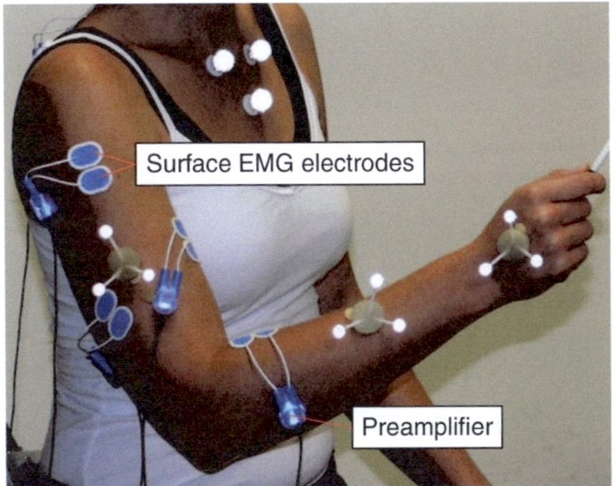

Fig. 6.8 Derivation of the surface electromyogram by means of surface electrodes (*blue*) for detecting the muscular coordination pattern of the upper extremity and marker arrangement for simultaneously detecting the movement execution

way provides information about which muscle was activated at which point in time during the movement execution [23, 24].

6.3.2 Muscular Coordination in Upper Extremity Movements

In the sense of an energy-efficient execution of movement, with slight variations synergistic muscles are activated at the same time in motions, while antagonistic muscles are activated so in time that the overlap becomes minimal.

Figure 6.9a shows the physiological coordination pattern of the two antagonists biceps and triceps as it occurs in the flexion/extension

Fig. 6.9 (**a, b**) Muscular coordination pattern of biceps and triceps during a hand-to-mouth movement (cookie test) (Fig. 6.5b). (**a**) Physiological coordination patterns. (**b**) Pathological coactivation of antagonistic muscles in a patient with obstetric plexus lesion.

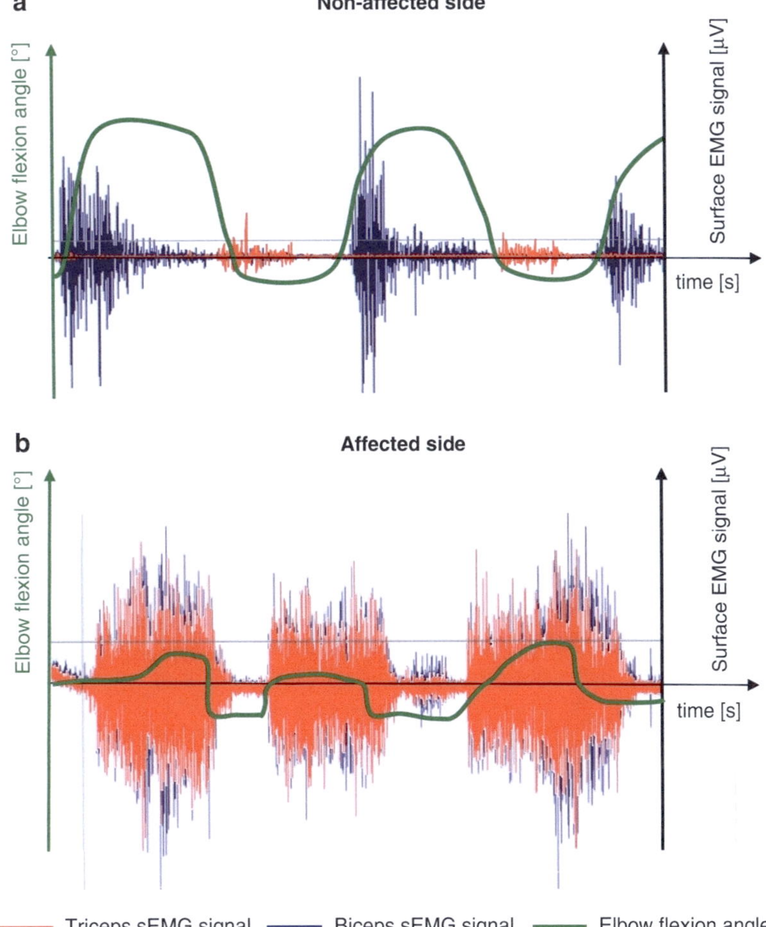

movement of the elbow. In accordance with its function as an elbow flexor, the biceps is activated by the central nervous system during flexion of the elbow, thus moving the forearm against the weight force. With complete flexion of the elbow, the biceps muscle only has a stabilizing effect, which requires less muscle strength and thus less activation by the central nervous system. The extension of the elbow is mainly caused by the weight of the forearm. For this reason, elbow extension is passive, and an active contribution of the triceps muscle is not required. The triceps is only activated when the elbow is overstretched in order to stabilize the joint.

Neurological diseases can lead to a pathological change in muscular coordination, which can be caused both centrally and peripherally. Central coordination disorders include the following above all **spasticity**. An example of a peripheral disorder is the patient from Fig. 6.5b with an obstetric plexus-brachialis lesion (Fig. 6.9b). Due to the obstetric plexus-brachialis lesion, active flexion of the elbow during hand-to-mouth movement was not possible. The cause of the movement disorder becomes clear through the method of surface electromyography. The two antagonists biceps and triceps are activated simultaneously by the nervous system. While the biceps bends the elbow joint, it is simultaneously extended by the triceps. The result is a remaining minimum active range of motion in the elbow.

The evaluation of the interplay between muscular activation, muscular coordination and resulting movement is still the subject of current research. The problem here is that neither the biomechanics of the movement of the upper extremities nor the principles of muscular force development are fully understood at present. The latter relates mainly to the role of the **titin** in physiological and especially pathological muscle contraction [25]. Many studies, especially in the area of the upper extremities, provide different results, which often lead to the entire methodology of surface electromyography being questioned. However, von Werder et al. were able to show that a systematic analysis of the signals in correlation with the execution of movement leads to significantly more reliable and comparable results [26], so that the diagnostic significance of surface electromyography and the muscular coordination pattern will increase in the future.

References

1. Rau G, Disselhorst-Klug C, Schmidt R. Movement biomechanics goes upwards: from the leg to the arm. J Biomech. 2000;33(10):1207–16.
2. Disselhorst-Klug C, Besdo S, Oehler S (2015) Biomechanik des muskuloskelettalen systems. In Kraft M, Disselhorst-Klug C: Biomedizinische Technik–Rehabilitationstechnik; De Gruyter, Berlin, S. 53–105.
3. Nigg BM, Herzog W. Biomechanics of the Musculoskeletal system. Chichester: Wiley; 1994.
4. Whittle MW. Musculoskeletal applications of three. Dimensional analysis. In: Allard P, Stokes AF, Blanchi J-P, editors. Three-dimensional analysis of human movement. Montreal: Human Kinetics; 1995. p. 295–309.
5. Williams S, Schmidt R, Disselhorst-Klug C, Rau G. An upper body model for the kinematical analysis of the joint chain of the human arm. J Biomech. 2006;39(13):2419–29.
6. Schmidt R, Disselhorst-Klug C, Silny J, Rau G. A marker based measurement procedure for unconstrained wrist and elbow motions. J Biomech. 1999;32:615.
7. Popovic N, Williams S, Schmitz-Rode T, Rau G, Disselhorst-Klug C. Robot based methodology for a kinematic and kinetic analysis of unconstrained, but reproducible upper extremity movement. J Biomech. 2009;42(10):1570–3.
8. Miltner O, Williams S, Disselhorst-Klug C. Dreidimensionale Bewegungsanalyse der oberen Extremitäten—eine klinische Anwendung. Orthopädische Praxis. 2003;39:272–6.
9. Miltner O, Williams S, Schmidt R, Siebert C, Rau G, Zilkens KW, Disselhorst-Klug C. 3D-Analyse der Armbewegung: eine neue Methode und erste klinische Anwendung. Orthopedics. 2003;141:171–6.
10. Bahm J, Meinecke L, Brandenbusch V, Rau G, Disselhorst-Klug C. High spatial resolution electromyography and video-assisted movement analysis in children with obstetric brachial plexus palsy. Hand Clin. 2003;19:393–9.
11. Bahm J, Becker M, Disselhorst-Klug C, Williams S, Meinecke L, Müller H, Sellhaus B, Schröder J, Rau G. Surgical strategy in obstetric bracjial plexus palsy: the Aachen experience. Semin Plast Surg. 2004;18(4):285–99.
12. Pauwels F. Grundriss einer Biomechanik der Frakturheilung. Verh Dtsch Orthop Ges 1940;34.
13. Wolff J. Das Gesetz der Transformation der Knochen. Berlin: August Hirschwald; 1892.

14. Pauwels F. Über die Bedeutung der Bauprinzipien des Stütz- und Bewegungsapparates für die Beanspruchung des Röhrenknochens. Acta Anat. 1951;12:207–27.
15. Bahm J, Wein B, Alhares G, Dogan C, Radermacher K, Schuind F. Assessment and treatment of glenohumeral joint deformities in children suffering from upper obstetric brachial plexus palsy. J Pediatr Orthop B. 2007;16(4):243–51.
16. Hogendoorn S, van Overvest K, Watt I, Duijsens A, Nelissen R. Structural changes in muscle and glenohumeral joint deformity in neonatal brachial plexus palsy. Bone Joint Surg Am. 2010;92(4):935–42.
17. Schewe. Biomechanik–wie geht das? Stuttgart: Thieme; 2000.
18. Kleiber T, Popovic N, Bahm J, Disselhorst-Klug C. A modeling approach to compute modification of net joint forces caused by coping movements in obstetric brachial plexus palsy. J Brachial Plexus Periphal Nerve Injury. 2013;8:10.
19. Zatsiorsky M, Seluyanov VN. The mass and inertia characteristics of the main segments of the human body. Biomechanics VIII-B. Champaign: Human Kinetics Publishers; 1983. p. 1152–9.
20. Winter DA, Patla AE, Rietdyk S, Ishac MG. Ankle muscle stiffness in the control of balance during quiet standing. J Neurophysiol. 2001;85(6):2630–3.
21. Basmajian JV, De Luca CJ. Muscle alive; their functions revealed by electromyography. 5th ed. Baltimore: William & Wilkins; 1985.
22. Ludin HP. Praktische Elektromyographie. Stuttgart: Enke; 1981.
23. Perry P. Gait analysis, normal and pathological function. New York: Slack; 1992.
24. Winter DA. Concerning the scientific basis for the diagnosis of pathological gait and for rehabilitation protocols. Physiother Can. 1985;37:245–52.
25. Herzog W. The role of titin in eccentric muscle contraction. J Exp Biol. 2014;217:2825–33.
26. von Werder S, Kleiber T, Disselhorst-Klug C. A method for a categorized and probabilistic analysis of the surface electromyogram in dynamic contractions. Front Physiol. 2015;6:30.

J. Schaumberg and D. Schwandt

7.1 Electromyography (EMG)

7.1.1 General Information

For doctors, the EMG with a concentric needle electrode is the most difficult neurophysiological examination and can, in our opinion, be learnt by adults and only to a limited extent by children. In contrast to electroneurography and evoked potentials, EMG should be performed by medical doctors, and in-depth knowledge of the anatomy and pathophysiology of peripheral nerves and muscles is required.

Needle EMG examinations are "random samples", only 1 mm^3 muscle per insertion can be assessed. The EMG findings must be correlated with the clinically collected findings. Pathological EMG findings should, if possible, be delimited "into the healthy". It is helpful to examine the same muscle on the opposite side.

A surface EMG with adhesive electrodes is pointless, since neither pathological spontaneous activity nor motor units can be assessed, and thus the question of neurogenic or myogenic damage cannot be answered.

For children and parents alike, the EMG is the most unpleasant neurophysiological examination because a thin needle electrode has to be inserted into the musculature.

It has proved successful to point out to parents and children, depending on their age, that the examination hurts in the short term and toddlers usually cry during it. An EMG is harmless and without side effects.

For important indications such as obstetric arm plexus paresis and hesitant parental consent, we perform a needle EMG examination on the mother or father for demonstration purposes. After that, the parents always agreed to the EMG examination of their infant. For us, the only contraindication is a blood clotting disorder.

EMG Indications Upper Extremity
- Traumatic nerve lesions due to fractures, cuts or pressure damage with the question of complete or incomplete nerve damage or question of reinnervation potential
- Paresis in the shoulder girdle area, neurogenic (e.g., spinal muscular atrophy) or myogenic (e.g., muscular dystrophy)
- Birth traumatic arm plexus lesions
- Myotonia clarification
- Muscle necrosis in compartment syndromes: silent EMG.

The domain of the EMG is muscle weakness or paresis.

Dr. Schwandt (Retired).

J. Schaumberg (✉)
Department of Neurology, Sana Kliniken Lübeck, Lübeck, Germany
e-mail: jens.schaumberg@sana.de

D. Schwandt
e-mail: dr.schwandt@hamburg.de

© Springer Nature Switzerland AG 2021
J. Bahm (ed.), *Movement Disorders of the Upper Extremities in Children*,
https://doi.org/10.1007/978-3-030-53622-0_7

7.1.2 Implementation

Needle insertion into the muscle should always be targeted, rapid and perpendicular to the surface. The loudspeaker must already be activated. Insertions should only be made tangentially to thin muscles such as the trapezius muscle or the facial.

The three examination steps of the EMG are:

- Evaluate spontaneous activity at rest
- Muscle action potentials with light muscle innervation
- Maximum innervation discharge frequency and interference pattern

These three examination steps are usually not possible separately for small children. For example, spontaneous activity in the EMG cannot be assessed in children's movements and often only a few motor units can be analysed in terms of amplitude, duration, shape, number of phases and discharge frequency.

Children sometimes have the remarkable ability to perform movements with pain-reflecting recess of the examined musculature. A passive movement of the extremity or a short push or tickle can then trigger an active defensive movement, a short innervation of the musculature, so that individual muscle action potentials can be analysed in the EMG.

Summary Principles of the Children's EMG (0–6 Years)
- Clinical examination, question, selection of as few muscles as possible.
- EMG as final investigation. Neurographs and evoked potentials are better tolerated.
- Instruction to parents and employees in front of the EMG on how to hold or passively move the extremities or, for example, how to tickle the sole of the foot in the EMG of the tibialis anterior muscle.
- No sedation. The EMG requires the movement and muscle activity of the child.
- "Arbitrary activity" is dropped in this age group. In the routine evaluation of motor units,

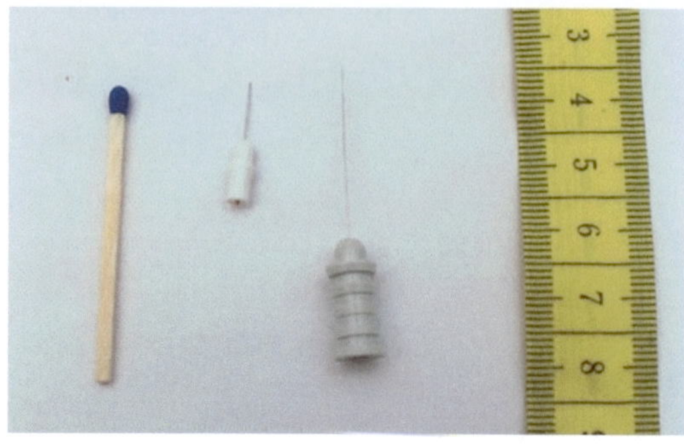

Fig. 7.1 Representation of the 10 mm × 0.3 mm needle electrode for deriving a cortical somatosensory evoked potentials (SSEP) (*on the left*) and a 25 mm × 0.3 mm concentric needle electrode for electromyography (*right*)

muscles should be selected that (contract pain-reflecting) during needle insertion, for example, the biceps brachialis muscle or the gluteus maximus muscle in prone position.
- Proximal limb muscles suspected of myopathy, distal muscles suspected of PNP.
- Selection of the thinnest needle electrode: 0.3 mm diameter (Fig. 7.1). Lidocaine patches are no longer necessary on the insertion site.
- Always turn on the EMG loudspeaker. Do not forget to ground the child with a ground electrode.
- Work quickly to keep the burden on child and parents short, that is, usually no longer than 5 min, no breaks, no 25 different motor units per muscle as in adults, 3–5 units are usually sufficient, and do not wait for minutes for pathological spontaneous activity, otherwise the patient/parents no longer come to control examinations.
- Friendliness and empathy of the examiner are particularly important at the EMG.
- Smiling toddlers at EMG are sick. They usually have paraphrased analgesia or analgesia syndrome. If possible, analgesic skin areas should be used for needle insertion, for example, if the ulnar nerve is injured, and the abductor digiti minimi should be examined first at the edge of the hand.
- In toddlers it is usually not possible to carry out a textbook electromyography.

7.1.3 Special Part

Identification muscles for **cervical root lesions** are:

- C5 syndrome: supra- and infraspinatus muscle, deltoid muscle
- C6 syndrome: biceps brachii m., brachioradialis m.
- C7 syndrome: M. triceps brachii, M. extensor digitorum communis, M. flexor carpi radialis, M. pectoralis major
- C8 syndrome: M. interosseous dorsalis I, M. flexor digitorum profundus ulnaris, M. abductor pollicis brevis

A radicular lesion or anterior horn damage can be supported by denervation activity of the respective segmental paravertebral musculature [1]. This examination is usually not possible for infants without sedation.

Identification muscles for **arm plexus lesions** [2, 3]:

- Upper arm plexus lesion: deltoid muscle, infra- and supraspinatus muscle, biceps brachii muscle, brachioradial muscle
- Lower arm plexus lesion: all forearm muscles except the brachioradialis muscle, all hand muscles, triceps brachialis muscle, pectoralis major muscle, latissimus dorsi muscle.

Pathological synkinesis of agonists and antagonists can be well diagnosed with a two-channel EMG. These synkinesies, for example, in the biceps brachialis muscle and triceps brachialis muscle, occur due to missprouting axons after plexus lesions and lead to considerable functional restrictions of the arm.

7.2 Electroneurography (ENG)

7.2.1 General Information

All neurographs are temperature and age dependent.

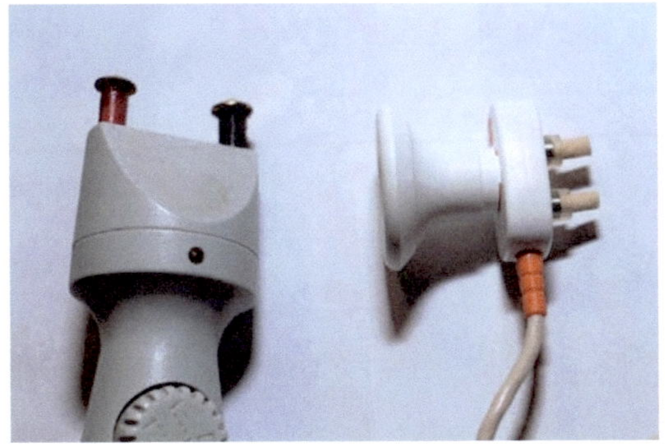

Fig. 7.2 Stimulation block for adults (*on the left*) with 2.2 cm electrode distance and for children (*right*) with 1 cm electrode distance

In children in the first and second year of life, the neurographic measurements are greatly reduced by the immature myelin sheaths [4].

A smaller stimulation block (Fig. 7.2) can be used for infants due to their small body size.

All neurographs have inherent measurement inaccuracies of ±0.1 ms when determining the potential loss and of ±5 mm when measuring the distance between two measurement points. This usually results in a measurement inaccuracy of ±2 m/s when determining the nerve conduction velocity (NLG).

The measurement inaccuracy of infants is greater because of the shorter distances. The distances between two measuring points should not be less than 8 cm [2]. To indicate the NLG with decimal places after the comma (e.g., 50.3 m/s) is nonsensical and pseudo accurate because of the measurement inaccuracy, but all devices indicate these decimal places.

ENG Indications Upper Extremity
- Chronic nerve compression syndromes (e.g., carpal tunnel syndrome, sulcus-ulnaris syndrome)
- Polyneuritides such as Guillain–Barré syndrome
- Polyneuropathies, hereditary and acquired
- Myasthenia syndromes: series stimulation with 3 Hz

The main area for ENG is sensitivity disorders.

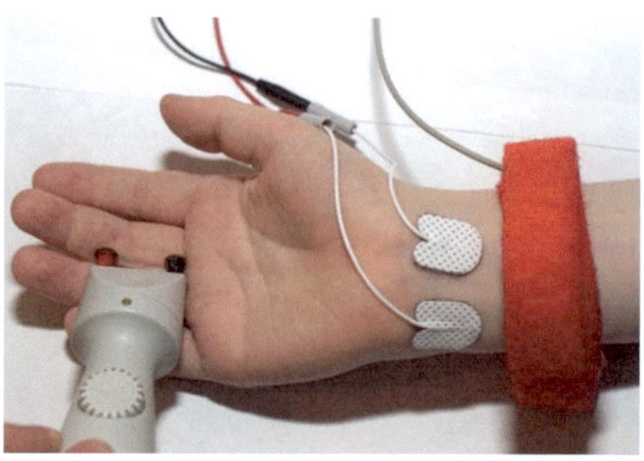

Fig. 7.3 Representation of a motor neurography of the median nerve with derivation via the abductor pollicis brevis muscle. Cathode (*black*) of the stimulation electrode above the median nerve at the wrist points to the derived muscle

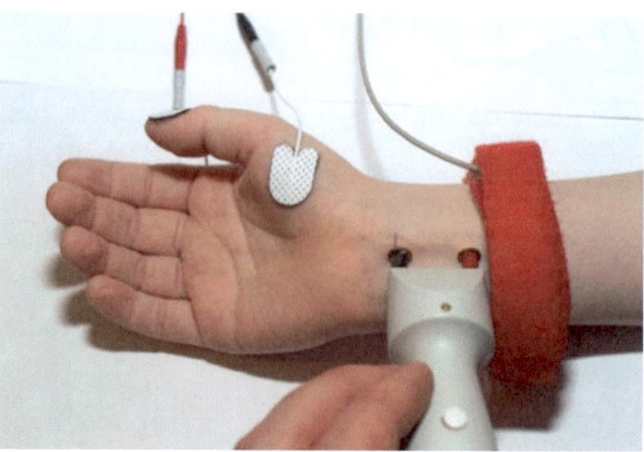

Fig. 7.4 Orthodromic sensitive neurography of the median nerve with stimulation at the proximal finger III and derivation over the wrist. Cathode (*black*) the stimulation electrode above the finger points proximal to the wrist

7.2.2 Sensitive Neurography

In sensitive neurography, due to the low amplitudes of the sensitive nerve sum potential, an accumulation by means of an average must take place [3]. The sensitive amplitudes (μV) are smaller by a factor of 1000 than the amplitudes of the motor responses (mV).

Sensitive neurography of peripheral nerves can be performed orthodromically from distal to proximal or antidromically from proximal to distal. In children, we recommend orthodromic drainage of the sensitive nerves (Fig. 7.3), since no disturbing motor responses occur at higher current intensities as with antidromic drainage. Orthodrome on the hand means a stimulation of the skin of the proximal fingers and a derivative with unipolar surface electrodes over the nerves on the wrist (median nerve and ulnar nerve). The radial ramus superficialis nerve is stimulated dorsally on the back of the hand in the spatium I and is derived superficially on the radial side of the distal forearm. Derivation by means of needle electrodes is more painful and usually not necessary. In case of strong motor restlessness no sum potential can be added up.

Sensitive neurography can be helpful in differentiating between sensitive root and plexus lesions and between supra- and infraganglionary damage. In purely infraganglionic arm plexus damage, the sensitive sum potentials are reduced or absent due to Waller's degeneration occurring 3–5 days after axonal lesion. In the case of purely supraganglionic lesions, such as root tears, the sensitive sum potential can be reliably deduced even though analgesia is clinically present.

7.2.3 Motor Neurography

In motor neurography, the motor nerve fibres are stimulated by means of a bipolar surface electrode. The cathode (usually black) points to the dissipating muscle (Fig. 7.4). The stimulation initially takes place with low current intensities and is increased with repeated stimuli until the amplitude of the response potential no longer increases [3]. The impulse should be announced before each stimulation.

In motor neurography, nerve conduction velocity (NLG), distal latency, amplitude and shape of sum potential are assessed.

The three main nerves at the upper limb:

- **N. medianus:** Stimulation of the wrist, elbow, if necessary in the axilla (painful). The derivation takes place at the M. abductor pollicis brevis.
- **N. ulnaris:** Stimulation of the wrist, distal and proximal to the ulnar sulcus. The derivation takes place at the M. abductor digiti minimi.

- **N. radialis:** Stimulation of the proximal forearm dorsally, ulnarly, on the distal upper arm and in the middle third of the upper arm laterally. The derivative is M. abductor pollicis longus [3].

In all three main nerves of the arm, electrical stimulation supraclavicular to the Erb's point is very painful and should be replaced by magnetoelectric stimulation (MEP).

The determination of **F waves** (follow-up waves) in proximal nerve lesions and especially in Guillain–Barré syndrome is another measurement method of motor neurography and is performed in a lateral comparison. The minimum F-wave latency is determined, from which the motor NLG can be calculated.

Principles of Electroneurography (ENG)
- ENG before EMG. Children are less uncomfortable with electrical impulses than adults, but the opposite is true for needle inserts.
- Announce each electrostimulation shortly before the patient.
- Parents are welcome to hold the child's hand, they do not get an electric shock.
- Higher current intensities can become very painful, therefore pay attention to the patient's face. Individual current tolerance.
- The more proximal a nerve is stimulated, the more painful it becomes.
- No pain reaction to high current intensities is pathological.
- If current intensities are too low, false pathological findings may occur if supramaximal stimulation was not used.
- Cold nerves conduct more slowly. Pay attention to the skin temperature, especially with sensitive neurography. Standard values were collected at 32 °C. Rule of thumb: Every degree less than 32 °C leads to a reduction of NLG by approximately 1 m/s.
- Slow NLGs are normal in newborns and infants [4].
- Consider the measurement inaccuracies of the method. NLG values have at least ±2 m/s range of variation. Observe sufficient distances of the measuring points, at least 8 cm.

7.3 Somatosensory Evoked Potentials (SEP)

The derivation, also known as sensitive evoked potentials, allows a functional test of the sensitive system. During stimulation, mainly thick, myelinated afferent nerve fibres of groups I and II (skin, muscle and joint receptors) are excited. In principle, SEP can be derived by nerve or dermatome stimulation [5]. SEP of the arm and leg nerves (Medianus-SEP, Tibialis-SEP) can also be derived regularly in infants from the first days of life. The latencies are prolonged by the immature myelinization of the sensitive nerve fibres, see electroneurography.

The upper extremity is usually affected by a **Medianus-SEP**. The median nerve at the wrist is stimulated (Fig. 7.5) and a three-channel SEP is derived over Erb's point homolaterally, HWK 2 centrically and over the cortical palm contralaterally at the head. Due to the considerable movement artefacts in child examinations, we only derive the cortical SEP (N20) and use needle electrodes with a diameter of 0.3 mm (Figs. 7.1 and 7.6). These are usually well tolerated and result in artefact-free and better pronounced curves than with surface electrodes. In infants, the needle must not be inserted in the area of the

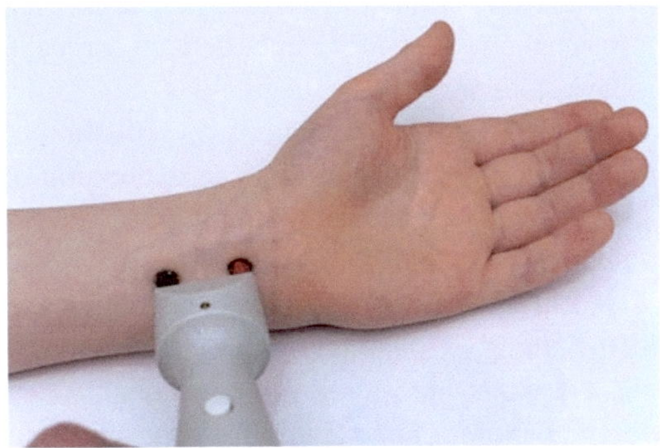

Fig. 7.5 Stimulation during Medianus-SEP. The process is equivalent to the motor neurography of the median nerve. Cathode (*black*) is directed proximally in the direction of the discharge electrodes

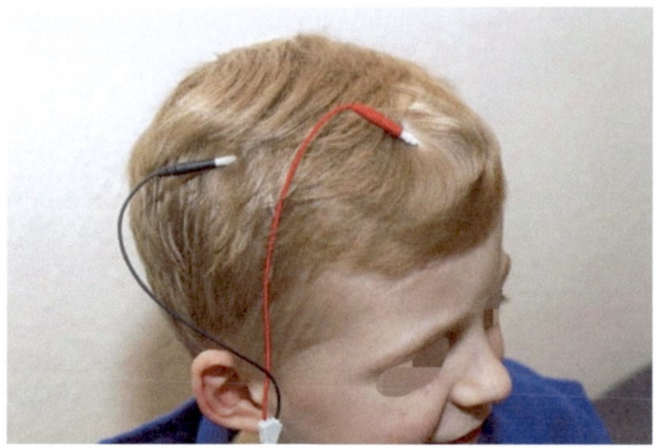

Fig. 7.6 Illustration of the derivation of a cortical medianus SEP with needle electrodes in left nerve medianus stimulation

open fontanelles. The indifferent electrode is placed over Fpz and the differential electrode contralateral over C3' or C4' [5, 6].

A note on the nomenclature: "right N20" or "N20 right" means that the right median nerve has been stimulated.

In the case of upper arm plexus damage, SEP can be performed by stimulation of the superficial nerve of the radial nerve (**Radialis-SEP**) [6]. In lower brachial plexus lesions, stimulation of the ulnar nerve (**Ulnaris-SEP**).

In the case of a purely supraganglionic nerve damage (e.g., root avulsion), an SEP can be derived analogously to sensitive neurography over Erb's point, since no Waller's degeneration occurs distally in intact spinal ganglia. In contrast, in the case of higher degree infraganglionic nerve damage (arm plexus lesions) no SEP can be derived from Erb's point. In both lesion types, supra- and infraganglionary, no SEP can be derived cortically if the lesions are of higher degree.

The assessment of an amplitude reduction of the SEP response potentials as an expression of axonal damage must be cautious due to many influencing factors [6].

In our experience, the yield of pathological SEP findings is particularly low in upper arm plexus lesions and is used more for diagnosis or differentiation of conduction disorders of sensitive nerve fibres of the spinal cord and brain.

SEP in sensory disorders of unclear genesis and to differentiate proximal from distal sensitive nerve lesions.

Like all evoked potentials, the SEP has lost much of its significance due to magnetic resonance imaging.

## 7.4	Magnetoelectrically Evoked Potentials (MEPs)

The principle of measurement, also known as motor evoked potentials, is based on electromagnetic induction [5]. For the upper extremity, a cortical, a cervical (HWK 7) and an arm plexus stimulation can be performed over Erb's point. For children aged 5 and over, reference values from adults can be used [6]. According to the literature, MEP stimulations can already be well deduced in newborns [6]. In our daily practice, however, in cortical magnetic stimulation and induction from the lower leg (tibialis anterior muscle) up to the age of 4 years, no MEP responses can usually be obtained. We attribute this to the still immature pyramid track in the first years of life.

Overall, the latencies of the MEP in the same child fluctuate by 1–5 ms in repeated measurements, as the pre-innervation in children cannot be kept constant. In the case of slightly delayed MEP latencies, interpretation should therefore be cautious.

For arm plexus lesions, we recommend cortical stimulation and stimulation over Erb's point and surface derivations from the arm or hand muscles. When stimulating over Erb's point, only the plexus transition times to the musculature should be evaluated in a lateral comparison [5]. The MEP has its advantages with additional central pareses or functional psychic "pareses" as well as with axonal lesions with clear amplitude difference in lateral comparison. From our point of view, amplitude differences <50% should first be considered pathological.

As with all other neurophysiological measurement methods, isolated pathological MEP values must always be critically interpreted and questioned without a clinical correlate.

MEP in pareses of unclear cause.

MEPs are indicated for central rather than peripheral motor nerve lesions.

References

1. Bischoff C, Schulte-Mattler W. EMG und periphere Neurologie in Frage und Antwort. Stuttgart, New York: Thieme; 2011.
2. Bischoff C, Dengier R, Hopf H. EMG NLG Elektromyographie und Nervenleitungsuntersuchungen. Stuttgart, New York: Thieme; 2008.
3. Stöhr M. Klinische Elektromyographie und Neurographie–Lehrbuch und Atlas. Stuttgart: Kohlhammer; 2005.
4. Ludin H-P. Praktische Elektromyographie. Stuttgart: Enke; 1993.
5. Maurer K, Eckert J. Praxis der evozierten Potentiale. Stuttgart: Enke; 1999.
6. Buchner H. Praxisbuch evozierte Potentiale. Stuttgart, New York: Thieme; 2013.

Central Neural Plasticity 8

Jörg Bahm

8.1 Introduction

If, as a non-neuroscientist, I have to contribute a small chapter on the adaptation capacities of the nervous system, then this is certainly a challenge. On the one hand, one could certainly write an entire book on this topic (from the competent side of "neuroscience"), on the other hand, our knowledge is very incomplete and the development of research in this area is very fast, comprehensive and actually unmanageable for non-insiders.

Nevertheless, we encounter central neural plasticity so frequently within our interdisciplinary work with children suffering from impaired mobility that it is necessary to define our position—also for the sake of completeness.

We may therefore be forgiven for a limited summary. Readers interested in further information will find in-depth current literature via the references given (e.g., [1, 2]).

In the past it was believed that the mature brain and nervous system could no longer be shaped after childhood. Today we know more and more about the high adaptability of the adult brain, especially after stroke, amputation of limbs and nerve injuries. Computer science has also shown us how the central computer is influenced by peripheral input and how such input from the environment adapts the functioning of the computer. This perspective and type of analysis also allows us to better understand the functioning of our brain and the flexibility of the cerebral cortex, called cortical plasticity.

Based on known clinical observations in our children, we will now define the essential terms and functions and end with known effects of the therapy procedures.

8.2 Empirical Observations

Children with movement disorders of their extremities show compensatory adaptation postures or compensatory movements depending on the severity of the impairment. In severe sensorimotor disorders of the upper extremity, such as complete plexus paresis, the arm is neglected in everyday activities ("neglect" or "learned disuse"). These are only two patterns of adaptation that demonstrate the existence of central neural plasticity.

During consultation it is common to talk about the presumed "laziness" of the children during the exercises or to observe that the arm is only used when verbally addressed: "I always have to remind my child to use this arm as well".

J. Bahm (✉)
Department of Plastic, Hand and Burn Surgery,
Section for Plexus Surgery, University Hospital,
Aachen, Germany
e-mail: jbahm@ukaachen.de,
jorg.bahm@belgacom.net

© Springer Nature Switzerland AG 2021
J. Bahm (ed.), *Movement Disorders of the Upper Extremities in Children*,
https://doi.org/10.1007/978-3-030-53622-0_8

After motor nerve transfers, there is usually a period of coactivation with the nerve donor target, such as synchronous breathing and muscle activity after intercostal nerve transfer, until an independent movement pattern develops.

8.3 Basic Concepts and Principles

Like any structure in the nervous system, the cerebral cortex is extremely adaptable and reactive to sensitive or motor changes in structure and function, on a biochemical, electrophysiological and cytological-histological level.

It is known that every sensory stimulus of a finger is directed via tactile corpuscles and the primary afferent pathway to the dorsal ganglion neurones, then into the spinal cord, from there into the contralateral thalamus and then the contralateral sensory cortex. All nerve nuclei involved have a specific somatotopic arrangement according to the body topography, both on the sensory and motor side. These arrangements can be severely disturbed by nerve injuries and trigger remodelling processes, which are modified by regeneration (see below).

Recovery after nerve reconstruction cannot therefore be assessed solely on the basis of local, microsurgical-technical aspects and nerve regeneration, but must also consider these central reorganization processes, which can be cooperative or counterproductive, for example, in the development of neuropathic pain.

8.4 Investigation Methods

In addition to **magnetic resonance imaging** (MRI) (analysis of damaged areas in cerebral palsy), specific non-invasive imaging techniques and brain stimulation techniques allow in vivo studies of neural plasticity:

Positron emission tomography (PET) uses three "tracers": water (measurement of regional blood flow in the brain, as an expression of neuro-nal activity); (fluorodeoxy)-glucose (measurement of brain metabolism) and radioactively labelled neurotransmitters (opiates, dopamine, serotonin and gamma-aminobutyric acid (GABA)).

Transcranial magnetic stimulation (TMS) allows studies of central motor control using low-frequency (inhibitory) and high-frequency (exciting) impulses.

Functional magnetic resonance imaging (fMRI) is based on the interaction between neuronal activity and oxygen supply from the blood flow–blood oxygenation level dependent (BOLD) contrast, voxel (**volume-el**ement, i.e., three dimensional data point)-based structural analyses of the grey matter and the diffusion tensor imaging (DTI) technique and tractography for the assessment of the white matter and thus the corresponding cerebral pathways.

8.5 Mechanisms

So far, two mechanisms are known that implement neural adaptability:

- A rapid process that takes place in minutes or hours after denervation, in which "sleeping" inactive synapses or nerve pathways are revived, unmasking or uncovering hidden functional pathways. One factor seems to be the loss of an inhibition process controlled by the neurotransmitter GABA.
- Another, much slower process is the formation of new nerve connections by collateral sprouting.

It may be asked whether these adaptation processes take place within a brain hemisphere or interhemispherically between the brain hemispheres. The latter has to be considered in contralateral nerve transfers and the question arises through which structural pathways a compensatory flow of information can take place between the two halves of the brain, since it is known that there is no anatomical bridge in the cerebrum itself outside the corpus callosum.

8.6 Cortical Reorganization After Nerve Damage

In experiments upon laboratory animals and in patients, cortical plasticity after nerve injury has been described in three situations, which we briefly summarize here:

- After a severe compression ("crush") injury with local demyelination and interruption of axons while the basal membrane envelopes remain intact (axonotmesis).
- After neurotmesis without repair.
- After neurotmesis with repair.

Already the **nerve compression** with subsequent axonotmesis leads to a "disturbance" of the cortical representation zone, which, however, is reversible: The deletion of the receptive fields is soon followed by an identical reoccupation, since an identical reinnervation and representation can take place due to the preservation of the endoneurial tubes.

It is different with a **substantial nerve damage**, which always involves some topographic reorganization, whether the nerve has been repaired or not. Here, in the area of cortical representation, it first comes to extinction, and then to the influx of the surrounding, uninjured nerves—which claim the vacated parking space: In the case of a fingertip injury of the index finger, the initially released representation field is taken over by corresponding parts of the nearby middle finger and thumb.

Since some local connections regenerate correctly over time, a puzzle of extinguished, invasively occupied and regenerated areas is created, which "improves" in the course of regeneration, but never reaches the original level of organization again. One then speaks of a **relative misattribution** ("missmatch"), which remains clinically conspicuous and can be further improved by targeted therapy.

All this applies to both sensory and motor fields of representation and is an extremely complex, progressive process that can continue for years.

An example of an insufficient end result after a complex sensory nerve injury is the permanent loss of one or more highly specialized sensory perception processes such as spatial sensitive perception called stereognosis.

It is also clear that these perceptions, and corresponding fine motor activities in the young child, cannot be easily tested in practice.

The structural and functional changes in the grey matter after these nerve injuries show similarities with the learning of fine motor skills, in which the corresponding fields of representation are primed by repeated exercise. There is functional adaptation and anatomical changes probably also occur. Whether the latter are causes or consequences of the learning process remains unclear at present.

Neuropathic pain is a typical example of "unsuccessful" cortical plasticity. I shall not consider this in detail here, as fortunately it is very rare in young children. Severe pain conditions in paralysed extremities after nerve damage are rare in children, in contrast to nerve root tears in traumatic adult plexus lesions, which can lead to terrible neuropathic pain.

Both in adults and children, other pain-enhancing mechanisms such as fear, depression and catastrophism do exist.

8.7 Adapted and Unmatched Plasticity

The example of neuropathic pain shows that adaptative plasticity can also be misdirected or unadapted, thus becoming counterproductive and harmful. In some cases such changes act as a central cause for a failure of treatment.

8.8 Special Adaptation After Nerve Transfers (Plexus Damage)

Nerve transfers as a reconstructive measure in severe proximal nerve damage have been described in detail in Chaps. 15 and 17. In three frequently used methods, cortical plasticity seems to play a major role in achieving a movement pattern that is independent of the nerve donor representation area:

- **Oberlin transfer** of N. medianus or N. ulnaris fascicles for elbow flexion activity: If the finger flexors innervated by the donor nerves have to be moved initially to get a response in the target muscle, over time elbow flexion is also possible with outstretched fingers.
- **Intercostal nerves:** after their repositioning on the motor branches of biceps muscle or brachialis muscle, initially muscle activation can only be achieved during breathing exercises or coughing. It sometimes takes years for the movement to become independent and truly volitional.
- **Contralateral C7 transfer**

It becomes even more complex when the initial control signal comes from a nerve of the uninjured extremity which is controlled by the ipsilateral hemisphere.

It remains uncertain, apart from the proximal muscle groups of the shoulder (where bilateral coactivation is also functional in healthy people), an independent, functionally significant, movement can really develop in the hand area in the long term.

Although the technical feasibility of these surgical procedures has been proven for more than 40 years, there seems to be limited, but definite, specific function gain. fMRI images show first ipsilateral, later bilateral hemispheric activity, and in the chronic stage some individual contralateral control activity. The validity of those results still has to be strengthened.

8.9 Adjustment After Central Nervous Damage

Cortical plasticity after acquired brain damage has been one of the most intensively researched topics in neuropaediatrics in recent years, but even a basal representation would go beyond the scope of this book.

8.10 Influence on Sensory and Motor Rehabilitation

Without wanting to anticipate the explanations in Chaps. 9 and 10, the findings described above can be incorporated into conservative exercise treatment:

> Motivation and enjoyment of movement are essential prerequisites for successful therapy. Meaningful therapy goals developed together with the child lead to a high level of motivation, which in turn results in a high repetition rate.

In addition to early sensitive training, sensory training involves other senses (acoustic and visual stimuli) and contralateral stimulation methods such as mirror therapy.

In muscle exercises, in addition to active movement exercises, electrostimulation of the denervated musculature and biofeedback methods are of considerable importance. Bimanual activities are very important as being integration exercises.

In the future, there is a hypothesis to directly promote adaptive plasticity and inhibit counterproductive plasticity by selectively intervening in biochemical regulatory processes at the level of neurotransmitters such as GABA.

We must closely monitor neuroscientific research in this area in order to identify new paradigms in good time and use them for the benefit of our patients.

References

1. Hendry SH, Hsiao SS. Somatosensory areas of the cerebral cortex (Chap. 25: The somatosensory system). In: Squire LR, Bloom FE, McConnell SK, Roberts JL, Spitzer NC, Zigmond MJ, editors. Fundamental neuroscience. 2nd ed. San Diego: Academic Press; 2003.
2. Knox ADC, Goswami R, Anastakis DJ, Davis KD. Cortical plasticity after peripheral nerve injury. In: Tubbs S, editor. Nerves and nerve injuries, vol. 2. Amsterdam: Elsevier; 2015.

Further Reading

Anastakis DJ, Malessy MJ, Chen R, Davis KD, Mikulis D. Cortical plasticity following nerve transfer in the upper extremity. Hand Clin. 2008;24:425–44.
Lundborg G. Nerve injury and repair. Philadelphia: Churchill Livingstone; 2005.

Part III

Conservative Treatment Methods

Physiotherapy

Jörg Bahm and F. Mecher

9.1 Physiotherapy from the Physician's Point of View

Non-operative therapy should support natural regeneration processes, rehearse postoperative functional goals and help to upgrade sensitive and motor functions and their cortical integration, while alleviating negative side effects such as pain.

> Physiotherapy and occupational therapy must always be considered with reference to the underlying disease and in addition to other, especially surgical treatment.

Therapy in children also has two other special characteristics:

- The child grows, meaning the anatomical structures change constantly (beware of joint dysplasia or the development of scoliosis in case of important muscle imbalances) and in infants the sensory-motor function has to mature after birth.
- In addition, children are "compliant" (eager to cooperate) depending on their age and daily condition, which is challenging for therapists and parents. Playful approaches are always the key to make a training programme attractive.

For children with neuroorthopaedic diseases, I highlight three points:

- The timing of nerve regeneration (either spontaneously in the developmental history of the child or after a nerve-reconstructive surgery): here the therapy must accompany the biological regeneration process along its time course (a speed of 1–2 mm/day from the repair site to the target organ) and bring it into meaningful, that is, functionally pragmatic, paths and thereby adapt cortical plasticity, that is, central learning. It is important that the biologically quasi "automatic" regeneration process is integrated as the basic motor for recovery, parallel to the need for therapy, both outlined to relatives, co-treaters and, above all, cost bearers.

> Physiotherapy is not a help for self-help, but an independent and specialized form of therapy with a scientific background.

J. Bahm (✉)
Department of Plastic, Hand and Burn Surgery, Section for Plexus Surgery, University Hospital, Aachen, Germany
e-mail: jbahm@ukaachen.de, jorg.bahm@belgacom.net

F. Mecher (✉)
Physiotherapeutic Group Practice, Mecher & Kollegen, Braunschweig, Germany

© Springer Nature Switzerland AG 2021
J. Bahm (ed.), *Movement Disorders of the Upper Extremities in Children*,
https://doi.org/10.1007/978-3-030-53622-0_9

– Support the growth of the child and thereby promote the functional integration of the affected extremity: Recognize and balance muscle imbalances, prevent contractures, facilitate everyday activities such as washing and dressing, think ahead.
– Specific work after secondary surgical corrections: Consider sensitive and motor reintegration of newly controlled functions within the time interval required for regeneration and corticalization. There is thus a "start" (usually after the postoperative immobilization period, about 6 weeks) and an end (e.g., 1 year after a muscle transfer, because during this period the morphological transformation of the target muscle in relation to its new task takes place). Exercising a muscle beyond this point has nothing to do with therapy, but means sport, fitness and personal responsibility.

In addition, the therapists are knowledgeable contacts for clinics and research in movement and sensory disorders, as they have studied the anatomy, biomechanics and neurophysiological basis as well as treatment methods, which details are foreign to us physicians. Also do they conduct clinical research about the relevance of functional improvement under therapy and about sensitive disorders (e.g., therapy of neuropathic pain).

Since physicians continue to bear the prescription sovereignty for physiotherapy and occupational therapy (without having sufficient knowledge and expertise) and since the insurance budget is limited, a constant and respectful exchange of ideas between the physicians and therapists remains extremely important (written reports, telephone update).

9.2 Physiotherapy from the Physiotherapist's Point of View

9.2.1 Introduction

In literature, the hand is described as the "sensitive wonder" [1], the "tool of the mind" [2] and the "stroke of genius of evolution" [3].

The differentiated possibilities which the hands have "acquired" in the course of evolution are almost immeasurable. The hands of our ancestors could handle coarse tools. Today we are able to play a virtuoso instrument or perform microsurgical procedures.

Movement disorders of the upper extremity, especially the hand, therefore have far-reaching effects on children, regardless of whether they are peripheral or central disorders.

> Undisturbed eye-hand coordination, as observed in children from the 2nd trimester onwards, is essential for perception (reception and processing of stimuli) and spatial orientation (position of the body parts relative to each other, position of the body in space). Skills that must be learnt in later life, such as cycling, writing, making music, build on them.

The hands grasp and about their hands the children learn. The child plays with his hands, touches himself and his body. The interplay of tactile (being touched) and haptic perception (touching something, holding it) is indispensable for capturing the stimuli from the environment. Through this constant interaction of grasping, touching and grasping, the body pattern is discovered and one's own body feeling is developed. The hands are our tools to grasp something, to put it in our mouths, to explore, to initiate the first processes of locomotion, such as turning and sealing, through the incentive to achieve something, and to gain experience in space. You can feed, care for, dress and protect yourself with your hands. The arms and hands can be used to stand up, support and move. Our hands enable us to write, paint, make music, construct and communicate.

Without an adequate hand-arm function one is dependent on help in many areas. An independence is, depending on the development, limited or not given. A limited or non-existent sensor motor function of the hand-arm function thus has a direct influence on the developing **body pattern**. The upper extremity is only integrated into the posture and movement patterns of the CNS via a well-developed hand function and is therefore available in spontaneous motor function.

An impairment of arm and hand in the form of deficits in coordination, mobility, strength and sensitivity has a direct influence on the **adjustment of spine and trunk** (vice versa of course also). The development of positional stability and erection cannot take place according to the developmental steps of postural ontogenesis in the first year of life.

9.2.2 Congenital and Acquired Movement Disorders

Movement disorders of the upper extremity in children can have various causes.

– In most cases, they are **congenital** or **acquired in early childhood** malformations (dysmelia, arthrogryposis multiplex congenita), obstetric injuries (upper and lower plexus paresis), muscle diseases as well as various forms of infantile cerebral palsy.
– In the majority of cases, schoolchildren and adolescents suffer from **traumas** to peripheral or central movement disorders.

Physiotherapy is an indispensable partner in the interdisciplinary team for the therapy of children's movement disorders, with a special focus on **early therapy**.

Very early on, the CNS is influenced, structured and differentiated in its maturation by corresponding stimuli. From about the sixth SSW onwards, the child reacts to tactile stimuli in the mouth and nose.

The disturbed afferents of a birth traumatic plexus paresis, arthrogryposis multiplex congenita (AMC) or other forms of malformation lead either directly after birth or already intrauterine to changes in the sensorimotor cortex and thus influence the central control of posture and movement. As a result, this not only affects the affected extremity, but also the shoulder girdle, spine and trunk.

Physiotherapy cannot cure plexus paresis, a malformation of the upper extremity or infantile cerebral palsy (ICP). Depending on age, findings and symptoms, the aim of physiotherapy is to integrate the affected extremity or hand into the developing body schema in order to enable the best possible restoration of the sensorimotor hand-elbow and shoulder function in terms of palpation, grasping, support and locomotion. Expected secondary problems are to be avoided or minimized.

According to the ICF-CY, participation is also a priority for infants and young children. It is always up to the individual to decide which compensation patterns and in which intensity are permitted in order to enable the child to perform the greatest possible functions (albeit limited) and thus to become independent.

While, for example, with a birth traumatic plexus paresis, with an AMC or other forms of the malformation, the restrictions and losses are immediately visible, one observes with a spastic threat the deficits with developing symptoms at the latest at the beginning of the second trimester.

9.2.3 Postural Development in the First Year of Life as a Basis for Findings and Therapy

9.2.3.1 Intrauterine Development

Irrespective of whether the problem is peripheral or central, knowledge of postural development in the first year of life is indispensable for the physiotherapeutic findings, the analysis of deviations and deficits, the definition of therapy goals as well as for the evaluation and assessment of the course of therapy.

In pictures (including [4]), the early development and differentiation of hand and fingers becomes visible.

Already 3–4 weeks after fertilization one can recognize arm buds. This still fin-like structure differentiates itself in the following weeks, so that at 12 weeks of age one can almost speak of an unfolded hand with an opposing thumb.

From the twelfth SSW onwards, development is characterized by perception and movement.

A genetic programme for touch, balance and self-awareness enables the child to perform, repeat, practise and "store" intrauterine movements.

Almost at the same time as the finger rays are differentiated, the first synapses are expected to form in the brain. The structuring and specification of the corresponding brain areas via intrauterine reactions to stimuli, movements and actions begins.

The newborn is born with a differentiated but still immature CNS. Through the growth of synapses, dendrites and their increasing connection to an interneuronal network, the brain increases in size over the next few months (years). Decisive for this development, however, are adequate and undisturbed stimuli and information from the environment.

The newborn has many abilities that must now be used and implemented under the influence of gravity.

9.2.3.2 Postural Ontogenesis in the First Year of Life

Supine Position

In the developmental steps in postural ontogenesis, we observe age-appropriate global patterns in the respective developmental steps that are directly related. Extremities and the spine are a condition of every locomotion.

Locomotion requires the control of the body position in space, the erection against gravity and a purposeful mobility.

In the following, the focus is placed on the development of upper extremity skills and functions related to feeling, touching, grasping and supporting. The relation to the spine and the lower extremity is only described to a limited extent.

In a newborn child, the upper arms are close to the body, the forearms are flexed, the wrists ulna-induced and the thumbs are included in light fist. In the event of sudden stimuli, the child reacts in the supine position in a full-body pattern with the **Moro reaction**.

Starting from the sixth week, we observe in the context of the motor establishment of contact the **fencing position**, wherein the posterior-facial extremities are in a loose flexing posture, the facial extremities in a loose stretching posture.

The global pattern of **hand–hand coordination** (touching the hands in front of the body) can be observed at about 8 weeks of age. The hands touch, are put into the mouth and briefly looked at. Prerequisite for this play with the hands is an age-appropriate posture background of spine and torso.

In the next few weeks, the upper arms are further removed from the body, shoulder joints and shoulder blades can be held centred, the hands show a slight radial reduction, the hands unfold and the thumb moves towards opposition. The spinal column is adjusted in the longitudinal axis, the pelvis is erect and the legs are "carried" in an age-typical way.

> The prerequisite for gripping is the eye and hand coordination.

The first targeted access takes place with approximately 4.5 months. In order to move an arm "isolated" to the side and grab an object, good control of the axis organ and trunk must be given.

Up to 4.5 months, the children grasp the offered object only on the side on which it is offered, after which it is possible to grasp it via the middle of the body ("split brain").

At the age of 5 months we expect a **hand-knee coordination** and objects are exchanged between hands.

About the **hand-foot-mouth coordination** (6/7 months), the child at this age is able to feel and understand its entire body, that is, to develop its own body image. It can turn from the back to the stomach, "spin" in the prone position and some children begin to crawl.

Prone Position

The arms are increasingly in the handle position. If the newborn turns its head in the stomach-layer, then a type of support on forearms or hand-root is to be observed fleetingly.

The arms did not move from the handle position towards the forearm support until they were about 6 weeks old. The ulnar duktion of the neonatal period has dissolved, the thumb is no longer inclined and through the goal of perceiving, seeing and fixating something, the first **erection on forearms** appears.

After another 6 weeks, at the end of the first trimester, the majority of the children show a **symmetrical elbow support**.

The head can be held and turned freely outside the support base, and the massive pelvic flexion has dissolved.

The support points of the upper extremity are ideally formed by the medial epicondyles of the humeri. The shoulder joint has centred itself, that is, in each section of movement the greatest possible contact surface of the joint partners is possible.

A first differentiation regarding supports and gripping begins about the fifth month to reach objects outside the support triangle (symmetrical elbow support). The supporting activity takes place on the backside arm, backside thigh and face side knee and the face side arm becomes "free" for an isolated gripping movement. This **gripping motion** is initially limited by duration and radius of action.

In **hand support** at the age of 6 months, the hand is unfolded, the thumb is abducted and support on the unfolded hands is possible. Vojta denotes the **tweezer handle** (7 months) as the starting stage of fine motor skills. At this time, the child can grab an object with only one hand and switch it back and forth between the hands. It is possible to strike hands or objects against each other.

From the middle of the eighth month on, the children are able to use the **pincer grip** The hand is unfolded. The thumb and index finger can approach each other in abduction and flexion and grip a small counterstalk between the fingertips.

Tenth-eleventh month: Most children are now able to reciprocate **scrabble** and begin to hold on to objects **straight**. The hand can be turned in an isolated manner, the first **hand games** (wave-wave) can be observed and the index finger begins to "point". The child begins to eat with the spoon (**use of tools**).

These basic fine motor skills will become increasingly differentiated in the coming months.

9.2.3.3 Boundary Stones of Development (Following Michaelis)

15 months

The child may place two blocks on top of each other at the pointing or prompting of the child. It wants to put keys in keyholes and eats with the spoon in the fist grip.

18 months

The child gives an object, which it holds, back on request, that is, it consciously opens the hand. The child prefers to use the index finger to explore, feel or press keys. More complex fine motor tasks such as unpacking a sweet succeed.

2 years

The tweezer grip with thumb and index finger succeeds safely. The child holds a crayon or similar with the first three fingers, that is, with "half" fist. Holding and working hands are characteristic.

3 years

The child can leaf through books individually. Smaller things are gripped with the fingertips. It can open/close zippers and close buttons.

4 years

The child can hold a pencil correctly (with the tips of the first three fingers).

5 years

The child can cut straight along a line with a pair of children's scissors, he can draw capital letters and first small things in a targeted manner.

6 years

The child holds a crayon or pencil just like an adult.

9.2.4 Clinical Reasoning

In physiotherapeutic treatment, different measures can be applied depending on the therapy goals, age and findings.

Within the framework of evidence-based medicine (EBM), proof of efficacy is repeatedly required in the form of corresponding studies. This proves to be very difficult for children. Especially in the first year of life there are no assessments that also take qualitative changes into account. And it is not ethically justifiable to compare therapy with non-therapy, etc.

However, through the differentiated documentation of the course of a treatment, parameters such as changes in mobility, strength and functional improvement in everyday life can be described.

Children are not small adults, therefore the therapy differs fundamentally from that of adult patients. For infants and small children, non-verbal forms of treatment on a neurophysiological basis are available: Bobath and Vojta therapy. It is an important task for therapists to empathetically accompany parents and find out which approach is best for them and their child.

Since the therapy can often take several years in the case of severe findings, it is a constant challenge to maintain motivation and cooperation with patience and creativity.

In the case of older children, additional or alternative interventions can be used. In play and everyday situations, it is always important to challenge and support the affected extremity in terms of grasping and supporting function. Wheelbarrow, bear stand, sloping level up and down crawling, with and without resistance, pulling, pushing, climbing, swings, handstand, ball games – there are no limits to your imagination (Fig. 9.1). The use of children's vehicles such as a running wheel, tri-

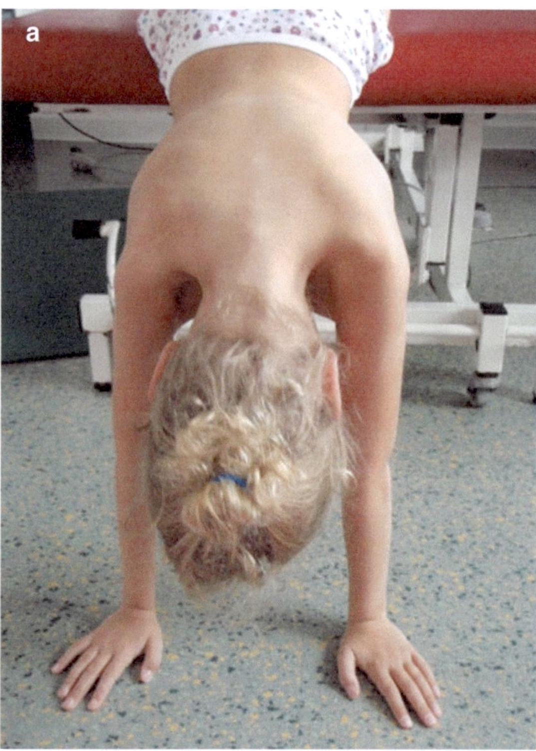
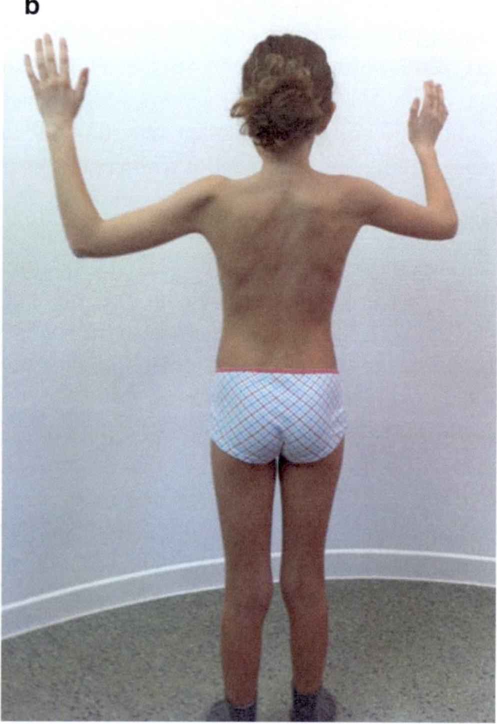

Fig. 9.1 (**a, b**) Dana, plexus paresis right. (**a**) At the age of six: Development of the symmetrical support function of the arms, reducing the weight of the legs (lying on the treatment table) and adjustment of the spine to the longitudinal axis. Dana is able to lean on her unfolded hands and stretch her elbows, which she does better on the left. The remaining deficits can be recognized by the increased protraction of the right shoulder, among other things due to insufficient function of the outer rotators in the upper arm and shoulder as well as limited adduction of the scapula. Compare distance shoulder-neck right/left. (**b**) At the age of 12: Testing the active shoulder mobility (external rotation) while standing. The right upper arm is increasingly in inner rotation, the right lower arm sinks more ventrally in the sagittal plane. The entire right arm or the right hand appear more slender. Unfortunately, the function of the outer rotators of the left shoulder (see "Hole"), for example, is also not optimal. Fortunately, there is no scoliotic deviation in the spinal column

cycle or Bobby Car can also support the therapy goals.

Together with the schoolchild, parents and doctor, the **therapy frequency** and regular monitoring is essential. In growth spurts or after diseases there can always be "regressions". The affected arm is no longer used "so frequently and so well", strength and extent of movement are reduced, and postural abnormalities in relation to the spine and shoulder girdle occur. With a short-term high treatment frequency, the structural findings have to be improved and the home programme checked, corrected and updated.

In adult therapy, there are studies that demonstrate the effect of task-oriented work, training therapy, repetitive practice, shaping and constraint-induced movement therapy (CIMT) (Taubsches Training). There is no evidence-based work for the children's area either. The principles of the above-mentioned interventions can, however, be applied to older children (school age). On the basis of everyday activities, the use of the affected extremity is worked out, many repetitions are "demanded" and the demand is increased (**shaping**).

With **CIMT** it is assumed that the "non-use" of an extremity can lead to "learned non-use" with corresponding cortical effects. During therapy, the unaffected hand is "immobilized" for several hours; it is put into a glove or wrapped around the body. This intervention is not possible without slight hand functions and the willingness of the children to cooperate. However, the basic idea of Taub's training can also be implemented in everyday life for a limited period of time by "skilfully" and playfully eliminating the hand that is not affected and thus making the use of the affected extremity unavoidable.

There have been attempts to improve the functions under treatment with a **Kinesio Tapes** to support the cause.

The use of **electrotherapy** is controversially discussed and is not used for infants and toddlers. It will certainly be necessary to increase the use of computer-supported **biofeedback process** to integrate.

A great challenge, also from a therapeutic point of view, is puberty (Fig. 9.2). A fitness stu-dio can then be the alternative to physiotherapy. The young people should be accompanied until they can deal with their limitations on their own responsibility.

If the posture deteriorates, the schoolchild should be questioned about sitting in class, looking at the blackboard.

Until the end of growth, supporting processes/exercises should be increasingly integrated into everyday life in order to provide the necessary incentives for growth and to keep the expected

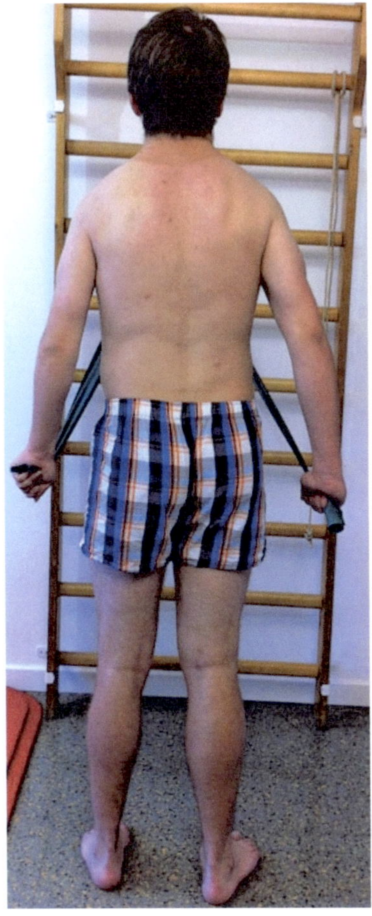

Fig. 9.2 Dennis, 19, Hemiparesis left. Instructions for the home exercise programme: In everyday life, the affected arm or hand is often only used as an auxiliary hand in bimanual handling. The Thera band, which must be held in place, can be used in different starting positions with different strengths and by different "suspensions" to bring the entire upper extremity in all directions of movement to use. Compensation mechanisms in the fuselage must be corrected

difference in length as small as possible. Threatening contractures require constant monitoring. Secondary problems in old age should be avoided as far as possible.

> Even with serious injuries, the aim is to achieve a hand that is suitable for everyday use.

A further field of activity of the physiotherapists is the **counselling of child and parents**. It is about play and everyday situations in the domestic environment, the day care centre and the school.

Sports

One-sided sports are negligible. Two-handed sports such as ball games, climbing and swimming are suitable (Fig. 9.3). Inline skating and

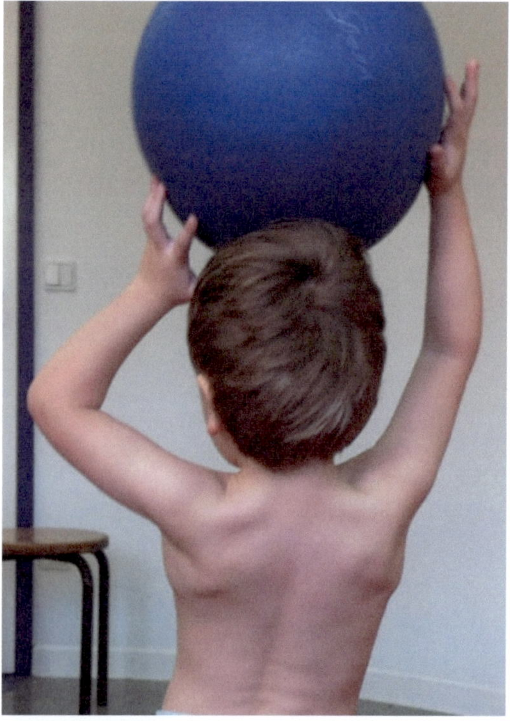

Fig. 9.3 Piet, 4 years old, plexus paresis left. Significant limitations of the upper arm and shoulder with respect to flexion, external rotation, abduction, missing scapula adduction and elbow extension. To lift and throw the ball over the head with both hands, Piet has to compensate in the trunk with increased extension, inclination and rotation. It can be assumed that functional deficits remain even after an operation with a severe plexus paresis. In order to achieve the use of the affected extremity in everyday life, the compensation patterns to be tolerated must always be weighed up

cross-country skiing also make sense, because here the reciprocal use of arms automatically occurs. However, the focus is on conveying to the child the joy of movement, even with its possible limitations.

Musical Instruments

Again the two-handed use is in the foreground (piano, flute, etc.). The transverse-flute and violin should not be used if necessary.

All leisure activities should never be about "top performance". The body should not be "forced" to unphysiological compensation patterns.

9.2.4.1 Approach of Vojta Therapy

Prof. Dr. Václav Vojta (1917–2000), a specialist in neurology and paediatric neurology, developed Vojta therapy and Vojta diagnostics.

In the reflex lotion according to Vojta, no functions are practised, but posture and movement patterns are derived from our innate motor programme. The entire skeletal musculature is activated and different switching levels of the central nervous system are addressed.

The basic positions of the human body, prone position (BL), supine position (RL) and lateral position (SL), are available for the therapeutic procedure. Movement sequences are initiated by triggering certain zones (the stretching receptors of muscles and tendons, the pressure receptors of the skin, the receptors of the internal organs and partly also the joint receptors). These zones are located on the trunk, arms and legs and, when stimulated in a certain way, are the "key" for the CNS (consisting of brain and spinal cord) and its ability to "control" innate movement programmes.

Information processing takes place partly on the level of the spinal cord and, via complex and differentiated switching and distribution processes in the afferent pathway system, in further sections of the CNS, also in the cerebrum. This also explains the "near" and "far" movement responses. These "programmes" form, among other things, the basis for the fact that humans can stand up from lying against gravity to walking in the first year of life via very specific posture and movement patterns. As these patterns are not consciously controllable, Vojta has defined them as **reflex lotion**.

Two main complexes are used in the therapy: **reflex reversal** (RU) and **reflex creep** (RC). They contain the three inseparable locomotion components: securing of the body position, erection against gravity and purposeful movement (gripping and supporting movement).

> Vojta therapy aims to activate innate movement programmes.

Assuming that the entire CNS and its nerve cells are connected via a network of synapses, the therapy is intended to influence the information processing of the synapses (state of the synapses, new formation of synaptic transmission sites, reactivation of unused connections). These are to be "stored" centrally in order to use them also in spontaneous motor function (**neuroplasticity**). The purpose of early therapy is to prevent abnormal patterns from fixing cortically.

The optimal dosage is four times daily, whereby a post-tracking (more effective transfer behaviour) of 4 h is assumed. The parents are guided within the scope of their possibilities to carry out the therapy with their children, whereby close monitoring, guidance, assistance and correction on the part of the therapists is indispensable.

The reflex locomotion creates conditions on which other forms of therapy (early intervention, ergotherapy) can build in addition or further (basic therapy).

9.2.4.2 Approach to Bobath Therapy

Physiotherapist Berta Bobath (1907–1991) and her husband, neurologist and paediatrician Karel Bobath (1906–1991) jointly developed this concept.

Parents also have an important role to play in Bobath therapy. Parental competence is to be strengthened. Parents have the task of integrating the therapeutic procedure into everyday life if possible, of not disturbing the self-regulation of the child (help to self-help) and of "demanding" the greatest possible independence. The instruction in handling enables parents to handle their child physiologically and age-appropriately in all everyday situations (lifting, carrying, feeding, etc.).

Bobath therapy uses optical, acoustic and tactile stimuli to stimulate the child to use the affected arm. However, this can only succeed if there is an activity of its own, if the arm can at least be lifted against gravity. Care must be taken to avoid massive compensation patterns.

With appropriate handling, the transitions back position → side position are initiated in the infant in order to initiate support on the affected shoulder joint. If the child lies on the healthy side in a lateral position, a decrease in weight may facilitate the operation of the affected arm by decreasing its own weight.

In the prone position, care must be taken to secure the shoulder joint well, that is, the humerus and shoulder joint must be positioned in such a way that maximum centring of the joint is achieved.

The initiation of the supporting function is particularly important in view of the growth stimulation of the affected arm and the differentiation of supports and movements necessary for locomotion.

There are no fixed exercises in the Bobath concept. The therapy is usually integrated into a game situation, which has to be adapted again and again to the developmental age and the respective interests (Fig. 9.4). The environment must be designed accordingly.

Depending on age, stage of development and symptoms, the aim is to motivate the child to develop its own strategies for coping with "tasks". Age-appropriate and everyday activities should be carried out and repeated as many times as possible. Through the learning of physiological movement sequences, the competence to act and consequently the independence is extended.

Elements from the principles "hands off" and "hands on" are used.

– **Hands off**: Movement sequences are initiated via daily life-oriented movement incentives and orders. The initially small sections of movement are then "initiated" into complex movement patterns in order to improve head-torso control, for example, to provoke

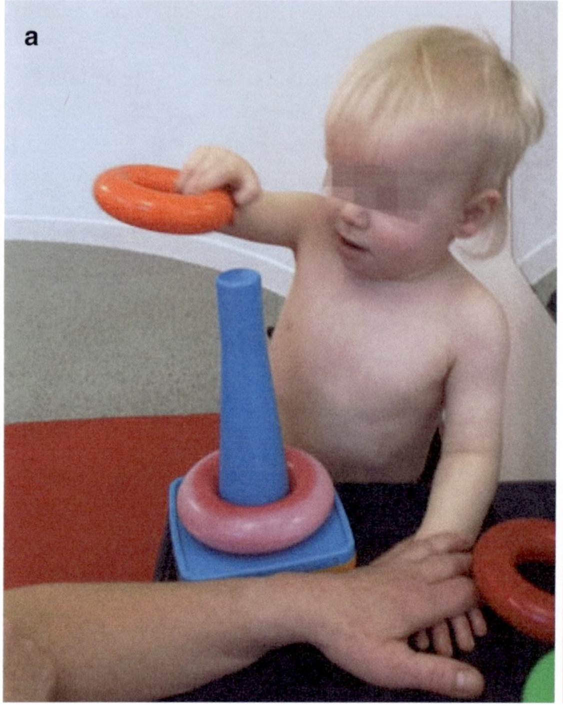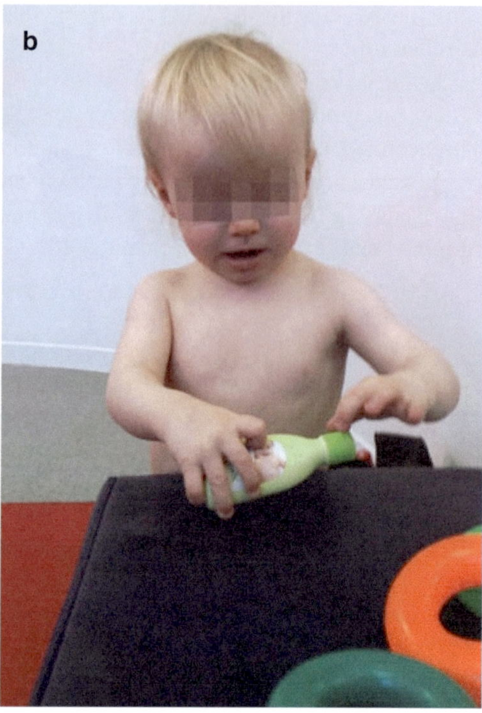

Fig. 9.4 (**a**, **b**) Luca, 2 years, hemiparesis right. Development of gripping, handling, eye-hand coordination via appropriate play materials. The non-affected extremity is "playfully fixed" to activate the right hand and the right arm. Development of the bimanual application of interesting materials suitable for children and suitable with regard to the size ratios

weight shifts and to initiate equilibrium reactions (support reaction).

- **Hands-on treatment techniques**: Inhibition (inhibition), stimulation (promotion) and facilitation (enabling the interaction of nerves and muscles) can facilitate the active coping with everyday situations if required.

The extent, use and duration of these techniques depend on the age, findings and cognitive and motor requirements of the child.

9.2.4.3 Manual Therapy Approach

Various measures are used to attempt to influence existing or developing limitations in individual joints and the resulting functional disorder. The treatment of the various structures thus not only has an effect on the joint in question but also on the central nervous control of the corresponding posture and movement patterns. Basic knowledge of joint mechanics and the various control loops is essential.

Active and passive mobilization of the joints and their surroundings as well as soft tissue techniques are available, also as preparatory measures.

9.2.5 Physiotherapeutic Therapy Management Using Early Childhood Plexus Paresis as an Example

9.2.5.1 General Handling of Children/ Infants with Plexus Paresis

Infants with plexus paresis are among the youngest patients in a physiotherapeutic department/ practice. In addition to physiotherapeutic therapy, great emphasis must therefore also be placed on empathetic accompaniment and information for parents. Due to the often long and difficult birth, the parents are massively burdened, they have received a drastic diagnosis, the consequences of which cannot yet be foreseen. They are still insecure in the handling with their newborn, and the fear around the affected arm strengthens this additionally.

During the examination and the resulting handling, the following points must be given special consideration during plexus paresis:

- Is the shoulder joint muscularly secured or is there a risk of dislocation?
- Is the epiphyseal fugue intact?
- Is there Horner syndrome (miosis, ptosis, enophthalmos)?
- What does the breathing movement look like in terms of direction and depth of breath (phrenic participation)?
- In which areas do sensory deficits (self-injuries) occur?
- Are there any abnormalities in the blood circulation, skin texture (poor healing process)?

Changes as a result of atrophy and contractures only become visible in the course of time. However, they should be documented from the beginning. Arm-circumference measurements in right-left comparison, angle measurement of all affected joints, photo/film documentation of spontaneous motor function.

9.2.5.2 The Physiotherapeutic Examination

In physiotherapy, the examination and findings are based on three pillars. In infants, spontaneous motor skills, reflexes and positional reactions are assessed. For older children, the cookie test and the AHA can be used.

The **assisting hand assessment** (AHA)—a new testing method to demonstrate the effectiveness of therapeutic interventions—measures and describes how effectively a child with a unilateral movement disorder uses the affected hand (assist hand) during the execution of bimanual play situations. The AHA is a standardized test procedure for children with hemiplegia or plexus lesion aged 18 months to 12 years. Unlike most procedures, this hand function test does not measure abstract performance at the body function level.

Spontaneous Motor Function

It is under investigation: What does the child do regarding his sensomotoric development, at what time and with what quality? The quality and quantity of the movement patterns are assessed. The contents of postural ontogenesis in the first year of life form the basis for the assessment.

Spontaneous motor skills in children with a movement disorder of the upper extremity are very quickly influenced by the respective symptoms, so that "similar" deviations in posture and movement can be expected in almost all children.

Supine Position

Age-dependent body position control is not possible. The child orientates himself towards the side not affected, forming an asymmetrical bald head at the back of the head. Also in the further course of development, a head rotation on both sides is not to be observed. The child does not manage to adjust and hold the head in the longitudinal axis of the spine, and symmetrical and isolated eye movements and orientation in space are not possible.

Depending on the damage, the affected arm lies in internal rotation with elbow extension or close to the body or in elbow flexion on the body. In lower plexus paresis, the hand falls into plantar flexion; in hemiparetic development, for example, we expect a firm fist (Fig. 9.5).

The development of hand–eye, hand–mouth, hand–hand coordination is disturbed, which has massive effects on the development of the entire body schema as well as on the development of grasping.

The spinal column is convex to the facial side, the pelvic axis is cranially and ventrally raised to the facial side, and the legs are not moved evenly; this often results in a delay in hip maturity on the affected side.

No matter whether it is a central or peripheral problem, hand–mouth and hand–hand coordination are not observed, and lateral gripping or gripping via the middle is not possible on the

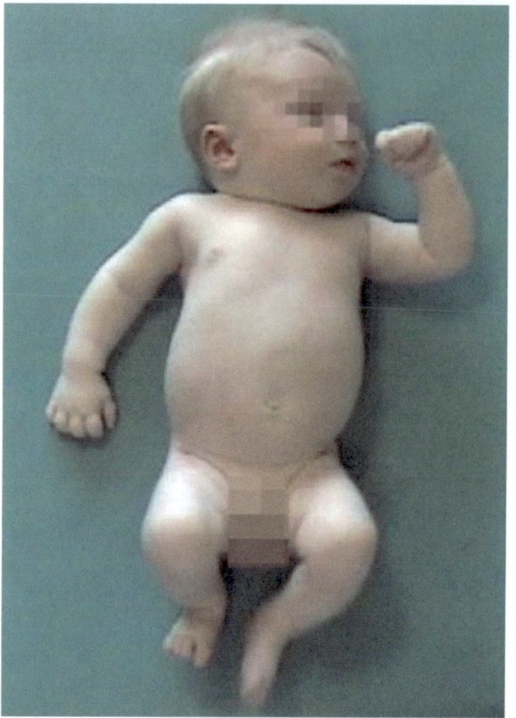

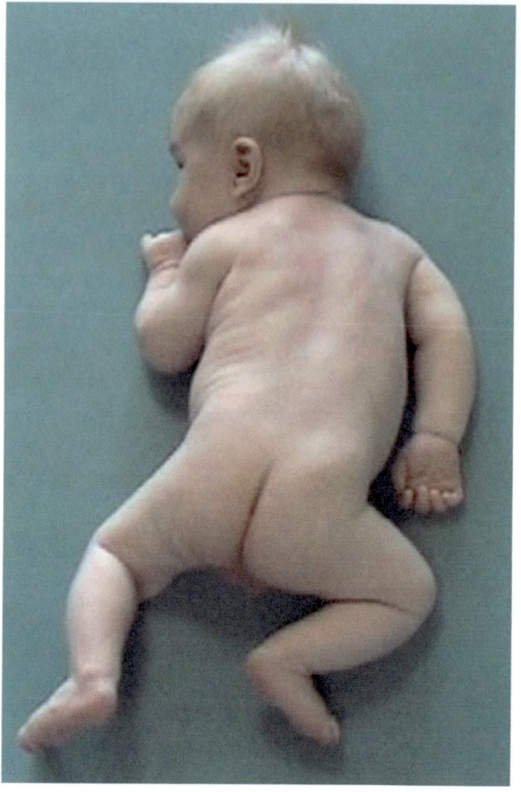

Fig. 9.5 Lennard, 4 weeks, right plexus paresis. Typical supine position of an infant with a plexus paresis: Depending on the damage, the affected arm lies more or less "motionless" in internal rotation with elbow extension close to the body. During lower plexus paresis, the hand falls into plantar flexion, the fingers are bent. The head is predominantly turned to the unaffected side (danger of plagiocephaly). The spine is convex to the facial side, the pelvic axis is cranial and ventral to the facial side, the legs are not moved evenly. This often leads to a delay in hip maturity on the affected side

Fig. 9.6 Lennard, 4 weeks, right plexus paresis. Typical prone position of an infant with plexus paresis: The head is turned to the unaffected side. The arm lies almost immovably next to the body. The affected shoulder is predominantly internally rotated and protracted. The spinal column deviates predominantly analogous to the head rotation. The hip of the affected side is restricted in abduction and external rotation. The erection over the arms is massively disturbed. The affected arm cannot be actively moved in front of the shoulder axis

affected side. Turning onto the abdomen is delayed, partly with compensation patterns. In most cases, the child rotates over the affected side because the unaffected arm initiates the rotation by grasping over the middle.

Prone Position

An age-dependent (age-appropriate) erection against gravity is not possible or only possible to a limited extent. The head is turned to the unaffected side. The arm lies almost immovably next to the body. The affected shoulder is predominantly internally rotated and protracted (Fig. 9.6).

The spinal column deviates predominantly analogous to the head rotation. The hip of the affected side is restricted in abduction and external rotation. The erection over the arms is massively disturbed. The affected arm cannot be actively moved in front of the shoulder axis. Therefore, neither a forearm support, a symmetrical elbow support, a single elbow support nor a hand support according to the contents of postural ontogenesis are possible.

The mentally awake child often tolerates prone position only for a short time, as the movement disorder severely restricts the child's erection and radius of action. It lies increasingly on the affected side, since it can take action at least with the unaffected hand. The spinal column does not come into the middle position in any movement sequence, and a free stretching and turning ability of the spinal column segments cannot be expected. The further milestones can therefore only be achieved and mastered with deviations.

It is amazing what compensation patterns the mentally healthy child is capable of when it wants to achieve something. Most children with a movement disorder of the upper extremity come, albeit significantly delayed, to a locomotion, a kind of seal and crawling.

This locomotion can never correspond to the ideas of a reciprocal locomotion pattern. The locomotion will always be one-sided. The spine will always remain asymmetrical, and the key joints cannot be centred (Fig. 9.7). In a seal, the affected arm lies under the body and the child pulls forwards over the unaffected arm. Head, spine and pelvis remain in asymmetry. When crawling, it is not possible to take on weight and thus support the unfolded hand.

The slanted seat is rarely observed in children with corresponding disorders. In order to reach this position, the child must lean up over the unaffected arms and rest on them. Since the affected hand is not available for playing etc., this

position does not bring any advantages to the child and is therefore not taken spontaneously.

In order to get to the standing position, the child pulls itself over the unaffected arm from the kneeling position over the one-bone kneeling position or also homologously at objects upwards. Depending on the side affected, this is also done unilaterally in relation to the pelvis and lower extremity.

All relevant primitive reflexes and positional reactions are still used in the physiotherapeutic findings to assess the developmental age and severity.

Primitive Reflexes

A check is carried out on very specific reflexes, which must be present or no longer present at a certain age in a precisely described manner. In plexus paresis, the focus is on the reflex of the hand, the reflex of the muscle itself and the reflex of the lid closure (optico-facial reflex).

Storage Reactions

The ability of the central nervous system (CNS) to respond adequately and promptly to changes in body posture is tested.

There are seven camp reactions available:

- Vojta reaction
- Traction reaction
- Peiper-Isbert reaction
- Collis-horizontalis reaction
- Collis verticalis reaction
- Landau reaction
- Axillary suspension reaction

The effects of a movement disorder of the upper extremity can be particularly clearly observed in the traction reaction, the Collis horizontalis and the Landau reaction.

> The securing of the affected shoulder joint must be absolutely taken into account when carrying out the procedure!

Joint measurements, circumference measurements, evaluation of sensitivity, trophy and blood circulation are naturally part of the physiotherapeutic findings.

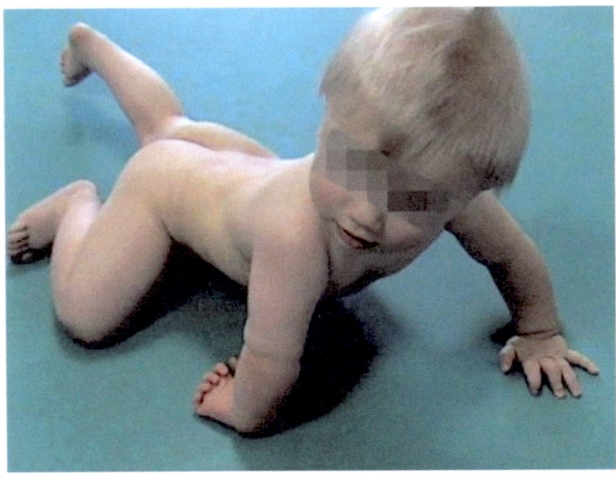

Fig. 9.7 Lennard, 9 months. Mentally awake children with plexus paresis also try to move and straighten up, to compensate them. The right arm remains in internal rotation and Lennard takes over the weight due to the missing dorsal extension on the back of the hand. An adequate support and step function of the right arm for crawling is not possible. The locomotion will therefore always be asymmetrical. A centring of the key joints of the unaffected extremities is therefore also not possible, the spinal column cannot adjust itself to the longitudinal axis

9.2.5.3 The Physiotherapeutic Therapy

Experience has shown that Vojta therapy, supplemented with handling according to the Bobath concept and mobilizing measures from manual therapy, is very effective for plexus paresis.

Interaction/Storage/Handling

Since plexus paresis has a great influence on the entire posture, the interaction between child and mother (caregiver) can also be impaired. The child finds it harder to keep his head in the middle, make eye contact, and interact with the parents, laugh at them and communicate with them. In order not to create a vicious circle here that massively unsettles the parents and the child ("my child does not smile at me, what am I doing wrong"), early information must be provided and parents must be provided with handling possibilities to help the child find its centre and to interact.

For example, the child can lie supine on the changing table, the legs are bent at the hips and lie on the belly of the mother standing over the child. The child is helped to find its "centre" and to adjust the head in the longitudinal axis by slight flat pressure on the chest. A gaze fixation and thus making contact is facilitated in this position.

During the first few days, the arm is immobilized in a plexus-relieving position, assuming that the oedema is resorbed after 7–10 days.

The child lies in **supine position**. The forearm lies at right angles to the abdomen, the hand is in the area of the navel. The sleeve can be fixed to the garment with a diaper, a baby safety pin or a Velcro fastener.

If a pronounced "fall hand" is present, an additional treatment with a "splint" may be necessary later. With the small infant this can be "tinkered" from spatula and skin-friendly tapes. The hand is thus held in the middle position to avoid contractures and overstretching.

If the child sleeps on its stomach during the day and only under observation (sudden infant death), the arm can lie next to the body in the zero position.

If the child is awake, you should spend 4–6 weeks with the **prone position** wait, because

only then a decrease of the pelvic bending posture and a beginning activity of the shoulder girdle musculature is to be expected by weight shift after caudal.

Since the child is not able to bring the affected arm forward in the frontal plane, the arms must be positioned in the forearm support (approximately 6 weeks) and in the symmetrical elbow support (approximately 12 weeks), depending on age, in order to offer a support function.

If the child lies on the **side,** the affected upper arm should be at right angles to the trunk in front of the body, and the blood circulation of the arm must be observed!

On the **non-affected side** when lying down, the arm can be fixed to the abdomen, to the side of the hip or to appropriate positioning material at eye level of the child.

> In general, the lateral position should only be taken under supervision and not for too long.

The plexus must not be exposed to unphysiological stretching during handling and therapy. Maximum contraction of the damaged musculature must be avoided. During the first few weeks of daily care (washing, dressing, etc.), it is essential to avoid additional stretching of the plexus.

The cervical spine should not be inclined to the healthy side, the affected arm should not be moved upwards, next to the head, the spreading of the arm should be avoided and a backward movement of the arm must not happen.

When tightening, the affected arm is first put into the sleeve, and when undressing, it is first pulled out.

When lifting and lying down, the child is taken over the unaffected side so that the arm is always in contact with the torso.

Vojta Therapy

According to ICF-CY, the "sites of action" of Vojta therapy in plexus paresis cover the areas of structure, function and participation. Due to nerve damage, arbitrary motor skills are not possible or only possible to a limited extent. The treatment goals are accordingly:

– **Structure level:** Stimulation of the not or only partially innervated musculature, promotion of reinnervation through activity, improvement of blood circulation, avoidance of contractures and atrophies.
– **Function level:** Development of a supporting function in order to influence the growth of length, avoid secondary damages such as positional deformations of the head, asymmetry of the spine, delay in hip maturation and changes of the shoulder joint.
– **Participation level:** Achievement of the milestones of postural ontogenesis, at least quantitatively.
– Integration of the affected extremity into the body scheme with transfer into spontaneous motor function.

The effectiveness of Vojta therapy in this clinical picture has also been proven electrophysiologically. During a series of examinations (27 children) in the Children's Centre Munich (1984—Dr. med. H. Bauer), an increase of the innervation frequency, a recruitment of motoneurons and a frequency stabilization of the activated motoneurons were determined during the treatment.

Myographic evidence of innervation compression was found in 22 children. Twelve children could be discharged as "cured" and ten children were still in treatment when the article was published, but they showed clear functional improvements and a good helping hand. In the remaining children there was a clear defect syndrome, and there was also no evidence of fasciculation electromyographically.

In the follow-up, an increase in the maximum arbitrary innervation and an increase in the density of innervation during facilitation could be demonstrated. This effect was also measurable after the end of the therapy.

Pizetti and Fredella (1984) report on a study of 110 children. Sixty-six were treated with conventional therapies and 44 with Vojta therapy. In 75% of the children who received Vojta therapy, a good improvement in function was observed. In the control group, however, the corresponding functional improvement was only 21%.

Procedure

After an exact analysis of the failed or limited muscles, the Vojta therapy selects starting positions (e.g., prone position, lateral position, supine position) in which the affected muscles are to be initiated. The activation always takes place in the pattern, since the CNS does not "know" any individual muscles.

By means of different zone selection and combination (spatial summation) and stimulation duration (temporal summation), the affected arm is activated in the overall pattern in support or gripping or step function.

During therapy, vegetative reactions often occur first. Smallest fasciculations of the musculature and changes of the skin (goose bumps, increased blood circulation, sweat), overactivated muscles and muscle groups are observed and evaluated as a first step of innervation. The goals of improving blood circulation, avoiding and/or reducing contractures and atrophy as well as influencing length growth are thus taken into account.

Even if movement is not observed at all or only incompletely in the periphery, it is assumed that the central response takes place in the pattern and that integration or maintenance of the function of the affected extremity in the body schema is achieved. If a regeneration time of 0.5–1 mm/day is taken as a basis, one can expect an incipient innervation in the shoulder girdle area after approximately 3 months in the case of incomplete damage.

In the case of stretch injuries, success can be observed after just a few days, sometimes even weeks, during therapy and a complete "recovery" of the arm and its functions can be expected at the end of the first trimester (even without therapy). However, therapy is also indicated here in order to provoke a "certain" deployment of the arms already during the recovery period, to avoid further secondary disorders such as symmetry disorders, positional deformities of the head, scoliotic changes of the spine, delay in hip maturation and to maintain central representation.

If after 3 months there is no activation with regard to hand function and elbow flexion, serious damage must be assumed and spontaneous recovery is no longer to be expected. Surgical intervention is indicated in this case. Another task of physiotherapy here is to provide advice and to get the parents to present the child to appropriate experts in order to clarify an indication for surgery or to determine the right time.

After a **nerve restoration** and/or corrective interventions (loosening of contractures), the activating and cautious mobilizing therapy must be restarted after wound healing and immobilization has been completed. Goals and priorities are the same as before the operation.

The central representation of the affected extremity on the sensorimotor cortex must be maintained until reinnervation and reintegration have taken place and active spontaneous movements can be observed.

For a **tendon or muscle displacement**, the children are older in most cases. Here, too, the same principles apply, but the possibilities of exerting influence over the cognitive level are added. After a resting period of approximately 6 weeks, the integration of the "new" motor and sensory functions is in the foreground. The control of the muscle in its now changed function (with regard to movement direction and muscle physiology) has to be worked out and integrated into the movement sequences. As long as the child has no "idea" of the changed function, it should only work in the muscle chain and without orders. If the "new" function is available again to some extent, all known physiotherapeutic interventions can be used with regard to coordination, strength and expansion of movement.

Reflex Creep with Respect to the Upper Limb

The locomotion complex reflex creep is activated in the prone position (head turned 30°). This is also a whole body pattern, with the following focus on the upper extremity and the shoulder girdle (Fig. 9.8).

In the area of the upper extremity, for example, we expect a supporting and straightening function in the shoulder joint above the facial arm. The acetabulum of the shoulder joint rotates over the head of the humerus, a loose flexion in the elbow joint with a support point of the medial condyle is to be activated. The scapula is held in

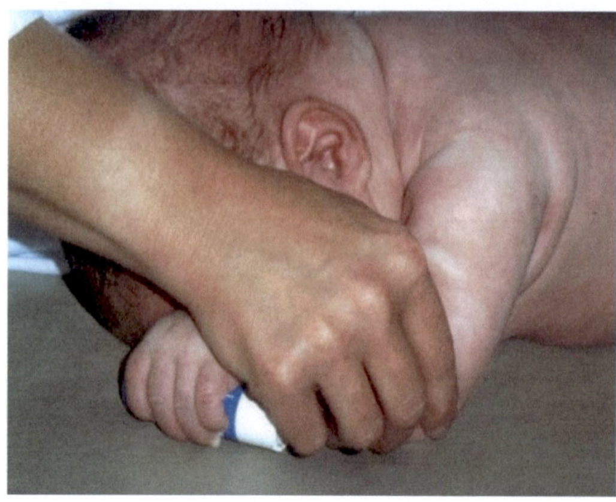

Fig. 9.8 Reflex creep, activation of the facial arm. Initial position: prone position, the zone at the medial humeral condyle is activated. We expect the facial arm to have a supporting and straightening function in the shoulder joint and a loose flexion in the elbow joint with a support point on the medial condyle. The forearm makes a pronation movement, the wrist is dorsally extended and radially reduced, abduction of the metacarpals and fist closure. The hands are made to grasp

a central position and the musculature of this section of the spinal column experiences a direction of action towards the punctum fixum epicondylus humeri. A dorsal extension and radial reduction in the wrist with abduction of the metacarpal bones and fist closure are part of this partial pattern. The hands are made to grasp.

In order to activate these movement responses, a differentiated synergistic interaction of the entire skeletal muscles is necessary. If there is only a partial neuronal connection, the affected muscles are activated as part of the coordination complex. The muscles not or only partially innervated during plexus paresis. Are integrated into this context.

On the back of the arm we expect a step movement forward. This time the acetabulum is punctum fixum, the arm punctum mobile. We observe a rotation of the scapula and an external rotation, abduction and flexion of the arm in the shoulder joint as well as a supination in the elbow joint. In the wrist, there is a dorsal extension and unfolding of the metacarpal bones with loose stretching of the finger joints. To achieve this, the corresponding muscles in the shoulder, elbow and wrist must be activated synergistically.

The effects of muscular imbalance in plexus paresis on the spinal column become immediately visible. The spinous processes of the thoracic spine cannot be adjusted in the direction of the supporting arm. Thus, it is not possible with a movement disorder of the upper extremity to control the entire spinal column physiologically and to adjust it in its longitudinal axis. This deficit can of course be observed in the reaction of the pelvis as well as in the reaction of the lower extremity.

Reflex Reversal with Respect to the Upper Limb

The posture and movement patterns that are activated in the locomotion complex are analogous to the muscle games that the child "uses" to crawl out of the supine position, the hands are made to support – muscle games that we cannot observe in either upper or lower plexus paresis.

The locomotion pattern of turning the reflex in the first phase is activated in the supine position by triggering the chest zone (rib space 7–8 rib), whereby the head is also turned by 30° here.

Among other things, we expect the facial arm to move across the centre of the body and the posterior arm to move towards the handle position (Fig. 9.9). The prerequisite for this abduction, external rotation and flexion movement in the shoulder joint is a differentiated interaction of the arm, shoulder, shoulder blade and trunk muscles, among others, with appropriate adjustment

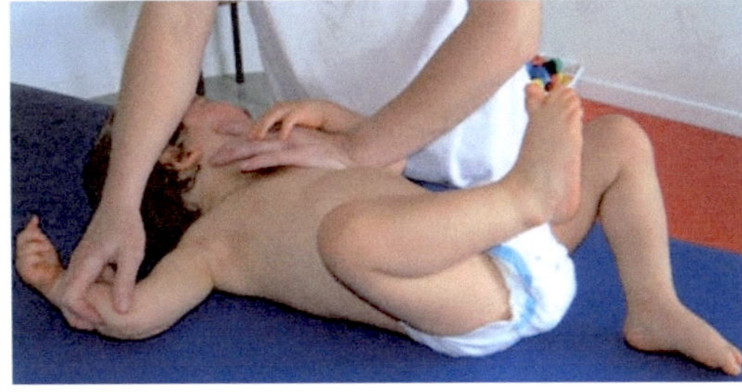

Fig. 9.9 Reflex reversal first phase. Initial position: supine position, the chest zone (space between ribs 7–8) is activated, additional stimulation at the medial humerus condyle on the occipital side. Among other things, we expect the rear-facing arm to move in the direction of the handle position. The elbow joint is flexed, the wrist goes towards the dorsal extension, the hands open, the middle hand unfolds and the thumb is abducted

of the spine. The elbows are bent slightly, the hands open, the middle hand unfolds and the thumb is abducted. The kinesiological contents of this pattern again encompass the entire body and condition themselves in their muscle function differentiation. Disturbances at the upper extremity thus automatically influence the control of the entire posture and movement pattern.

Manual Therapy

Since the child's spontaneous motor skills are severely restricted, regular and timely **mobilization therapy** is indispensable. During the first 3 months, it must be strictly observed that the plexus is not overstretched during mobilization.

However, modified and differentiated joint and soft tissue techniques from manual therapy must be used as early as possible to counteract impending contractures on the shoulder, elbow and wrist.

At the **upper plexus paresis** the danger of an internal rotation contracture (subscapularis muscle) in the shoulder joint exists due to an imbalance of the rotator cuff (weakly innervated external rotators). This evolving problem must be observed and addressed from the outset.

The small child should lie on its back and the shoulder is carefully mobilized into the external rotation with the elbow close to the thorax. Possible evasive movements (e.g., lateral inclination and twisting of the thoracic spine, reclination and lateral inclination of the cervical spine, protraction of the shoulder joint) must be avoided.

In older children, this mobilization is also possible while standing or sitting, but the danger of evasive movements increases.

In addition to the functional problems, an internal rotation contracture can lead to a dysplastic change of the humeral head in the long term; this is a feared secondary problem of upper plexus paresis.

Due to a disbalance (contracture of teres major and latissimus muscle, limited function of the serratus anterior muscle), the shoulder blade moves prematurely with every flexion and abduction movement.

At the **lower plexus paresis**, it is essential to avoid a contracture in plantarflexion (**falling

hand). The wrist must be mobilized in dorsal extension, a good and strong fist closure can only be performed when the dorsal extension has been completed (passive and active insufficiency). The elbow joint is mobilized in extension as well as pro- and supination. The mobility of the finger joints and the opposition of the thumb must be passively developed and maintained.

An increase in contractures can be expected over time. The muscular disbalance leads to an increased use of the still innervated musculature in spontaneous motor function. An automobilization of the affected joints through physiological use with regard to support and grasping is not to be expected or only to a limited extent. The realistic therapeutic goal is therefore to minimize the contractures rather than to avoid them.

The treatment of a movement disorder of the upper extremity can take many years. It is up to the child and parents to decide when and if there are breaks in therapy.

References

1. Rigos A, Engeln H, der Kampe J. Das sensible wunder. Geo Kompakt. 2013;34:77–86.
2. Wehr M, Weinmann M. Die Hand. Werkzeug des Geistes. Heidelberg: Spektrum; 2008.
3. Wilson FR. Die Hand, Geniestreich der Evolution. Stuttgart: Klett-Cotta; 2000.
4. Nilson L. Ein Kind entsteht. München: Mosaik; 1990.

Further Reading

Ambühl-Stamm D. Früherkennung von Bewegungsstörungen beim Säugling. München: Urban u. Fischer; 1999.

Aschersleben G. Erste Gedanken-Was im Kopf eines Säuglings vor sich geht. Gehirn und Geist Serie Kindesentwicklung. 2014;1:50–5.

Bahm J, Uphoff R, Mahler M. Der geburtstraumatische Plexus brachialis Schaden. plexuskinder.de. 2010.

Bauer H, Vojta V. Behandlung der geburtstraumatischen Plexusparesc. Sozialpädiatrie in Praxis und Klinik. 1984;11:596–602.

Biedermann H. Manuelle Therapie bei Kindern. München: Elsevier; 2006.

Hollenweger J, Kraus de Camargo O. ICF-CY. Bern: Huber; 2011.

Hüter-Becker A, Dölken M. Physiotherapie in der Pädiatrie. Stuttgart: Thieme; 2005.

Kienzle-Müller B, Wilke-Kaltenbach G. Babys in Bewegung. München: Urban u. Fischer; 2008.

Orth H. Das Kind in der Vojta-Therapie. München: Elsevier; 2011.

Pizzetti M, Fredella D. Terapia Incruenta: Confronto Tra Metodo Tradizionale E Nuovo Metodiche Di Facilitazione Neuro-Musculari. Bologna: Aulo Gaggi; 1984.

Rosenkötter H. Motorik und Wahrnehmung im Kindesalter. Stuttgart: Kohlhammer; 2012.

Spitzer M. Lernen Gehirnforschung und die Schule des Lebens. Heidelberg: Spektrum; 2003.

Steding-Albrecht U. Das Bobath Konzept im Alltag des Kindes. Ergotherapeutische Prinzipien und Strategien. Stuttgart: Thieme; 2003.

Vojta P. Das Vojta Prinzip. Berlin, Heidelberg/New York: Springer; 2007.

Vojta V, Schweizer E. Die Entdeckung der idealen Motorik. München: Pflaum; 2009.

Occupational Therapy for Children and Adolescents

A. Haegele

10.1 Contemporary Occupational Therapy

Due to restrictions in everyday activities, occupational therapy is very often one of the remedies prescribed by doctors for children and adolescents with a movement disorder of the upper extremity. These include children with unilateral or bilateral cerebral palsy, acquired hemiparesis and plexus palsy.

> Occupational therapy supports and accompanies people of all ages who are restricted in their ability to act or whose ability to act is in danger of becoming restricted. The aim is to empower them to carry out activities that are meaningful to them in the areas of self-care, productivity and leisure in their environment.
>
> Specific activities, environmental adaptation and counselling serve to enable people to act in everyday life, to participate in society and to improve their quality of life [1].

The current view of occupational therapy is based on process and content models that describe the subject of occupational therapy and the procedural approach in treatment. The client-centred, activity-centred, and evidence and context-based approach forms the foundation [2].

The procedure within occupational therapy can be divided into a process with the elements evaluation, intervention and outcome. As a process model, the **Canadian Practice Process Framework** (CPPF) can be named, which divides the treatment process into eight steps [3]. This process model describes the process based on the Canadian Model of Occupational Performance and Engagement (CMOP-E) content model. The **Canadian Occupational Performance Measure** (COPM) assessment, which was developed by a Canadian working group, is very frequently used in occupational therapy. Due to its semi-structured interview, it is highly suitable for the diagnosis and evaluation of the treatment process.

There are many other occupational therapy models that can be used by occupational therapists, which provide a structure in the treatment process and can recommend assessments or facilitate the decision on the selection of suitable assessments. Another process model is the **Occupational Therapy Intervention Process Model** (OTIPM), which is a model based on a client-centred, activity-based, top-down approach that can be used to plan and implement assessments and interventions [4].

Due to the client-centred perspective that is common today, clients and their caregivers are actively involved in the therapy and actively shape the treatment process with the associated decisions. This refers, for example, to the joint agreement of the therapy goals and is also reflected by the fact that the share of counselling

A. Haegele (✉)
Kinderneurologische Ambulanz, Sana Kliniken
Duesseldorf, Duesseldorf, Germany
e-mail: anke.haegele@sana.de

© Springer Nature Switzerland AG 2021
J. Bahm (ed.), *Movement Disorders of the Upper Extremities in Children*,
https://doi.org/10.1007/978-3-030-53622-0_10

within the intervention has increased, so that the transfer into everyday life is guaranteed and the clients/caregivers gain more understanding of interrelationships.

Never before have therapists had so much knowledge at their disposal as they do today. The latest findings from international studies can be accessed on the Internet and, above all, via searches in databases (PubMed, Cochrane, LIVIVO, OTseeker, etc.). Although they must be examined for their transferability to the respective context, the gain in knowledge is often significant. Also, other databases such as the EBP database of the German Association of Occupational Therapists/Deutscher Verband der Ergotherapeuten (DVE) provide access to translated study summaries. This database is unique in the German-speaking world and has been developed by the DVE in recent years exclusively for its members. It contains well over 2000 German summaries of studies from all over the world, and examines the efficacy, effectiveness, costs and benefits of occupational therapy and occupational therapy-relevant interventions [5].

10.2 Approaches in Therapy

Children with movement disorders of the upper extremity often avoid using their affected arm or their more severely affected arm. In children with unilateral cerebral palsy, this phenomenon is called "learned non-use". It is often easier for the children to use their more skilful arm, and they usually automatically use strategies for themselves that are as economical as possible. It is, of course, possible for a child to act independently and skilfully in everyday life with just one arm. So why should it be important for the child to use both arms or hands? There are some arguments for that. Countless actions in everyday life require the use of both hands, for example, eating with cutlery or closing the zip of a jacket (Fig. 10.1). It is often noticed that the affected arm and the affected hand are significantly shorter and smaller than the other arm. This and the resulting trunk posture can in turn influence the growth of the spinal column. Increased use of the affected hand as an assisting hand can stimulate growth in the

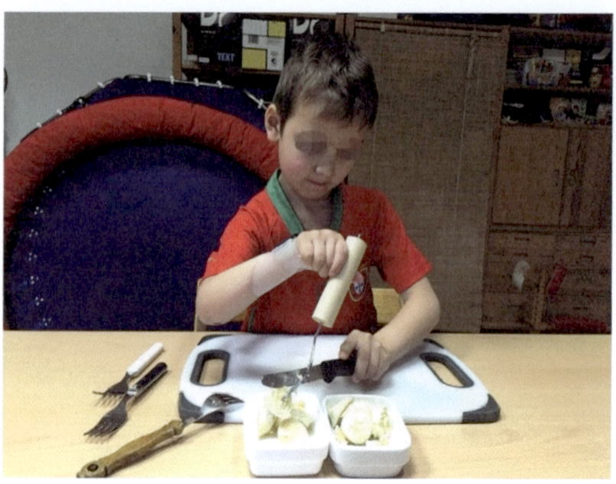

Fig. 10.1 Testing adapted cutlery

arm and hand, and also have a beneficial effect on the overall posture. Adolescents often report that it bothers them that the arm is shorter and the hand is smaller. With increasing age, intrinsic motivation often increases, and children and adolescents voluntarily address their difficulties in everyday life and want to use their affected hand more in everyday life. It is then easier for them to name their goals in concrete terms, especially if they are important to them.

A concept that starts at an early age can often prevent or minimise consequential effects and secondary damage, and the children can thus learn to use both hands at an early age. In the meantime, there are already several studies that prove this and call for early intervention to prevent learned non-use [6–8].

> One goal in the treatment of these children should be to stimulate the use of both hands in everyday life from the very beginning and to automate bimanual use at meaningful activities, if it is possible.

The aim is, for example, to analyse the difficulties and abilities of the children in everyday life by means of targeted assessments and/or an activity analysis, and to subsequently enable them to perform the desired activities. In the toddler age, the children should be given the opportunity to play games (according to the interests of the child) and carry out activities that are typical for their age. In this age group, the objectives should be specified after interviewing the parents, for example, using the COPM. For some children, it may also be important to develop **compensation**

strategies as an approach to therapy, in order to achieve more independence in everyday activities. The use of **aids** or an adaptation of the environment can also be a strategy to achieve more independence in the child's actions. Some children may show clear evasive movements, and some sitting postures may also be unphysiological due to reduced posture control in the trunk. These side effects should also be taken into account during occupational therapy.

Children with a plexus paresis can have various limitations. Often, their experiences of movement in the first years of life are not comparable with those of healthy children. In most cases, the affected arm is used less—this is comparable to the learned non-use in children with unilateral cerebral palsy. These children, too, can show deviations in the development of the body schema. Just like the restrictions imposed by central paresis, this has an impact on action and movement planning. A further approach for these children is the **strengthening of targeted muscle groups** depending on the findings, clinical picture and degree of limitation. It should always be checked whether an increase in muscle strength is possible; with increasing age, children/adolescents can be very receptive to doing self-exercises.

A further component of occupational therapy intervention is the **instruction and advice for parents and other caregivers**. This counselling often refers to assistive equipment and suggestions for the use of both hands in everyday life and while playing (Fig. 10.2).

> Occupational therapy for children and adolescents with a movement disorder of the upper extremity should always be individually adapted to the child and its needs. The aim of occupational therapy is to maximise the children's independence and ability to act in everyday life.

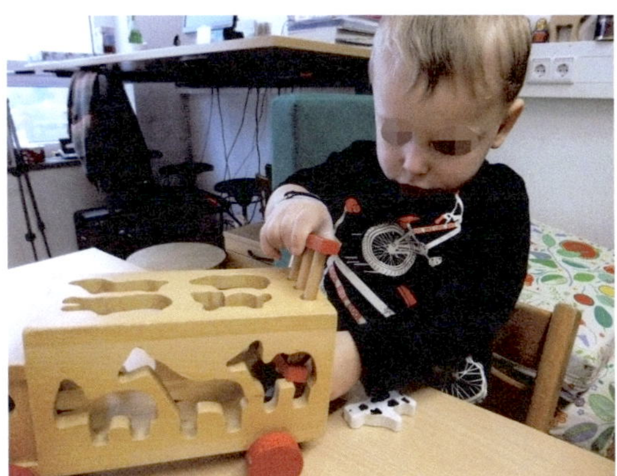

Fig. 10.2 Playing with both hands

the therapist, the caregiver or the physician. The principle here is to use standardised and validated assessments as far as possible. However, these are not always accessible or their use is not possible, as the performance of certain assessments requires certifying training. This effort is often only worthwhile if the assessments are frequently used in practical activities. Depending on the case, it can also be useful to refer the child for diagnosis in a special paediatric centre, where assessments are used frequently. It is also possible to use self-evaluation tools such as questionnaires, interviews and checklists. On its website, the DVE provides a very good overview of established assessments and their target groups (www.dve-info.de). In addition, video and photo documentation can be recommended and used for diagnosis and evaluation.

10.3 Appropriate Assessments and Their Application (Selection)

When using assessments, the purpose and goal of their use must be clarified. They are to be applied specifically to the specific question of

10.3.1 Assessments for Children with Unilateral CP, Hemiparesis or Plexus Paresis

10.3.1.1 Assisting Hand Assessment (AHA; www.ahanetwork.se)

The AHA was developed in 2003 by Krumlinde-Sundholm et al. at the Karolinska Institute in Sweden [9]. The purpose of the AHA is to measure and describe how effectively children with a unilateral impairment use their assisting hand for bimanual actions.

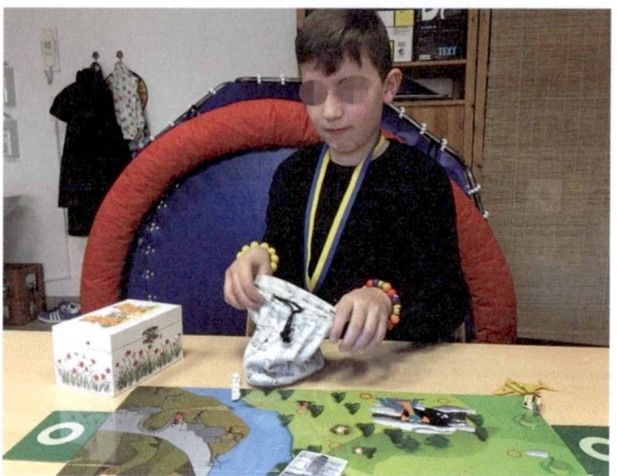

Fig. 10.3 AHA

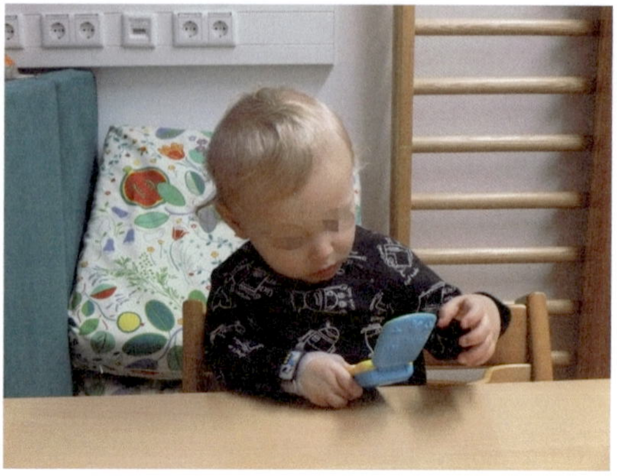

Fig. 10.4 Mini AHA

This hand function test measures actual performance at the activity level rather than abstract performance at the body function level. It is used for children from 18 months to 12 years of age with hemiparesis, unilateral cerebral palsy or plexus lesion.

It is carried out within the framework of a semi-structured game situation with provided game material (Fig. 10.3). The evaluation is standardised, and the result is an Excel file with the item hierarchy and the individual profile of the child. It then becomes clear where the child stands in this item hierarchy and how effectively it uses its hand in bimanual game activities. With the result, one can analyse which abilities the child still needs or which abilities should be strengthened so that the child can develop a more effective assisting hand. The AHA is standardised and valid; it measures the performance of the child in the use of its assisting hand. Thus, it can be used for the planning, implementation and evaluation of an activity-oriented therapy. The assessment can show the effectiveness of therapeutic interventions. The prerequisite for carrying out the AHA is a two-and-a-half-day certification course. In 2016, the age group in the AHA was extended. Adolescents aged 12–18 years are observed performing one standardised everyday activity (making a sandwich) or at playing a short strategy game [10]. This closes a gap, and a standardised survey can also be carried out for this age group.

10.3.1.2 Mini-AHA

Like the AHA, the Mini-AHA measures and describes the performance of the affected hand in bimanual playing actions. It evaluates changes over time and differentiates among children with unilateral movement impairment aged 8–18 months with different degrees of impairment (Fig. 10.4). It supports the planning of clinical interventions [11]. A course with certification is also required for this assessment.

10.3.1.3 Children's Hand-Use Experience Questionnaire (CHEQ; www.cheq.se)

The CHEQ is an online questionnaire that records children's experiences with their affected hand in activities that are normally carried out with both hands [12]. Parents and/or the child answer questions about 29 typical bimanual everyday activities. It is designed for children and adolescents from 6 to 18 years with a functional limitation of one hand, for example, hemiparesis or unilateral cerebral palsy. It serves the purpose of defining treatment goals and evaluating the effects of treatment. The final report after completion of the questionnaire shows on two pages how the children and adolescents cope with these typical activities and provides information about the use of the assisting hand. It is highly recommended as it is free of charge and provides a good overview of the execution of typical everyday actions. Recently, it has been supplemented by the Mini-CHEQ for the age group 3–8 years (www.cheq.se/miniquestionnaire).

10.3.1.4 Manual Ability Classification System (MACS; www.macs.nu)

The MACS is a classification of manual skills for children aged 4–18 years with cerebral palsy [13]. The MACS classifies how children with cerebral palsy use their hands in everyday use of objects. It is a functional description that serves to complement the diagnosis of cerebral palsy with its subtypes. It assesses the general ability of the child to use everyday objects, without taking the lateral differences in hand function into account. It is free, easy to use and provides a common language for all professionals involved with the child.

10.3.2 Additional Assessments (Cross-Diagnostic)

10.3.2.1 Canadian Occupational Performance Measure (COPM)

The COPM is based on the Canadian Model of Occupational Performance and Engagement (CMOP-E) [3]. It was first published in Canada in 1990 and the first German translation was published in 1998 [14]. Since 2007, there has been an adapted version of COPM in Germany for primary school children aged 6–10 years, the COPM a-kids [15]. For children up to the age of 6 years, the parents are the main interviewees.

The COPM is a semi-standardised interview that measures occupational performance problems at the level of activity and participation according to the International Classification of Functioning, Disability and Health (ICF). It is a client-centred and activity-related assessment, which refers to typical activities mentioned by the child, records occupational problems and checks their achievement. It has high validity and reliability, and mainly serves the report and evaluation.

10.3.2.2 Pediatric Evaluation of Disability Inventory (PEDI)

The PEDI was developed in the USA by Haley et al. in 1992 [16]. It is a research method for measuring skills and performance in the areas of self-sufficiency, mobility and social functions. It also records the support from caregivers and the frequency and type of aids needed. It can be used for children from 6 month to 7 years and 6 month, possibly also for older children if there are delays. It is suitable for many diagnostic groups.

The parents or caregivers are questioned in writing and orally. It can be used easily by multidisciplinary teams, but also by occupational therapists in practices working with physically and mentally disabled children. It is valid and reliable, can be used for report and evaluation, and is related to the ICF. It is an internationally recognised assessment; the German translation and revision by Schulze and Page was published in 2014 [17].

10.3.2.3 Goal Attainment Scale (GAS)

The GAS was developed in 1968 by Kiresuk and Sherman. While it was originally used in the area of psychiatry, it was later also used in rehabilitation [18].

The scale is a semi-standardised procedure that is ideal for formulating objectives and evaluating the course of therapy. It can be used to measure the individual goals of the client and the therapist. These goals can be activity goals, structural/functional goals or participation goals, and can be qualitative or quantitative. The objectives should be formulated as concretely as possible so that they are verifiable. The GAS can be adapted individually and is oriented towards the goals of the children and adolescents. It is a reliable, sensitive and substantial assessment.

10.3.2.4 Paediatric Occupational Therapeutic Assessment and Process Instrument (PEAP)

The PEAP (Pädiatrisches Ergotherapeutisches Assessment & Prozessinstrument) consists of two elements. The first element is a standardised assessment for child activity [19] that records and measures the performance status of a child in its age group from different perspectives. The second element is a process instrument that supports the whole therapeutic process. The process instrument can be used, as necessary, partially or in its entirety. The assessment is standardised and based on 15 age-typical fields of activity. It is currently designed for children between 5.0 and 8.11 years. What is new is that this assessment combines several client perspectives and the therapist's perspective. Various aspects of activities related to the environment are standardised and systematically recorded [20]. Both elements support the client-centred and activity-oriented approach in occupational therapy. Further training is recommended for practical use. It is until now, only published in Germany.

10.4 Therapy Concepts and Interventions (Selection)

10.4.1 Therapeutic Concepts

10.4.1.1 Therapy According to the Bobath Concept

"The Bobath concept requires a sound knowledge of the complexity of development and developmental disorders as well as central movement disorders, and the comprehensive ability to perceive the individuality of patients in a differentiated way and to develop therapeutic solutions to problems that promote the activities and participation of patients in their social context. This also includes the anticipation and prevention of typical secondary complications" [21].

In the Bobath therapy, the focus is on the child with its individual abilities and difficulties in the context of its individual environment. The aim of the therapy is to support children and adolescents in their autonomy, development and rehabilitation, thus enabling them to participate more and to become more active (Fig. 10.5). Working professionally with the concept means the competent application of specific methods and techniques. "The Bobath concept commits us to the interdisciplinarity of professional action and continuous learning. The constant search for knowledge as well as the conceptual further development are integral components of the Bobath Concept" [21].

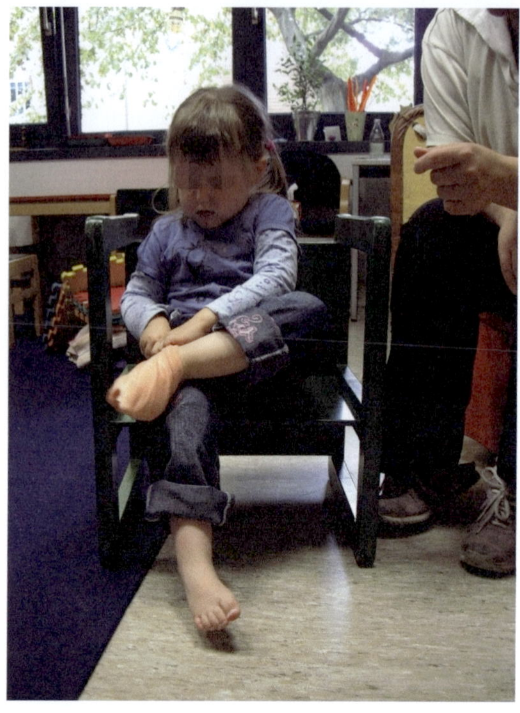

Fig. 10.5 Put on socks independently on a special chair

10.4.1.2 Sensory Integration According to J. Ayres

As children and adolescents with a movement disorder of the upper extremity can, depending on the findings and degree of limitation, also show sensory abnormalities or abnormalities in perception processing, the approach of sensory integration therapy may also be indicated.

10.4.2 Interventions

10.4.2.1 Intensive Training

In recent years, numerous approaches to intensive therapy for cerebral palsy and hemiparesis were published and have become well known in the research literature. Numerous study results make it possible to get a comprehensive picture of the various programmes, their indications and their possible applications. It can be useful to carry out an intensive programme instead of or in addition to regular therapy; this procedure also makes sense for children with plexus paresis. It is essential to check the indication for this form of therapy. If possible, there should be a realistic individual, activity-oriented goal.

10.4.2.2   Constraint-Induced Movement Therapy (CIMT)

The main features of CIMT are the restriction of the less affected hand, for example, with a glove or another form of restriction (bandage, sling, cast or splint) as well as intensive practice and exercises. There are different types of CIMT, each of which is described in more detail in studies; modified CIMT [6], for example, is a child-friendly variant. Studies have shown that CIMT is more effective than the usual approach, but not necessarily better than structured bimanual training. All types of CIMT have shown a positive effect [22]. Recent study results show that the dosage (in terms of duration of intervention and therapy per day) is not as high as in previous years. CIMT involves the repetitive practice of movements and actions with the affected hand, aiming purely at the unimanual capacity. If the child already uses the affected hand spontaneously, bimanual training should be considered [23].

10.4.2.3   Bimanual Upper Limb Therapy

Bimanual training (BIT) is not new but has not yet been sufficiently defined [24]. Hoare describe 2017 a new definition of bimanuel therapy: "The process of learning bimanuel skills through the repetive use of carefully chosen, goal related, two-handed activities that provoke specific bimauel actions and behaviours" [25]. Conventional occupational therapy typically involves a bimanual approach. BIT includes components of motor learning and cognitively based theories [24]. The therapist is the teacher, the focus is more on the task and the environment, and less on the movements. The principles are active problem solving, repetition and challenge. In contrast to CIMT, BIT ensures intensive training of bimanual coordination (Fig. 10.6). It uses a targeted, activity-based framework using the principles of motor learning. Specific practical tasks promote problem solving (Fig. 10.7) [22].

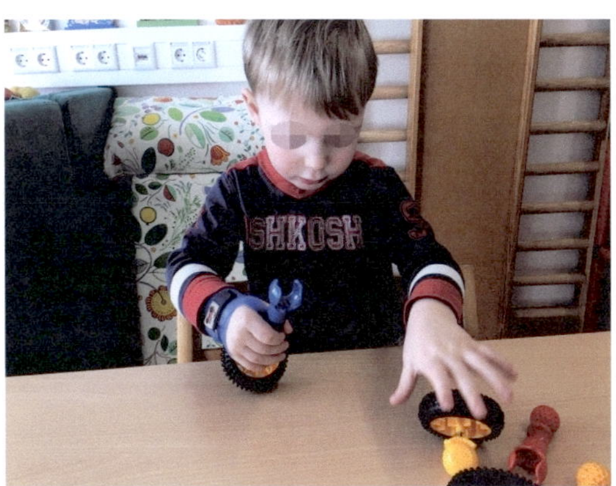

Fig. 10.6   Play with structural material

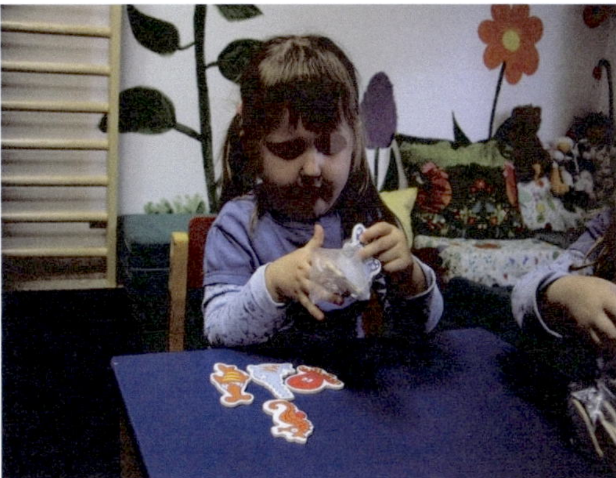

Fig. 10.7   Playing with both hands

10.4.2.4   Goal-Directed Training

Goal-oriented training can be used from 5 years of age if concrete goals can be formulated. It is a typical top-down approach with the motto "you learn what you practise". Active problem solving takes place, for example, if a child wants to learn how to tie his or her shoelaces; this has to be analysed and elaborated concretely. It is important that the goals are named by the child, showing there is intrinsic motivation (Fig. 10.8). The goals should be meaningful for the child within the context of his or her life (Fig. 10.9). The principles of goal-oriented training are the adaptation of the activity, supportive hints (physical, verbal, …) and repetitive practice to consolidate and automate the activity [23].

In the meantime, there is a large number of evidence-based therapeutic interventions to choose

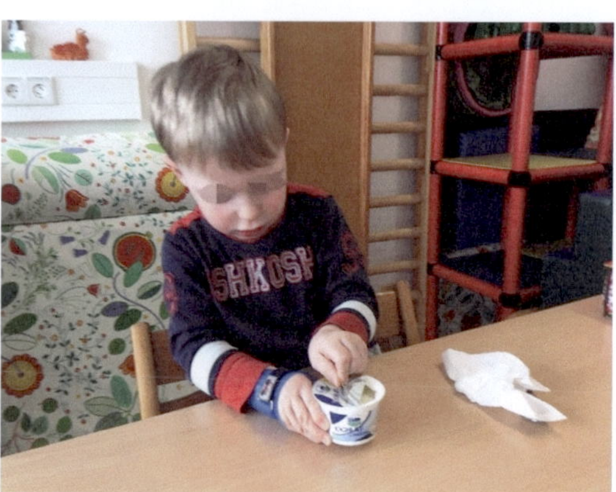

Fig. 10.8 Opening a yoghurt pot

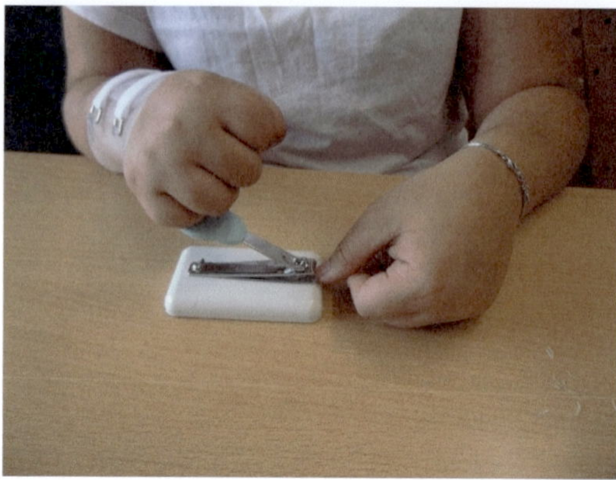

Fig. 10.10 Clipper for cutting fingernails

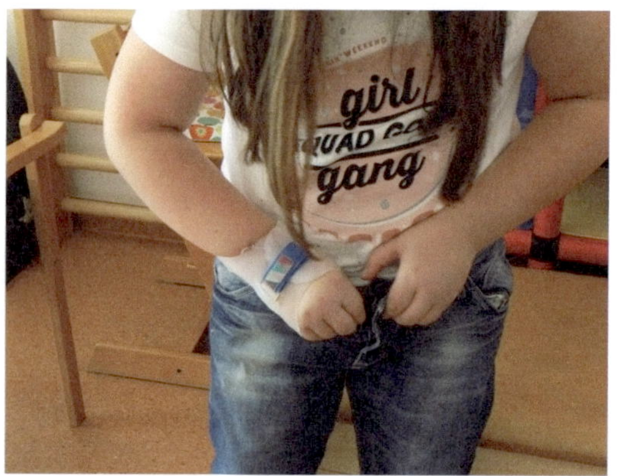

Fig. 10.9 Closing a button

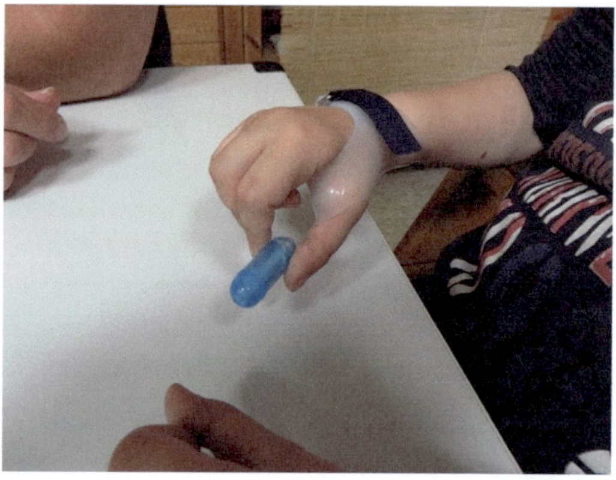

Fig. 10.11 Dynamic hand orthosis

from for children with a unilateral movement impairment; hybrid forms, that is, combinations of individual approaches and home programmes, are also described. There are several aspects to be considered in the selection process, such as the age of the child. A meta-analysis concludes that intensive, activity-related, targeted interventions (as mentioned above) are more effective than standard therapy in improving unimanual use and the achievement of individual goals [26].

10.5 Assistive Equipment and Adaptation of the Environment

Assistive equipment can support children and adolescents in their daily activities and thus lead to increased participation (Fig. 10.10). They should be individually selected and adapted, and the pro-

vision of care should follow a commonly agreed objective. There are many everyday tools, such as breakfast boards, non-slip foils or adapted cutlery, which give the children more independence in everyday life. Dynamic hand orthoses made of silicone can be a way of changing the child's hand position, thus enabling the child to perform a bimanual action in the first place (Fig. 10.11).

Silicone is gaining ground in the use of hand orthoses due to its dynamic properties. Acceptance among children is very high, which means that a long wearing period during the day can be guaranteed. A study carried out as part of a bachelor's thesis shows that 3–7-year-old children with unilateral cerebral palsy participate more and are better able to act in everyday life—this is what parents report in interviews. The acceptance of the silicone hand orthosis by children mainly depends on the material properties and the quality of the process [27].

10.6 Case Study

A case study with an inpatient illustrates the practical application of the theories: Lisa, 6 years and 4 months old before starting school in 2015.

10.6.1 Diagnoses

- Development/intelligence: no known symptoms.
- Physical findings: **upper plexus paresis G54.0.**
- Psychological findings: awareness of deficits; attention-related problems for further assessment.
- Social background: nothing of specific relevance for the disorder.
- Aetiology: obstetric traumatic lesion.
- Participation: endangered; specific therapy required.

10.6.2 Anamnesis During the First Outpatient Presentation in 2014

At the presentation, Lisa has a congenital right-side plexus paresis after shoulder dystocia at birth. A nerve transfer operation took place in January 2010. She is presented in our clinic by her parents with the question regarding the indication for inpatient intensive therapy. Lisa and her parents report restrictions in everyday life, which at the time refer to the area of self-care (washing hair, tie hair and putting on tops).

10.6.3 Brief Description of the Findings from a Medical Point of View

There are no contractures at the right-side upper extremity, the active external rotation in the shoulder is 2/5 MRC (force degree) and the active mobility is limited (described in the detailed findings). Hand function is good, but Lisa shows clear signs of a learned non-use.

10.6.4 Hand-Intensive Therapy Concept

This concept includes a 2-week intensive goal-directed training based on target agreements at the levels of activities/participation and body functions/structures.

The interdisciplinary concept includes physiotherapy, psychomotor therapy, occupational therapy, a pedagogical group activity and therapeutic or nursing support during meals. Some characteristics are:

- Consideration and design of environmental factors.
- Operationalisation of the occupational goals and evaluation on the basis of COPM and GAS.
- Guidance and counselling of parents regarding environmental factors and their influences.
- Suggestions and support for everyday life.

10.6.5 Lisa's Occupational Goals during Admission

Tie bows with both hands, braid her hair with a scrunchie, put on tight tops on her own and cut solid foods.

10.6.6 Assistive Equipment

None.

10.6.7 Occupational Therapy

Within occupational therapy, Lisa has pursued and developed the goals of "putting on and taking off tight tops", "tie a firm bow" and "cutting firm meat with a knife and fork". She was motivated to pursue her goals. She sometimes needed support in focusing attention on the agreed action. In the process, she acted more and more skilfully when putting on and taking off her tops. The development and implementation of new strategies were carried out together with the therapist.

Table 10.1 COPM survey table

Occupational request All goals have the importance of 10 (= very high) for Lisa	Self-assessment of the execution at the time of admission (1 = does not work, 10 = very good)	Self-assessment of satisfaction at the time of admission (1 = not satisfied, 10 = very satisfied)	Self-assessment of execution at the time of discharge	Self-assessment of satisfaction at the time of discharge
1. Tying bows tighter with both hands	3	8	10	10
2. Tying hair more tightly with a scrunchie	5	8	7	10
3. Putting on tight tops	1	1	6	6
4. Cutting firm meat	1	1	9	10

To consolidate and automate her achieved abilities, frequent repetitions of the actions in the daily routine were important. Lisa lacked practice and exploration in dealing with cutlery. Within the first week, she was quickly able to use cutlery variably for various foods in the therapy unit. She was accompanied during meals and quickly reached her goal of cutting meat. At the time of her discharge, she was able to hold the fork with her right hand or the knife to cut. In this case, the use of a sharp knife can be cited as an example of the environmental adaptation aspect. The tying of a bow, which she had learnt shortly before the stationary admission, became automated during her stay. In functional terms, a higher level of strength endurance was developed when it came to tightening bows. At the time of discharge, she could actively use her forearm in the mid-position, but frequently still compensated automatically through increased lateral abduction in the upper arm and internal rotation in the shoulder. She has become aware of this automatism and can temporarily stop it. After 2 weeks, she has largely achieved her goals to her satisfaction. The COPM was performed with her within the occupational therapy on the first and last day of her stay.

10.6.8 Physiotherapy

In the physiotherapy, besides movement activities (e.g., ball games) and games (holding cards), which Lisa chose according to her preferences, manual therapy was the main focus. Getting changed for therapy and, if necessary, braid her hair in a ponytail were further contents of the physiotherapy.

10.6.9 Psychomotor Therapy ("Motopädie")

The contents of psychomotor therapy[1] mainly referred to her goals "dressing quicker for sports" and "tying a ponytail". It was possible to give Lisa good support in increasing her attention and endurance. Lisa also chose climbing as her medium, as this was something she wanted to learn. The functional goals were integrated well and she was able to improve her abilities.

10.6.10 Outcome Measurement

Lisa's goals and their achievement were specified according to COPM and assessed independently (Tables 10.1 and 10.2).

10.6.11 Progress Summary

Lisa was motivated and cooperative in the pursuit of her goals; at the time of her discharge, she was more skillful and independent in executing the activities than at the beginning of the intervention. She has made significant progress at both

---

[1] The therapy concept "Motopädie" is not well known in English-speaking countries.

Table 10.2 Active range of motion (neutral-zero method)

	Time 1	After 2 weeks	After 4 months (follow-up)
Abduction in the shoulder joint IR/AR	70/30/0	70/0/30	70/0/45
Held close to the body IR/AR	70/30/0	70/0/0	70/0/0

the structural and the activity levels and has achieved her goals to her satisfaction (Table 10.1).

10.7 Conclusion

Occupational therapy, which is individually oriented to the needs and goals of the children, and includes all important contextual factors and integrates evidence-based praxis, is an important component in the therapy of children with a movement disorder of the upper extremity. Through an activity-centred and client-centred therapy, the participation of the children can be increased, and more self-activity as well as greater independence can be achieved.

References

1. Deutscher Verband der Ergotherapeuten-DVE. Definition ergotherapie. 2007. https://www.dve.info/ergotherapie/definition.html. Accessed 15 Dec 2015.
2. Le Granse M, van Hartingsveldt M, Kinébanian A. Grondslagen van de ergotherapie. Amsterdam: Reed Business; 2012.
3. Townsend EA, Polatajko HJ. Enabling occupation II: advancing an occupational therapy vision for health, Well-being, & justice through occupation. Ottawa, ON: CAOT Publications ACE; 2007.
4. Fisher A. OTIPM occupational therapy intervention process model (translated by B. Dehnhardt). Idstein: Schulz-Kirchner; 2014.
5. DVE. EBP database. 2015. https://www.dve.info/ergotherapie/ebp-datenbank.html. Accessed 15 Dec 2015.
6. Eliasson AC, Shaw K, Berg E, Krumlinde-Sundholm L. An ecological approach of constraint induced movement therapy for 2–3-year-old children: a randomized control trial. Res Dev Disabil. 2011;32(6):2820–8.
7. Eliasson AC, Sjöstrand L, Ek L, et al. Efficacy of baby-CIMT: study protocol for a randomised controlled trial on infants below age 12 months, with clinical signs of unilateral CP. BMC Pediatr. 2014;5(14):141.
8. Nordstrand L, Eliasson A-C, Holmfur M. Longitudinal development of hand function in children with unilateral spastic cerebralpalsy aged 18 month to 12 years. Dev Med Child Neurol. 2016;58(10):1042–8.
9. Krumlinde-Sundholm L, Eliasson AC. Development of the Assisting Hand Assessment: a Rasch-built measure intended for children with unilateral upper limb impairments. Scand J Occup Ther. 2003;10:16–26.
10. Romein E. Klientenzentrierte Ergotherapie: AHA-Assisting Hand Assessment Version 5.0. 2015. http://www.klientenzentrierte-ergotherapie.com/Instrumente-und-Methoden-in-Ergotherapie/aha-assisting-hand-assessment-kinder-und-jugendlichen-mit-hemiparese-plexusparese-von-18-monate-bis-18-jahre.html. Accessed 30 Dec 2015.
11. Graeves S, Krumlinde-Sundholm L. Manual Mini AHA English Version 1.2. 2014.
12. Sköld A, Hermansson L, Krumlinde Sundholm L, Eliasson AC. Development and evidence of validity for the Children's Hand-use Experience Questionnaire (CHEQ). Dev Med Child Neurol. 2011;53(5):436–42.
13. Eliasson AC, Krumlinde-Sundholm L, Rösblad B et al. MACS brochure. 2005. www.macs.nu (in English and German).
14. George et al. (COPM-Team Deutschland). Derzeitiger Entwicklungsstand rund um das kanadische Modell in Deutschland. In: Jerosch-Herold C, Marotzki U, Stubner BM, Weber P, editors. Konzeptionelle Modelle für die ergotherapeutische Praxis. Heidelberg: Springer Verlag; 2009. p. 156–70.
15. Gede H, Kriege S, Strebel H, Sulzmann-Dauer I. Kinder zu Wort kommen lassen (COPM a-kids). Idstein: Schulz-Kirchner; 2007.
16. Haley SM, Coster WJK, Ludlow L, et al. Pediatric Evaluation of Disability Inventory (PEDI) Version 1.0: Development, standardization and administration manual. Trustees of Boson University, Center for Rehabilitation effectiveness, Boston, 1992.
17. Haley SM, Coster WJ, Ludlow L, et al. PEDI-D: Pediatric Evaluation of Disability Inventory –Assessment zur Erfassung von Aktivitäten des täglichen Lebens bei Kindern mit und ohne Beeinträchtigung (übersetzt und bearbeitet von C. Schulze, J. Page). Schulz-Kirchner, Edition Vita Activa, Idstein, 2014.
18. Schädler S. Assessment: goal attainment scale. Subjektive Ziele objektiv messen. Phys Ther. 2006;4(9):34–5.
19. Kraus E, Romein E, Weise U. PEAP Pädiatrisches Ergotherapeutisches Assessment & Prozessinstrument. Idstein: Schulz-Kirchner; 2015.
20. Romein E, Kraus E, Weise U. Den Betätigungsstatus bei Kindern standardisiert erheben. Ergotherap Rehabilitat. 2015;4:26–31.

21. Gemeinsame Konferenz der Deutschen Bobath-Kurse e.V. (G.K.B.). Curriculum Bobath-Kurs für die berufliche Arbeit mit dem Bobath-Konzept. 2014.

22. Sakzewski L, Ziviani J, Abbott DF, et al. Radomized trial of CIMT and bimanual training on activity outcomes for children with congenital hemiplegia. Dev Med Child Neurol. 2011;53(4):313–20.

23. Hoare B. CP teaching—course manual: functional hand use in hemiplegia. 2014.

24. Hoare BJ, Imms C, Rawicki HB, Carey L. Modified constraint-induced movement therapy or bimanual occupational therapy following injection of Botulinum toxin—a to improve bimanual performance in young children with hemiplegic cerebral palsy: a randomised controlled trial methods paper. BMC Neurol. 2010;5(10):58.

25. Hoare BJ, Graeves S. Unimanual versus bimanual therapy in children with unilateral cerebral palsy: Same, same, but different. J Pediatr Rehabil Med. 2017;10(1):47–59.

26. Sakzewski L, Ziviani J, Boyd RN. Efficacy of upper limb therapies for unilateral cerebral palsy: a meta-analysis. Pediatrics. 2014;133:175–204.

27. Hirsch M, Jekel K, et al. wie beeinflusst der Einsatz einer Silikonhandorthese die Partizipation bei Kindern mit infantiler Cerebralparese. Bachelorarbeit der Hoogeschool Zuyd, Heerlen, Niederlande, 2011. silikonorthesen@googlemail.com.

M. Schäfer

11.1 Provision of Aids for the Child's Upper Extremity

The orthopaedic treatment options for movement disorders of the child's upper extremities are very complex in nature, extent and function. Depending on the diagnosis, congenital and acquired disorders such as lesions of the central and peripheral nervous system as well as traumatic and posttraumatic disorders of the musculoskeletal system are differentiated. Furthermore, a distinction is then made between the extent and severity of an existing limitation of movement and ultimately also between the specific characteristics and the resulting therapeutic goals of the treatment.

The latter should comply with the Code of International Classification of Functioning (ICF) with the following objectives [1]:
- Promoting active participation in life
- Promoting independent active movement
- Improvement of communicative and receptive skills
- Improvement of capacity to act

M. Schäfer (✉)
Orthopädie-Technik, POHLIG GmbH,
Traunstein, Germany
e-mail: m.schaefer@pohlig.net

In the orthopaedic technical supply of everyday life, mainly *orthoses* and *assistive devices* are proven.

Orthoses are substitutional aids which support tasks such as function assurance, relief, stabilization, guidance, immobilization and preoperative conditioning of incorrectly positioned and functionally impaired parts of the body. According to the ISO standard, they serve to modify the structural and functional properties of the neuromuscular and skeletal systems [2].

In interdisciplinary dialogue, orthoses are often referred to as splints, whereby splints—similar to a plaster cast—fulfil exclusively static and immobilizing tasks. They therefore represent only a restricted part of orthotics. With regard to the beneficial influence on movement disorders of the upper extremities, aids are most likely to have growth-controlling, dynamically correcting and function-giving properties. Everyday aids, on the other hand, are tools which are used to carry out specific activities and which attempt to facilitate non-existent or no longer existing bodily functions or related everyday activities.

Due to progress in reconstructive surgery of the upper extremities, the focus of orthotic care has increasingly shifted from conservative care alone to pre- and postoperative measures of function-giving surgical interventions [3].

An orthotic supply of aids to the upper extremities only makes sense if it prevents malpositions and their progression, promotes function, prevents or

© Springer Nature Switzerland AG 2021

J. Bahm (ed.), *Movement Disorders of the Upper Extremities in Children*,
https://doi.org/10.1007/978-3-030-53622-0_11

alleviates pain, relieves body situations mechanically or supports and accompanies a postoperative result early-functionally.

For this purpose, all disciplines involved in the supply process must be aware of the possibilities and limitations of the respective methods. Best results can only be achieved in a closely coordinated interdisciplinary teamwork between doctor, therapist and certified orthotist.

After the explanation of the areas of application and the types of orthoses, the following section describes orthotic fittings and everyday aids oriented from distal to proximal indications, their constructive functional principles as well as the objectives of the respective aid provision.

All aids pursue the functional improvement and expansion of the application possibilities of the upper extremities. The focus of this care must be the improved participation of the child in its environment.

11.2 Fields of Application

Movement restrictions can be caused by a wide variety of clinical pictures.

One differentiates between *lesions* and *injuries to the central nervous system* such as spastic paralysis and cerebral insults. On the other hand, there are the *lesions* and *injuries to the peripheral nervous system*. These are often caused by compression damage to the nerves and can be accompanied by flaccid forms of paralysis and the resulting sensorimotor deficits. Typical representatives of this group are the nerve damage of the brachial plexus as well as the radial, ulnar and median nerves.

The orthotic restoration of *congenital malformations* is mostly focused on the hand and in a few cases, e.g. in the case of radial clubhand, also on the forearm.

The *juvenile chronic arthritis* is rather rare with a prevalence of 0.1% [4]. The focus here is on joint protection and pain-relieving stabilization of the affected joints.

Upper limb orthoses are increasingly being used to improve the function of children with neuromuscular diseases and forms of paralysis such as infantile cerebral palsy.

Based on the pathomechanics of the respective form and function disorder of the CP, the goals of the orthotic fitting must always be defined in advance. These can lie in stretching the musculature, improving the joint position, stabilizing effects, preoperative testing or even the postoperative protective function [5]. When monitoring the results and assessing a spastic-paralytic deformity, both the comparison with the initial findings (never the normal condition) and the sustainability of the therapeutic effect should be taken into account [6].

11.3 Orthotic Types and Material Selection

Orthotic fittings of the upper extremities can be systematically recorded according to various criteria. First of all, the application area for the orthotic treatment should be determined. For this purpose, the international classification according to ISO 8549-3, which also includes orthotic types of the upper extremity [7], is used (Table 11.1).

The task of the orthosis should then be described, i.e., whether the orthosis fulfils at minimum one of the following criteria:

Table 11.1 International classification of orthoses according to ISO standard

Shorthand	Meaning
FO	Finger orthosis
HO	Hand orthosis
HFO	Hand finger/thumb orthosis
WHO	Wrist hand orthosis
WHFO	Wrist hand finger orthosis
EO	Elbow orthosis
EWHO	Elbow wrist hand orthosis
EWHFO	Elbow wrist hand finger orthosis
SO	Shoulder orthosis
SEO	Shoulder elbow orthosis
SEWHO	Shoulder elbow wrist hand orthosis
SEWHFO	Shoulder elbow wrist hand finger orthosis

– Static working principles, such as immobilization and fixation, postoperative securing of a defined position and protection for sections of the extremities.
– Dynamic principles of action, i.e., exerts mobilizing and redressing forces in the direction of correction by means of dynamic elements such as joints, springs or cables.
– Serves as a functional replacement orthosis for functional failures, whereby a secure functional position is usually aimed for.

Important information about the use of materials and the determination of design features is given by the description of the functional disturbance and the resulting requirement for the orthotic effect.

The orthoses are always constructed according to the laws of orthotic biomechanics [8]. These include the 3-point correction principle acting in the frontal and sagittal planes (Fig. 11.1) as well as the laws of leverage and torque, which have a considerable influence on the design of the orthoses.

The determination of the wearing time of the orthosis also influences the material selection. You must define whether an orthotic fitting is to be performed for the *day* or for the *night* or even to 23-h therapy. In the context of full-time use, a modular orthosis system must be considered in many cases, which can be upgraded and dismounted for the respective requirements of the time of wear (Fig. 11.2).

Day orthoses should always allow the best possible functional use of the orthosis for the child and must not limit physiological functions still existing in the joints.

The wearing comfort of the aid is also of great importance, as its acceptance depends to a large extent on it.

With nighttime orthoses, on the other hand, the best possible correction effect that is tolerable for the child is in the foreground.

Here, proximal limb sections must often also be integrated into the corrective construction. Orthoses with dynamically acting components should introduce the correction forces as gently as possible, that is why flat constructed correction zones are preferred here.

The corresponding *choice of materials* [9] for the aids is oriented towards:
– The biomechanical requirements for the required strength (levers and forces) (thermoplastics, fibre composites (FC), carbon-fibre prepregs, silicones).
– Technical design: e.g. adaptive properties, flexible orthotic edges (silicones); lowest weight (FVW), highest strength and modular design (FVW, C-fibre prepregs; polyamides).
– Re-adjustments (C-fibre composites, silicones) and growth adjustments.
– A specific weight as low as possible, since the affected children often have weak muscles

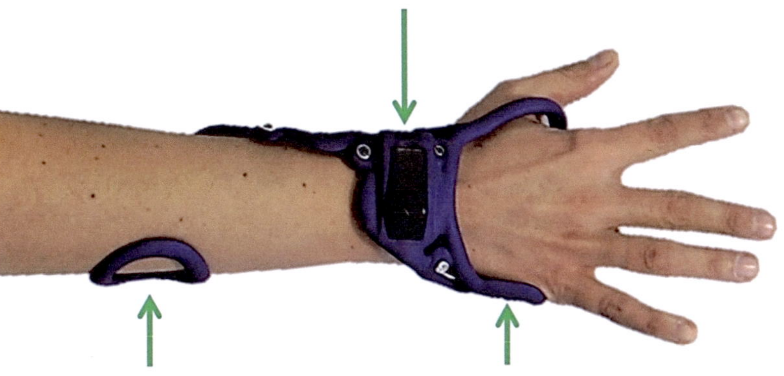

Fig. 11.1 3-point principle for correction of ulnar deviation using the example of a forearm spiral print orthosis

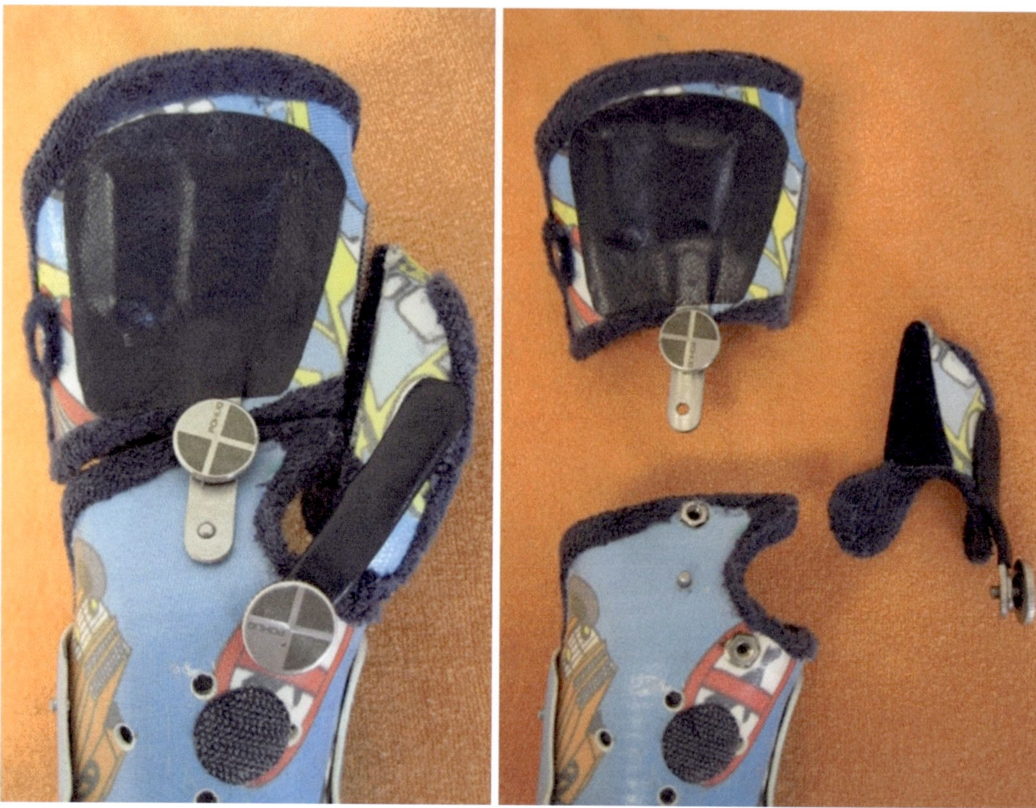

Fig. 11.2 Modular orthotic system for using the orthosis 23 h

(fibre composites, polypropylenes, C-fibre prepregs, polyamides).

- High wearing comfort and adaptive properties (silicones, leather, flexible thermoplastics).
- Resistance to dirt and moisture (silicones, thermoplastics, fibre composites, C-fibre prepregs).
- The wearing time of the orthosis (short-term treatments up to 4 weeks postoperatively: with low-temperature thermoplastics; long-term treatments with PE/PP plastics and FVW).

In many cases the materials are used in combination, whereby the positive properties of the individual material are shown to advantage in the material composite.

Most of the finger and hand orthoses shown here were made of high-temperature cross-linked silicone [10], as both the elastic bedding and the high wearing comfort lead to a high acceptance of the handorthetic treatment. Starting with the wrist-integrating middle hand forearm orthoses (WHO) up to the shoulder-length variants (SEWHO), modern fibre composites and thermoplastic 3D-printed materials are increasingly being used.

11.4 Orthotic Fittings

The orthotic types described in the following are exclusively custom-made, which were adapted to the specifications of the interdisciplinary rehabilitation team after individual shape recording. The orthotic treatment of the child's upper extremity is presented as an example for various movement disorders of different genesis.

11.4.1 Finger and Thumb Orthoses (FO)

Malpositions and deformities in the area of the fingers can be of different kinds. Especially in children with neuromuscular disorders, such as infantile cerebral palsy (CP) or arthrogryposis multiplex congenita (AMC), it is important to recognize whether there is a causal structural malposition in the finger or whether the cause of the malposition is secondary. For example, swan neck deformities and boutonniere deformities can occur and are muscular compensatory in nature.

These deformities can be caused by spasms of the affected musculature (CP) or by muscular imbalances and weaknesses of major proportions (AMC), which adversely affect the muscle balance and thus also the range of motion.

> Compensatory instabilities, such as those that occur in children with neuromuscular deficits, must therefore not be treated with classic finger-length orthoses, but must take into account the proximal joint sections involved causally by the musculature (see also the WHO orthosis section, long finger recording).

In congenital malformations, malpositions can occur in the area of the finger joints in both the frontal and sagittal planes. The *camptodaktyly*, another form of congenital finger deformity, describes a congenital flexion contracture in the area of the PIP joint; usually the small finger is affected, which can be accompanied by over-stretching in the end joint. The *clinodaktyly* describes, according to Tamplin (1846), the lateral angulation of the finger in the mid-link region or of the thumb in the terminal region. Both malformations are surgically corrected in the case of progressive progressions and pronounced findings and should be treated postoperatively with a stabilizing splint and intensive hand therapy.

In the conservative as well as in the postoperative phase, a silicone orthosis with palmar correction element up to the metacarpal joint row has proven successful in camptodactyly. This can be manufactured either with or without a locking element. When the finger is tightened, some ultrasonic gel is applied to it so that it slides easily into the partially elastic part of the silicone orthosis. Due to the high adhesion of the material, the finger guidance remains stable and in the correct position on the finger, even with small children's hands. The silicone also has a smoothing effect on the surgical scar in the postoperative phase (Fig. 11.3).

> The orthotic treatment most frequently used in the area of children's movement impaired fingers is probably due to the thumb-in-palm deformity.

It is used both in children with neuromuscular diseases and in children with congenital malformations and has the task of securing the thumb in a physiologically abducted position (Fig. 11.4). This is a functional orthosis for improving hand function in everyday use. Children with AMC and CP are particularly affected by this deformity. Since the acceptance of orthoses in the hand area depends to a decisive degree on the function and wearing comfort of the aid, the fabrication of the orthosis using silicone technology was able to gain outstanding significance. The elastic properties of the material allow in many cases a closure-free and flexible-adaptive design of the orthosis, whereby the other functions of the hand can freely unfold. The orthosis is only equipped with an additional high-shore silicone stabilizer in the effective area of the required abduction, so that the thumb is stabilized in the functional gripping position.

In the postoperative condition after a **thumb-in-palm surgery**, the positioning orthosis should have the best possible abduction of the thumb with simultaneous palmar flexion ($40°$) and radial abduction ($20–30°$). The thumb abduction can be adjusted by an integrated thermoplastic prepreg if necessary. The thumb should be positioned completely in an extended position with this orthosis variant and accompanies the child after the operation for a period of 3–6 months.

11.4.2 Hand Orthoses (HO and HFO)

Hand orthoses (HO) and finger hand orthoses can contain all construction variants in the supply

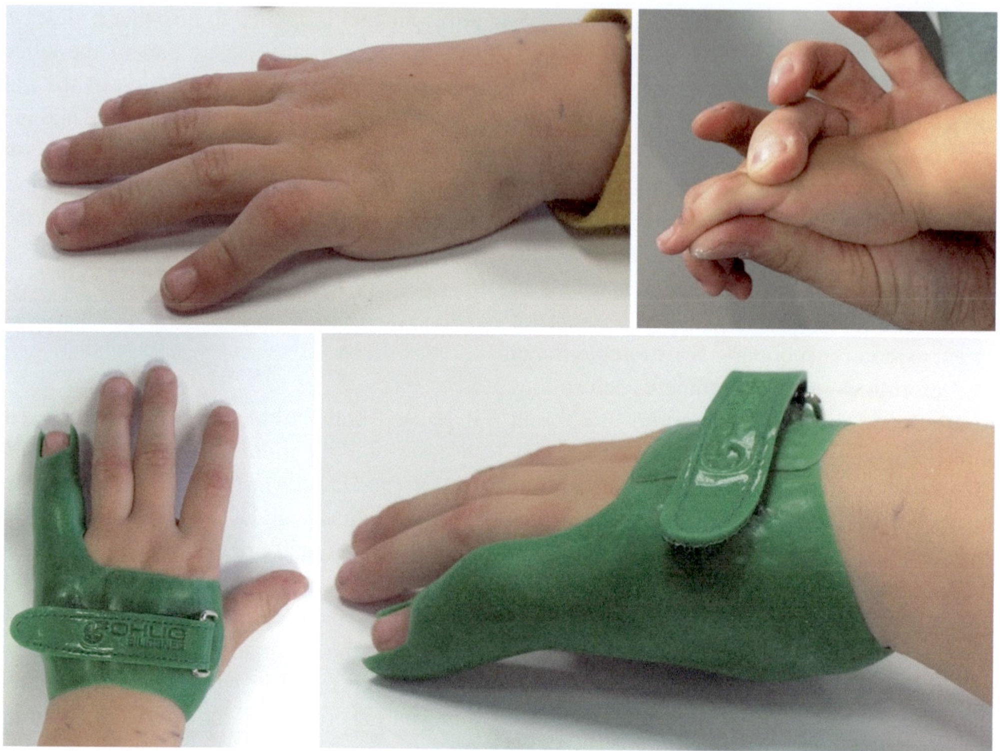

Fig. 11.3 Silicone finger orthosis (FO) for camptodactyly DV left

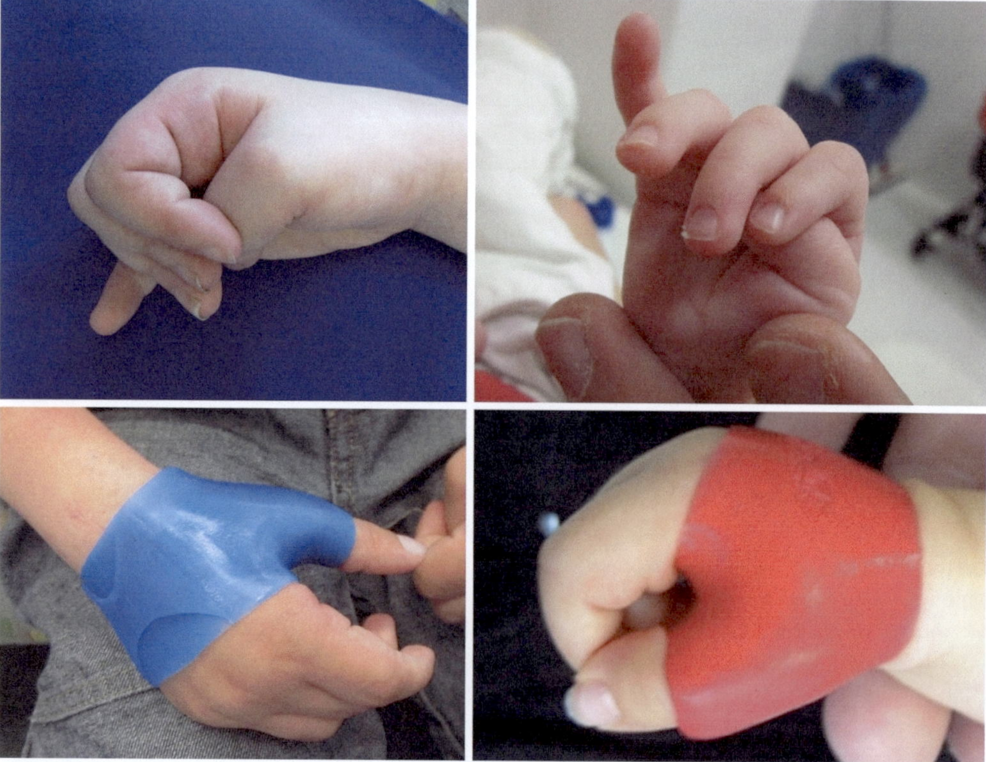

Fig. 11.4 Silicone thumb abduction orthosis (FO) for thumb-in-palm deformity

length from the fingertips to the final wrist, with and without integration of the fingers.

Functional orthoses in the hand area are used either for malpositions in the MCP joints or for existing muscular imbalances and functional deficits of the stretching and flexing muscle groups of the fingers.

Static orthoses are preferably used to control growth and avoid compensatory malpositions in the finger and metacarpal joints.

Based on the design of a dorsal middle hand splint described by [11] to strengthen the transverse curvature of the hand, a circular middle hand splint made of silicone, for example, can provide a very functional input to avoid consecutive hyperextension in the metacarpal joints of a claw hand. This malposition is mainly due to damage and motor deficits of the ulnar nerve. The clinical signs for checking ulnaris paralysis are described in a lack of fist closure on the ulnar side, an impossible small finger specimen

of the thumb and the formation of a claw hand with hyperextension in the MCP joints [12]. These deformities can also be observed in neuromuscular diseases such as CP. Based on a sagittal 3-point correction, the hyperextension is usefully inhibited in the MCP joints of the fingers, whereby the hand can be used in a physiological position with improved function (Fig. 11.5).

> Functional deficits in the case of neurological deficits in the finger-moving musculature can be accompanied by dynamic orthoses both during preoperative testing and postoperative after reconstructive function-improving interventions.

In the area of the hand, typical motor failures can be observed, e.g. as a result of obstetric plexus lesions. Depending on the degree of severity, it can happen, for example, that the finger-flexing musculature can realize active finger flexion, whereas the finger extensors have failed completely.

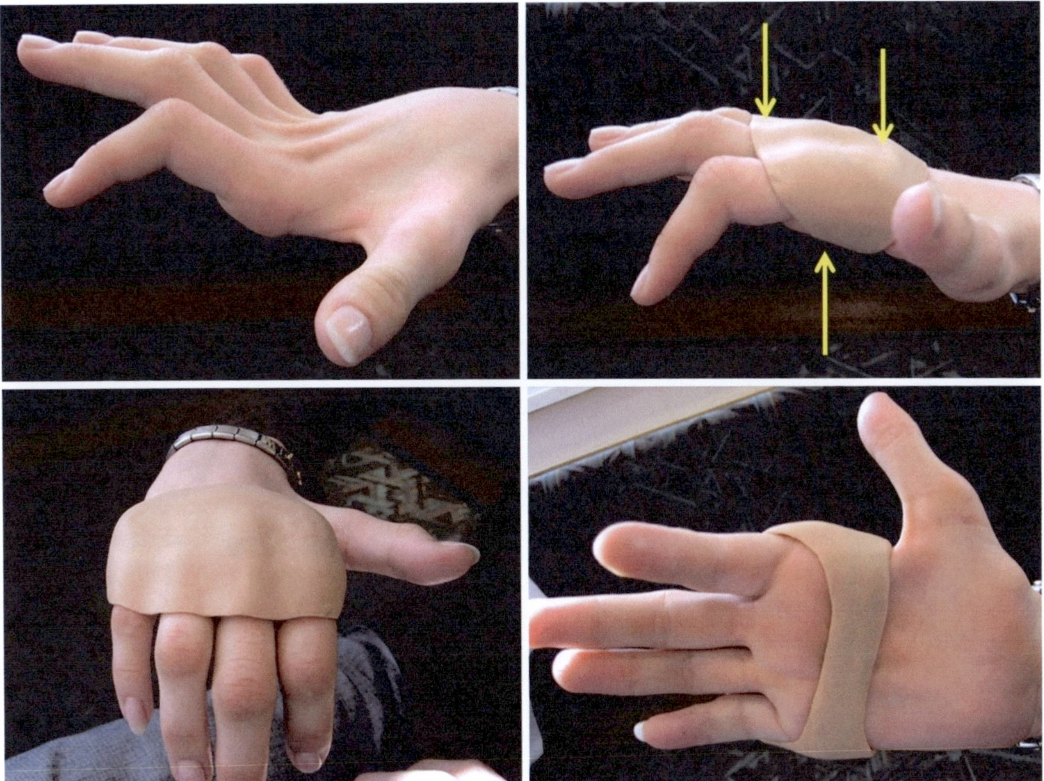

Fig. 11.5 Consecutive hyperextension in the MCP joints in a 16-year-old patient with CP

Here, a dynamic orthosis made of the elastic basic material silicone can at least support a stretching function of the fingers. Silicone alone can be sufficient to initiate active stretching from flexion. If the extension of the glove-like silicone functional orthosis alone is not sufficient, elastic extensions of varying strength can be applied to the dorsal side of the fingers, which strengthen the extension movement out of flexion (Fig. 11.6). Alternatively, in the case of asymmetrical failures, this supply can also be carried out only for the ulnar or radial fingers (Fig. 11.6 bottom right).

Congenital flexion deformities that are difficult to correct, such as those frequently occurring in arthrogryposis, should be treated orthopaedically during the first few months of life if possible, as this is the best time to prognosticate conservative treatment success. Orthotic care should always be accompanied by physiotherapeutic treatment. If these so important first months of life were missed, a good result is hardly possible any more in a conservative way.

Finger hand orthoses are successfully used in preoperative conditioning as well as in postoperative treatment, which enable an adjustable stretching effect on the affected fingers due to exchangeable spring elements.

11.4.3 Hand, Metacarpal and Forearm Orthoses (WHO and WHFO)

Wrist overlapping deformities or deformities, which arise due to the functionality or dysfunctionality of wrist overlapping muscle groups, require in almost all cases also wrist overlapping orthosis or splint constructions.

With *flaccid paralysis* the splint or orthosis should at least fulfil the task of stabilizing the hand in a physiological position. If these motor deficits affect, for example, the radial nerve, the extensor apparatus with finger and wrist extensors is affected. Depending on the severity of radial paralysis, motor damage of lesser severity

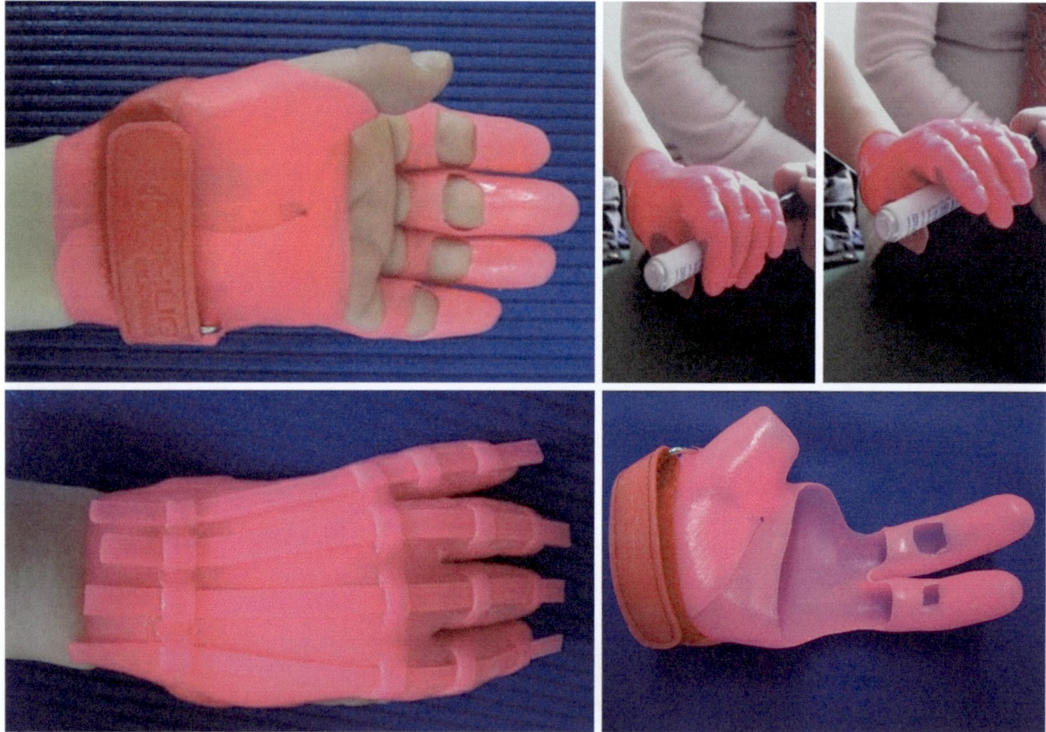

Fig. 11.6 Dynamic silicone hand orthosis (HFO) with adjustable elastic bands to support the stretching function

may occur, e.g. failure of thumb abduction or extension of the metacarpophalangeal joints, up to the well-known *drop hand deformity* which no longer shows active extension in the finger and wrist. If, however, this falling hand is passively balanced, intact functions of the ulnar nerve and median nerve often appear.

It is therefore recommended to stabilize the wrist in a physiological position at least with a palmar splint and correction zones close to the wrist joint (3-point principle, Fig. 11.7). The minimalist design leaves plenty of room for the hand and can be equipped with flat correction zones in the end areas if required and, e.g. in the event of more severe deformities. Although the splint cannot create a hand function by correcting it, in many everyday cases, it allows the hand to use it passively in a more functional way.

Serious functional and aesthetic impairments following an obstetric brachial plexus injury can affect the entire upper limb. In addition to motor deficits, these cases often show joint limiting movement restrictions in the large joints. Particularly if such movement restrictions exist over several years, they can lead to pain in addition to functional impairments. These are often due to the one-sided stress and strain situations of the body.

Adequate orthosis care should prevent imminent contractures (Fig. 11.8) and deformities in these cases.

- In night-time orthoses, if necessary with dynamic support.
- In everyday life orthoses, allow a minimally restrictive orthotic support into the physiologically neutral joint positions.

Conservative and postoperative orthotic care after traumatic lesions of nerves must promote the attainment of physiological joint positions with all available possibilities.

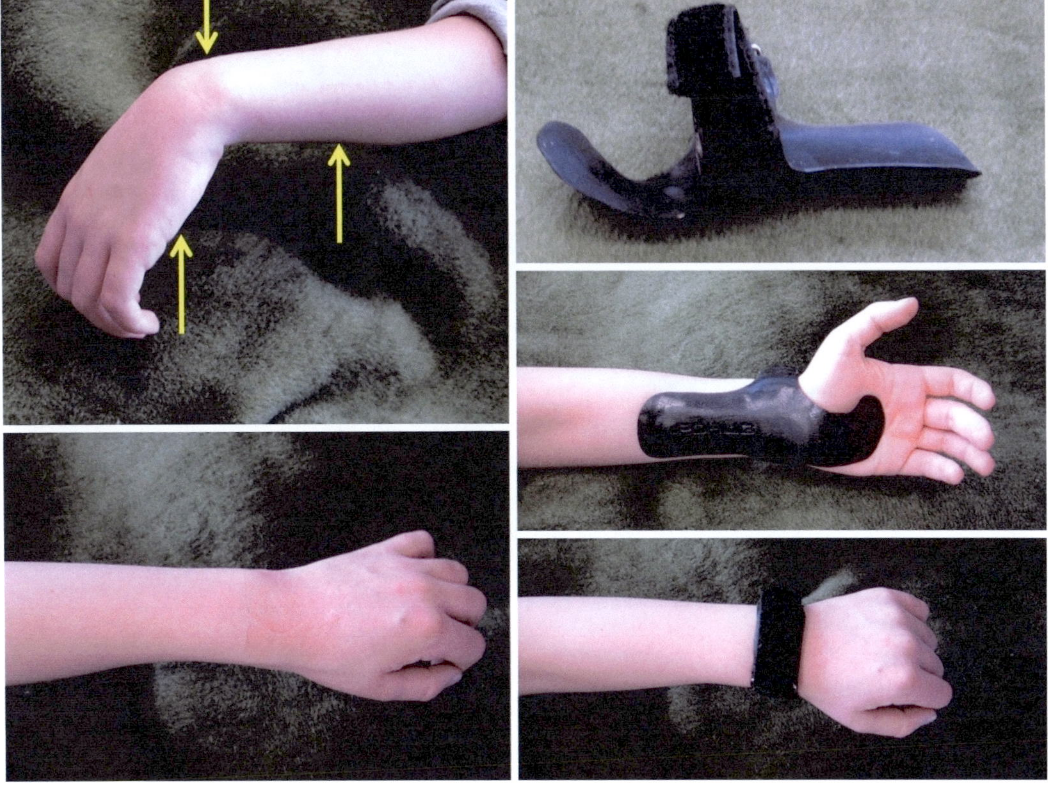

Fig. 11.7 Palmar wrist splint in 3-point principle for stabilization of the wrist in the sagittal plane

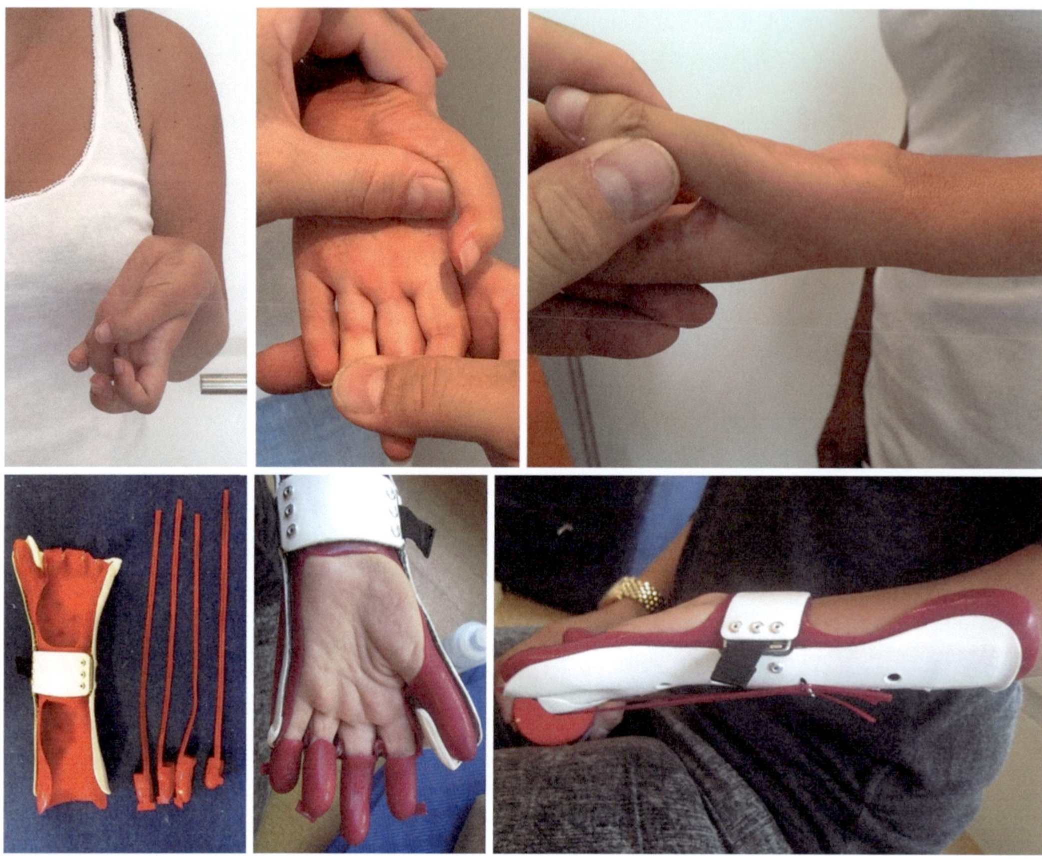

Fig. 11.8 Forearm correcting orthosis (WHFO) for the night with elastic finger imbedding and extension bands, positioning the wrist in neutral position

For children with *cerebral palsy (CP)*, typical pathological patterns can be observed during the initiation of different gripping functions, which impair the gripping functions. In the wrist, the hand describes the spontaneous movement into volar flexion and ulnar abduction, whereby the hand only grasps inaccurately and slowly. Similar malpositions can also be observed in children with AMC. If these malpositions can be corrected manually, a forearm spiral orthosis is recommended (Fig. 11.9). Depending on the severity of the malposition and size of the extremity, this can be made of different materials and is worn in everyday life with a function-improving effect. At best, the full correction of ulnar deviation is achieved in the frontal plane. The adjustment of the correction in the sagittal plane in spasticity depends on the behaviour of the hand and finger-flexing muscles. Ideally, a functional position in

the wrist is desired. However, if this is accompanied by a compensatory fist closure and if the thumbs cannot be opened anymore actively, the dorsal extension in the wrist needs to be adjusted into a neutral position.

Alternatively, partially elastic circular silicone orthoses can also be used in situations with increased muscle tone. These distribute the pressure more evenly and are therefore perceived as more pleasant by many children. However, due to the enlarged orthosis surface, a greater loss of sensitivity in the area of the orthosis is also accepted.

For children with *AMC*, partial contract situations may exist so that a functional position in the wrist cannot be achieved. The maximum achievable correction position should be set here. In both clinical pictures, compensatory malpositions can occur in the fingers during conservative

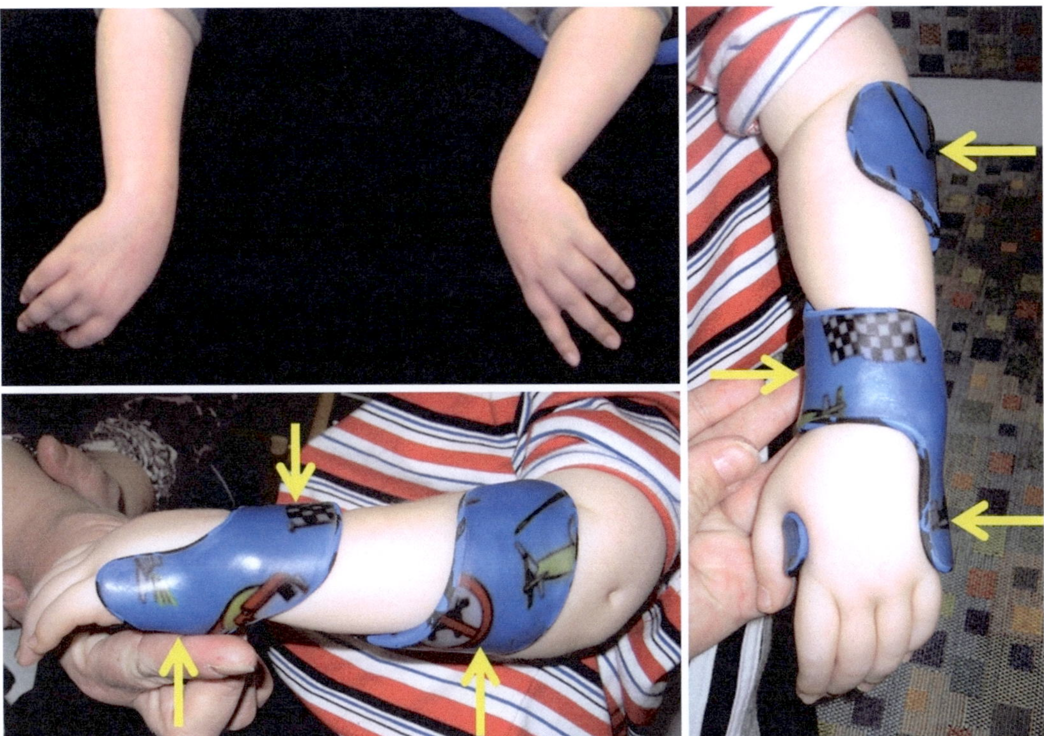

Fig. 11.9 Forearm spiral orthosis (WHO) for correction of ulnar deviations and palmar flexion malpositions of the hand in everyday use

correction treatment in the wrist and metacarpophalangeal joints. In these cases, the stabilizing restoration with a finger-length metacarpal forearm positioning orthosis with individual finger bedding and possibly a full-surface counterpressure plate (Fig. 11.10) is recommended both for the growth-guiding restoration and for the preoperative conditioning of the muscle and ligamentous apparatus (Fig. 11.10).

As a classical forearm orthotic treatment in the case of congenital malformations, the forearm orthosis for correction of the radial clubhand can be described. The orthosis often accompanies the children over a longer period of time and is used for preoperative conditioning and progression brake as well as after surgical correction. Depending on the shape and severity of the radial clubhand, various surgical methods can be taken to centralize and radialize the ulna [13]. Even after pollicization of the second finger [14], a static orthosis is indicated (Fig. 11.11). The orthosis must imitate the axial adjustment of the

hand to the forearm in both the frontal and sagittal planes. A pollicizated finger should be guided in the best possible abduction with a slight radial position to the counter-grip to the remaining long fingers, so that the largest possible gripping volume can be imaged.

11.4.4 Arm-Based Orthoses (EWHO, EWHFO, SEWHFO)

The higher the level of care required, the more carefully the functional benefits of orthotic care must be weighed up in everyday life.

Functionally correctable *elbow flexion deficits* can initially be conservatively fitted with dynamic arm-based extension orthoses. The dynamically correcting effect comes either from spring joints or, better still, from gas pressure springs with adjustable force (Fig. 11.12). In the dynamic correction of bending or extension deficits, the distally following joints must also be

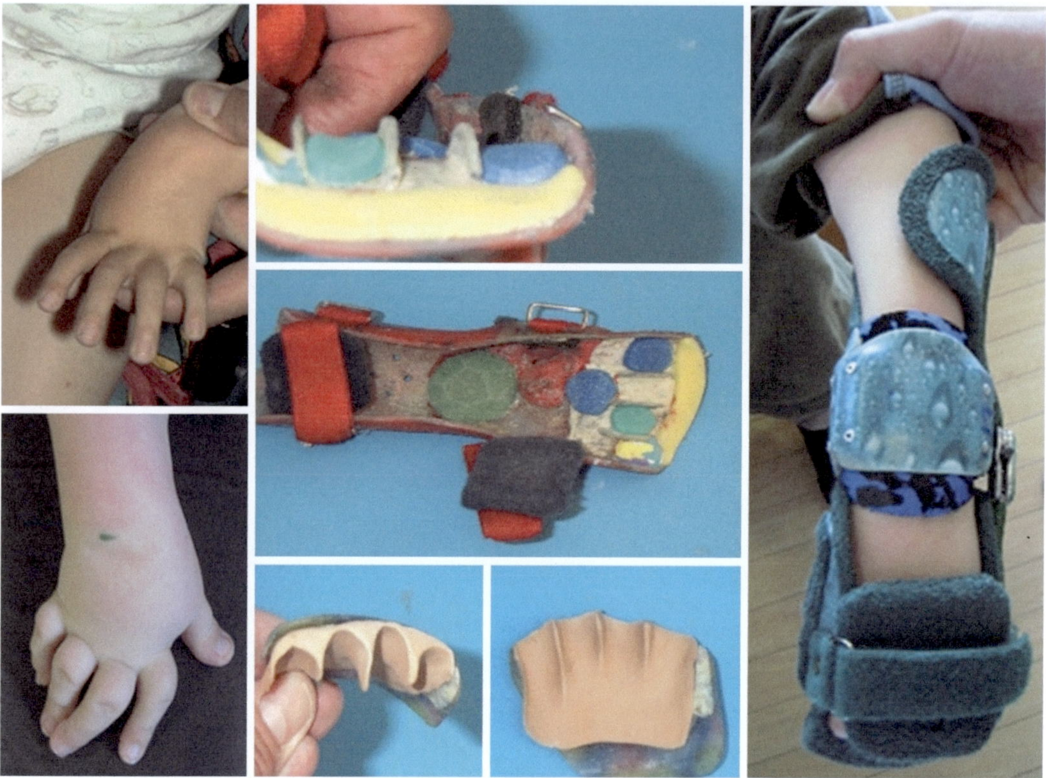

Fig. 11.10 Midhand forearm orthosis with long finger guiding zone, individual finger correction with level embedding of the fingers and flat counterpressure plate

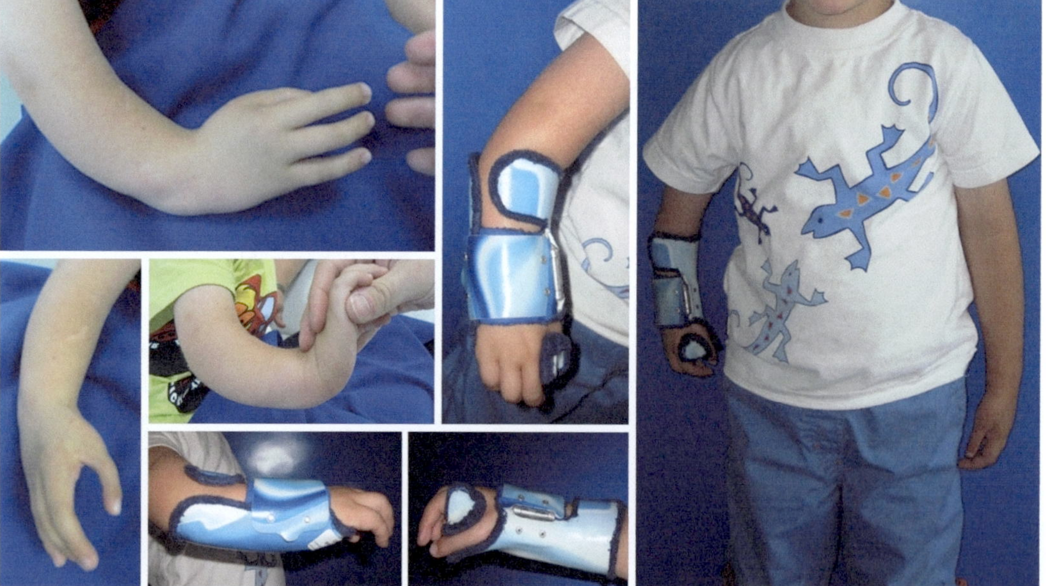

Fig. 11.11 Midhand forearm orthosis (WHO) after surgical correction and pollicization of the radial clubhand, orthosis in fibre-composite technique with carbon fibres

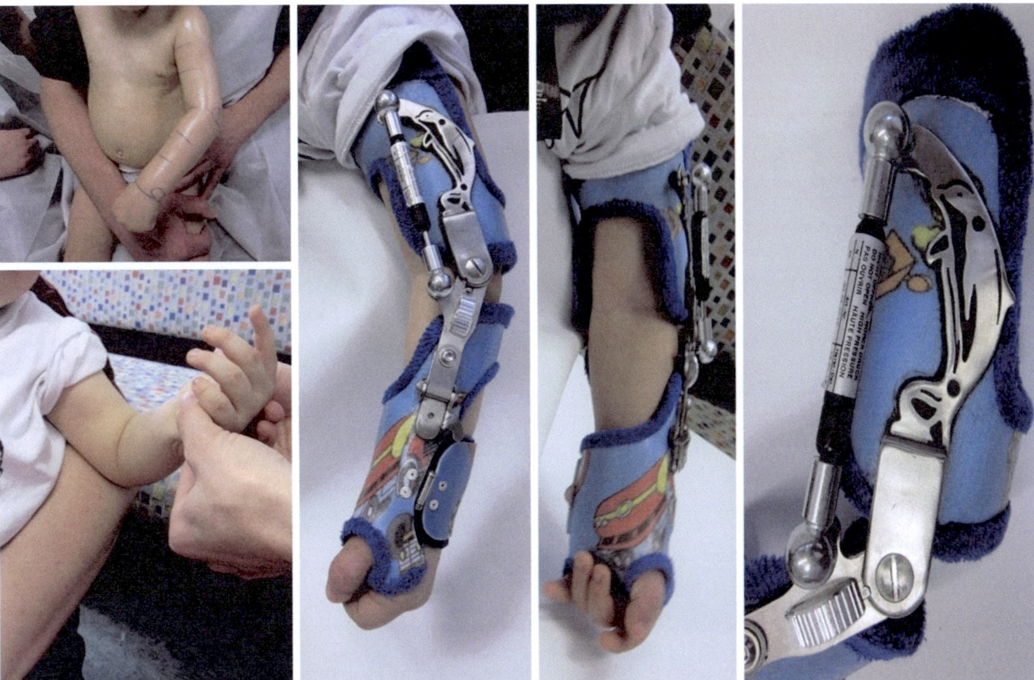

Fig. 11.12 Dynamic arm-based orthosis (EWHO) with gas pressure spring system for dynamic correction at the elbow

taken into account. It makes sense to secure the wrist plane in the correct position with a dynamic arm-based extension orthosis.

For children with CP, various surgical methods are used under given conditions to improve function and—in the case of severely affected children—to facilitate care. These include tendon transfers, tenotomies, capsulotomies, bony procedures and arthrodeses. The possibility of joint locking allows dynamic pauses to be taken (Fig. 11.12).

> In early functional postoperative use, the protective orthoses should be equipped with dynamizing joint units that support the surgical corrective measures in a functionally appropriate manner.

Essential function-enhancing procedures are, for example, corrections of restrictive forearm pronation contractures as well as the extension of the elbow flexor and the ventral capsulotomy of the elbow joint with existing contractures. In the postoperative phase, adequate early functional orthosis care is expected to ensure that the direction of movement to be practised

– For correction of pronation contracture—in supination direction
– For correction of the flexion contracture—in extension direction

is dynamically supported.

Combined corrections can also be made during an operation, so that the early functional and protective orthosis must dynamically promote both directions of movement (Fig. 11.13). The plaster casts that are otherwise common in many places are completely dispensed with, whereby the already muscularly weakened CP children do not have to accept unnecessary atrophy and can benefit significantly faster from the functional improvements of the operation.

The situation is different with the *peripheral traumatic nerve damage*. Posttraumatic plexus lesions can range from isolated damage to individual nerve branches with incomplete failures to complete paralysis of the arm with complete functional failure. Spontaneous regeneration or incomplete paralysis with the potency for spontaneous regeneration will continue to be observed, while poor prognoses with complete lesions (C5–T1) will require surgical revisions as early as pos-

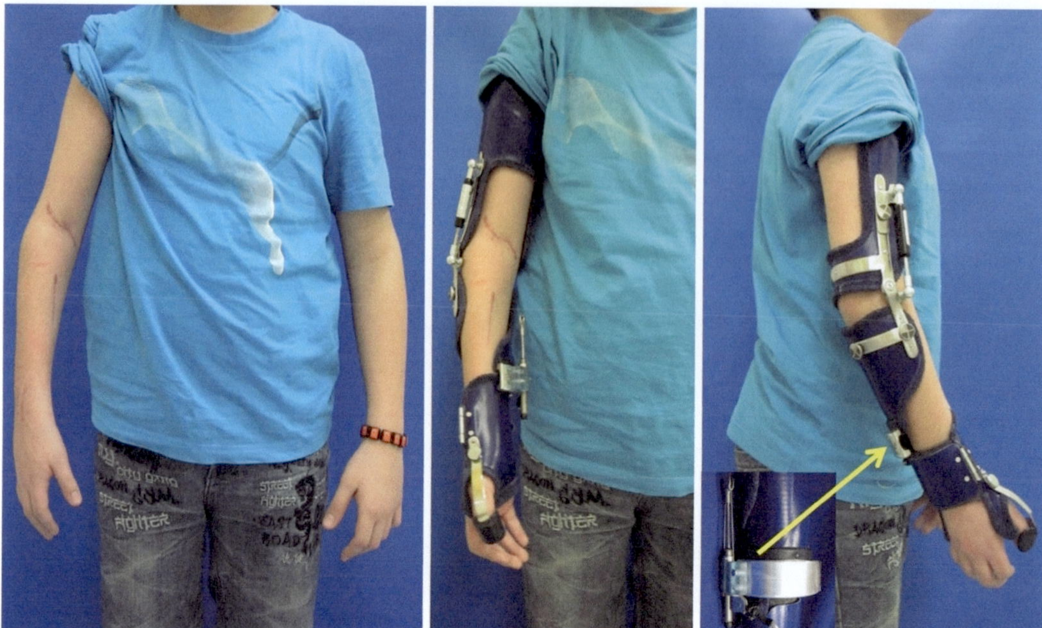

Fig. 11.13 Dynamic arm-based orthosis (EWHO) with gas pressure spring system for dynamic stretch correction in the elbow as well as for dynamic correction in supination direction (Pohlig slide system)

sible [11]. The focus here is clearly on surgical measures with nerve reconstructions, muscle replacement operations, neurolysis and nerve transplants.

If required, orthopaedic technology should provide orthotic fittings in teamwork that support these measures or at least passively provide functions that no longer exist through external functions. Remaining conditions after traumatic plexus lesions should be stabilized in the orthosis according to the body axis. Starting in the hand area—due to frequent volume fluctuations, the elastic silicone technique is predestinated for these hand situations—a position-adjustable elbow joint can secure flexion positions of the arm in various degrees. It also makes sense to use a unilateral swivel-bearing guide that allows the upper arm to rotate. Since in many cases the shoulder joint is at risk of subluxation or even luxation, we recommend the weight-bearing flexible integration of the shoulder section, which is held in position by a narrow chest bandage with contralateral counterpressure plate (Fig. 11.14). These orthotic fittings must be segmentally designable so that functional areas of the orthosis

can be trained within the framework of spontaneous regeneration or successful surgical interventions.

In principle, these complex orthotic variants should also be designed according to the supply principle "as little as possible and as much as necessary".

11.5 Assistive Devices

Assistive devices are unfortunately given far too little consideration in everyday care, although the different function-oriented aids can mean significant functional gains in everyday life.

> Assistive devices are used as an alternative to orthoses when there is little prospect of an improvement in the situation, sections of the extremities are strongly limited in movement and important recurring activities of everyday life cannot be carried out functionally or only poorly.

Such situations can occur after nerve lesions with accompanying flaccid paralysis and corresponding fine and gross motor deficits. The children

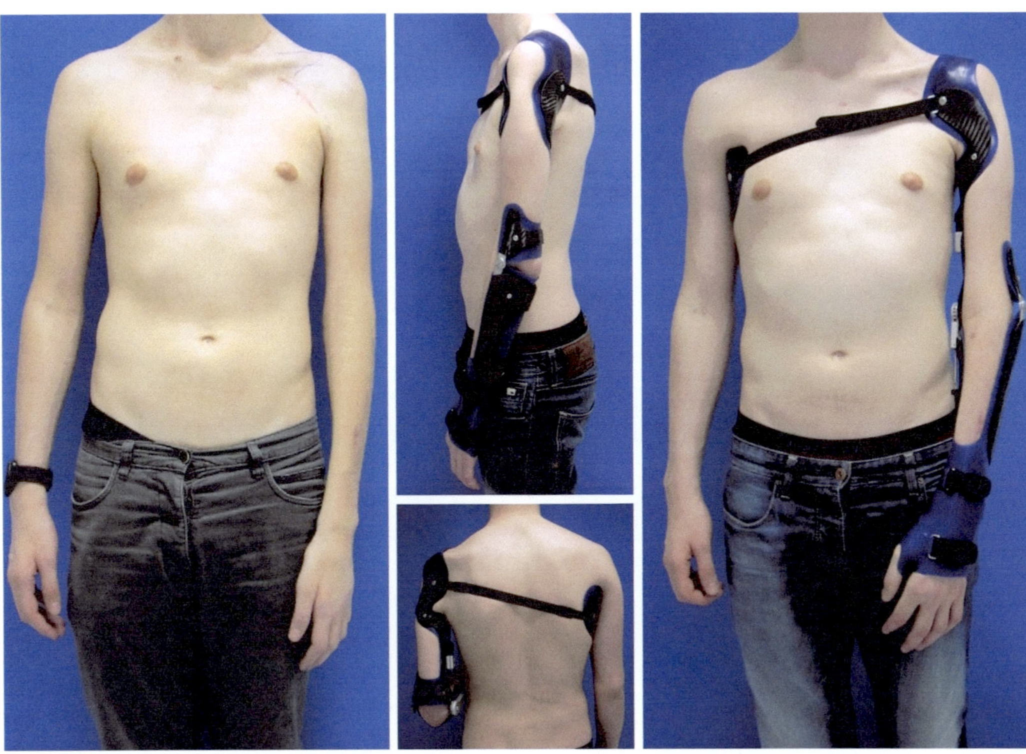

Fig. 11.14 Arm-based orthosis with silicone shoulder clip element, silicone hand orthosis (SEWHO), lockable elbow joint, rotation joint in unilateral upper arm splint

will then not be able to actively grasp or even hold everyday objects and tools.

This is illustrated by the example of the bicycling. For children with no active gripping function, function-oriented gripping aids can be used (Fig. 11.15 left), which enable the child to grip the handlebar and thus help to increase safety when riding a bicycle. Shortened or restricted upper extremities can also be compensated by an appropriately adapted bicycling aid (Fig. 11.15 right).

Everyday aids are usually named according to their function, such as individually adapted gripping aids, eating aids, writing aids, cleaning aids, button aids, etc., so that the everyday functional benefit is already anchored in the name of the aid.

11.6 Innovations and Future Trends in Orthotics

The electronics and microprocessor technology has already taken place in the orthotic treatment of the lower extremity. Today, load-dependent motion cycles and electronically controlled swing phase controls of orthotic joints can already influence the motion control of modern orthotic fittings.

In the area of orthotics of the upper extremity, this step is still to come. With motor deficits with flaccid paralysis, we seem almost helpless. How tempting it would be to gain an active gripping function. The promising future development of an active motor orthosis to support the gripping function is already in the starting blocks at the

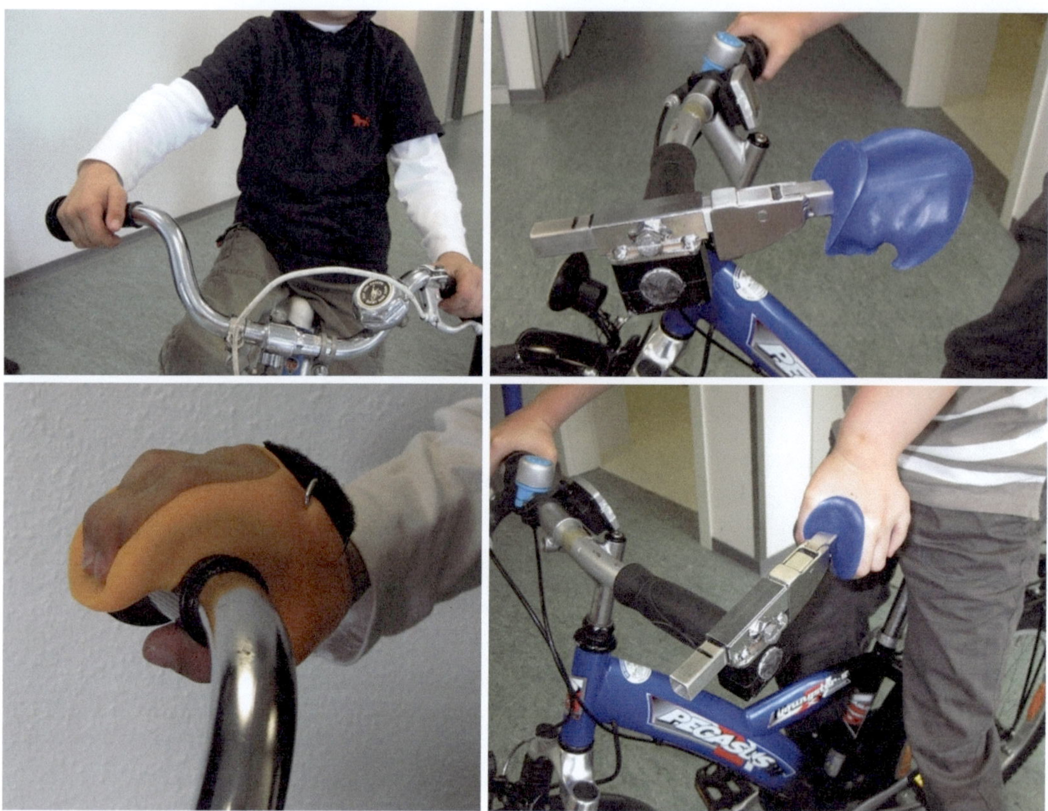

Fig. 11.15 Silicone bicycling aid for functionless hand (*on the left*) and shortened arm (*right*)

German start-up Vincent Systems with the external power orthosis Grip Assist. The US-based company Myomo Inc. has already gained initial experience with a motor-driven myo-orthosis in the elbow. At the end of 2015, this system was supplemented by an active gripper unit. It remains to be seen which functional gains patients can actually achieve with these systems in everyday life.

A no less attractive trend for the future lies in the virtual design of orthetic constructions on the PC as well as the subsequent realization of the design in the selective laser sinter printing process. The use of this technology enables the orthopaedic technician to find completely new ways of designing. Through the use of print technology, complex three-dimensional structures can be implemented in orthotic constructions. In addition to the load-bearing orthotic correction areas, this production technique can also take into account breathable orthotic zones [15], for example, which are then produced from polyamides and other materials using a three-dimensional printing process (Fig. 11.16). Unfortunately, the usual variety of materials still leaves something to be desired in this manufacturing process. However, the many design possibilities that this technology permits in the realization of specific requirements could also enrich orthopaedic technology in the future.

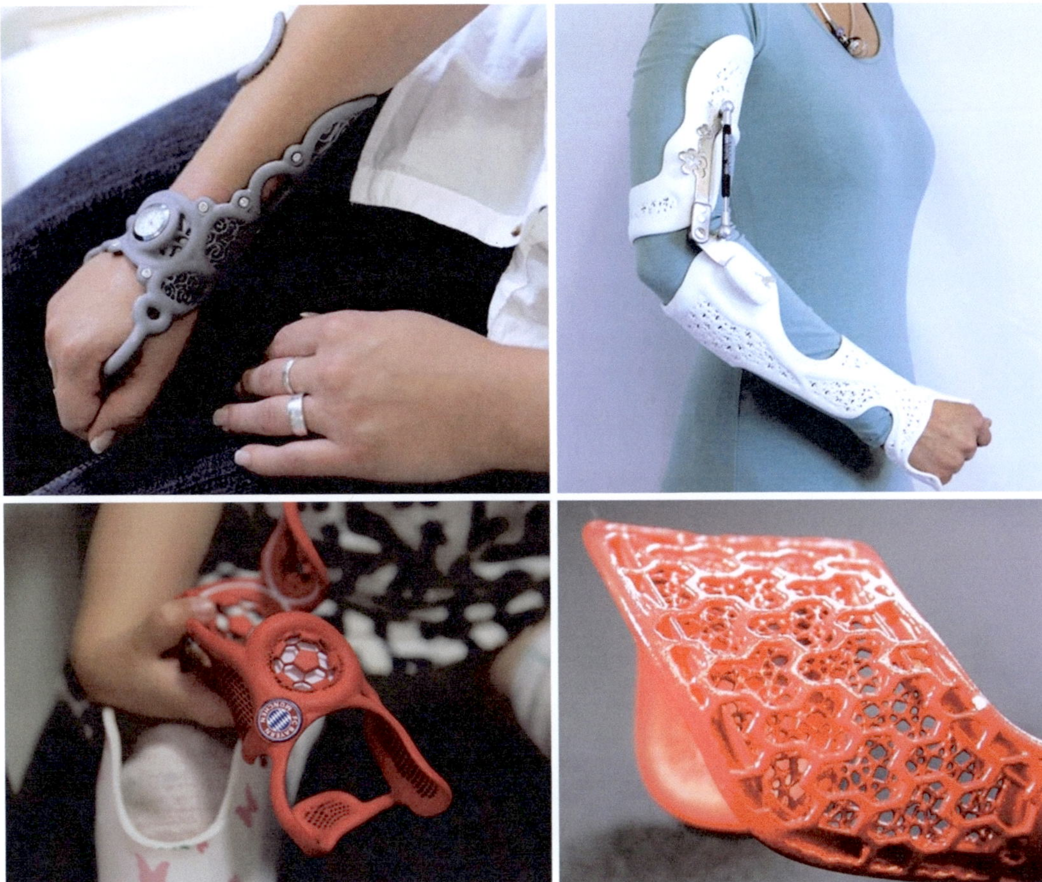

Fig. 11.16 Future trend: Design orthoses made of polyamide, manufactured using selective laser printing technology

References

1. WHO. How to use the ICF—a practical manual for using the international classification of functioning, disability and health (ICF), Exposure Draft for Comment. Geneva. 2013
2. ISO 8549-1. 1989(en) Prosthetics and orthotics-vocabulary-part 1 general terms for external limb prostheses and external orthoses, ISO International. 1989.
3. Hohmann D, Uhlig R. Orthopädische Technik, 9. Aufl. Stuttgart: Thieme; 2005. p. 334–87.
4. Minden K, Niewerth M. Rheumakranke Kinder und Jugendliche, Kerndokumentation und Prognose. Monatsschr Kinderheilkd. 2012;160:237–43.
5. Tonkin MA. The upper limb in cerebral palsy. Curr Orthop. 1995;9(3):149–55.
6. Döderlein L. Infantile Zerebralparese, 2. Aufl. Berlin, Heidelberg: Springer; 2015. p. 341–61.
7. Disselhorst-Klug C. Orthesen, Schienen und Bandagen. In: Kraft M, Disselhorst-Klug C, editors. Biomedizinische Technik-Rehabilitationstechnik, Band 10. Berlin: Walter de Gruyter; 2015. p. 284ff.
8. Bähler A, Bieringer S. Orthopädietechnische Indikationen, 2. Aufl. Bern: Huber; 2004. p. 19–27.
9. Schäfer M, Baise M. Orthetische Versorgung der oberen Extremitäten bei Kindern mit neuromuskulären Erkrankungen. Verlag Orthopädie-Technik. 2011;62(3):174–83.
10. Schäfer M. Silikone in der technischen Orthopädie, Medizinisch orthopädische Technik. Tischler Verlag; 2008, p. 7–16.
11. Malick MH, Baumgartner R. Lagerungsschienen für die Hand. Stuttgart: Thieme; 1977. p. 66.
12. Towfigh H, Hierner R, Langer M, Friedel R. Handchirurgie, Band 1. Berlin, Heidelberg: Springer; 2011. p. 502–3.
13. Buck-Gramcko D. Congenital malformations of the hand and the forearm. London: Churchill-Livingstone; 1998. p. 433–47.
14. Blauth W, Schneider-Sickert F. Handfehlbildungen. Berlin, Heidelberg: Springer; 1976. p. 312–30.
15. Schäfer M et al. "30Reasons"-Orthesenprojekt zur funktionellen Verbesserung der Handfunktion eines Fliegenfischers. Verlag Orthopädie-Technik. 2019;70(3):46–9.

Botulinum Toxin

12

T. Becher

12.1   Indication

The benefit of botulinum toxin (BoNT) in reducing upper extremity spasticity is undisputed.

The syndrome of the first motoneuron consists of three main components: spasticity, paresis and reduced control. Spasticity is often the leading symptom that interferes with the arbitrary motor function of the muscle.

Due to the frequently occurring co-contraction, typical patterns also occur in the arm, which become visible especially during motorically demanding tasks or during faster activities. The activation of all flexor muscles leads to inclination of the thumb, flexion of the fingers, flexion and usually ulnar deviation of the wrist, flexion in the elbow as well as adduction and internal rotation in the shoulder. Hand and arm are no longer in the child's field of activity; motor impairment is accompanied by invisibility—this increases the learned non-use of the hand. Many children also experience the bending of the elbow or the abduction in the shoulder when walking as very unpleasant. Both processes reinforce the asymmetric body experience.

With this typical finding and the resulting disability, there is a medical indication for treatment with BoNT if there is sufficient dynamic in the sense of an increase in resistance to rapid stretching. Contractures that have already occurred cannot be treated with BoNT.

An international consensus statement [1] states Grade A evidence (definitely effective) for the use of BoNT A to achieve individual therapeutic goals in the treatment of paediatric upper limb hemiplegia, Grade B evidence (possibly effective) for tonus reduction after BoNT A injections and Grade U evidence (ambiguous) for improvement in upper limb activity and function.

Ten studies in 2010 met the inclusion criteria for a Cochrane Review update [2], according to which a combination of BoNT A and occupational therapy is more effective than occupational therapy alone in reducing impairment, improving activity levels and achieving goals, but not in improving quality of life or self-efficacy. The systematic review found strong evidence for the use of botulinum toxin as additional therapy to aid upper extremity management in children with spastic cerebral palsy. However, botulinum toxin should not be used alone but in combination with planned occupational therapy.

In children and adolescents with very good functionality, limited supination and difficulties generating and modulating strength are strongly related to limitations of the hand function; 74% of variance in actual use is explained by the

T. Becher (✉)
Kinderneurologisches Zentrum Gerresheim,
SANA Kliniken Düsseldorf, Duesseldorf, Germany
e-mail: thomas.becher@sana.de

© Springer Nature Switzerland AG 2021
J. Bahm (ed.), *Movement Disorders of the Upper Extremities in Children*,
https://doi.org/10.1007/978-3-030-53622-0_12

combination of supination and strength—this was the conclusion of a Norwegian working group [3]. In a group of children with unilateral cerebral palsy and MACS levels 1–3, they found, among other things, that strength in elbow, forearm and hand; tone in elbow flexors and forearm supinators; and active range of motion in elbow extension and supination correlated with AHA and Melbourne Assessment scores. Treatment of pronators and elbow flexors with BoNT can improve supination and elbow extension.

The additive effect of botulinum toxin combined with occupational therapy has been shown in various studies, most recently by a Swedish working group [4]. Ten children were each treated with either occupational therapy or occupational therapy plus botulinum toxin for 1 year. The primary outcome was the Assisting Hand Assessment (AHA); the secondary outcome was the range of motion (ROM) and the Canadian Occupational Performance Measure (COPM), measured after 3, 6, 9 and 12 months. The AHA showed a superior effect in the ergotherapy/BoNT group. The authors conclude that repeated injections with BoNT A combined with occupational therapy are superior to ergotherapy on its own in terms of bimanual performance. The active ROM and targeted performance improved in both groups.

Agreeing on verifiable therapy goals both on the level of structure and function (spasticity reduction, ROM) and on the level of activities in consultation with patient, parents and therapist should be the rule. Obligatory follow-ups during the effective period as well as the use of the Goal Attainment Scale are particularly suitable to evaluate the therapy (GAS, Chap. 4).

12.2 Treatment Techniques

12.2.1 Sonography-Assisted Injection

The superiority of sonography-assisted injection is undisputed and has been a generally recognised standard in Germany since 2007 [5, 6] and in Europe since 2009 [7]: The safe localisation and injection of the muscles (especially in the case of structures altered by spastic paresis), painlessness and the possibility of dynamic images with active or passive movement of the target muscle are the greatest advantages over the EMG or palpation. Very good atlases are available as well as a very informative website: http://www.munichultrasoundcourse.com [8].

As a rule, 27-gauge needles with a length of 20 or 40 mm are used. With regard to the volumes and production of the BoNT A solution, reference is made to the technical information provided by the various manufacturers. The injection volume should be less than 1 mL per injection site. Low doses are often sufficient at the beginning and prevent the most probable side effect: the excessive weakening of the muscle and thus of the hand function. The injection intervals are sometimes increased as successful therapy progresses, because the effect lasts longer. With dystonic disorders, the dose should be chosen very carefully.

12.2.2 Sedation

Fortunately, medical measures are now, as a standard, largely pain-free in all paediatric departments, which is why intervention under sedation is carried out on children who are incapable of consenting. Rectal sedation with midazolam, often in combination with ketamine, has proven particularly effective in cases of unilateral spasticity in which the number of injections is lower.

In the case of an indication for deeper sedation, IV sedation with the aforementioned drugs or with propofol and ketamine (Ketofol®) could be considered under appropriate conditions—propofol alone is not analgesic and thus makes pain memory possible. In some facilities, a fixed mixture of nitrous oxide and oxygen is also used for inhalation (Livopan®). For children of school age, it is possible to "negotiate" with the children about an injection without sedation; with the consent of the child, an attempt can be made, but the child should have the possibility to ask for sedation at any time. Mild anxiolysis with lorazepam can also be helpful.

12.3   Target Muscles

Spasticity can be modulated with botulinum toxin: If the tone increase of the (bending) antagonist decreases, the weaker (stretching) agonist can become more active when it can be controlled and can thus be trained specifically. The muscular imbalance in the functions performed by the child is of decisive importance. Here, spasticity in the elbow (which withdraws the hand from the field of activity of the child), the ulnar deviation of the hand, the pronation posture and the adducted thumb have proven to be essential target structures. The reduction of spasticity can have a significant effect, especially with regard to supination and dorsal extension of the wrist—this is the only way to make any existing control visible and training of the agonist possible.

The indication for the injection of finger flexors must always be made cautiously, as grip strength and spasticity are influenced at the same time, which can lead to a loss of gripping ability. Initially, the first injection should assess the effects of the treatment of the wrist flexors and thumb; the finger flexors can only be treated in a second step. By means of sonographic control, it is possible to identify individual fascicles and inject them selectively, if, for example, the flexion spasm of the index finger represents a recurring obstacle in the gripping function (Fig. 12.1).

The injection of the biceps muscle leads to a reduction of the flexion spasm in the elbow joint. Thus, the forearm and the hand often remain

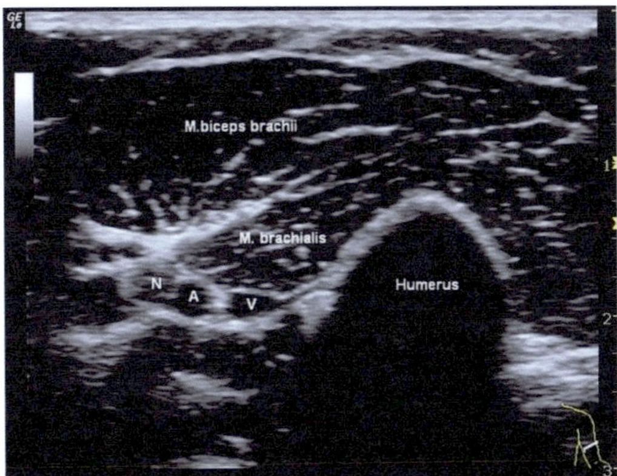

Fig. 12.1 M. biceps. (Courtesy of Ulf Hustedt)

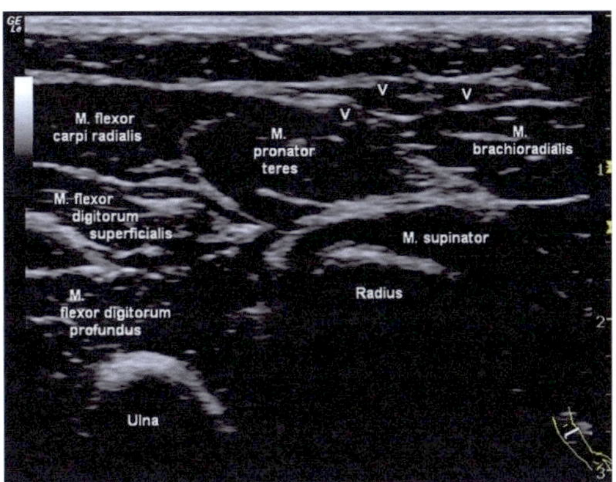

Fig. 12.2 M. pronator teres. (Courtesy of Ulf Hustedt)

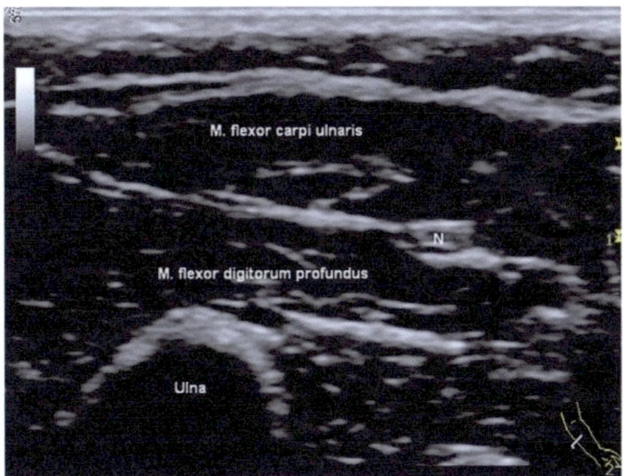

Fig. 12.3 M. flexor carpi ulnaris. (Courtesy of Ulf Hustedt)

more in the field of activity during activities at the table, and the visual perception of the hand improves. Also, the extension of the arm improves, the flexion of the arm when walking is reduced, and the sense of symmetry increases (Fig. 12.2).

The pronator teres is the most important pronator of the forearm. Its treatment often makes it possible to assess the remaining strength and to control the supinator. Thus, effective training of supination becomes possible (Fig. 12.3).

The flexor spasm of the hand and the ulnar deviation of the hand are often caused mainly by the flexor ulnaris muscle. Therefore, this muscle should always be injected first. If necessary, the M. flexor carpi radialis can also be treated additionally if the effect is insufficient. Especially if a functional hand orthosis is used for paresis therapy at the same time, a significantly improved position of the wrist can be achieved (Fig. 12.4)

The inclined thumb is often a major obstacle to gripping. A low-dose injection of the muscle opens the hand, which also improves the use of the other fingers as well as support and gripping.

12.3.1 Special Indications

Many children find the abduction of the arm when walking very stressful, because it attracts attention and considerably impairs the symmetry experience and disturbs in terms of function. A low-dose injection of the pars acromialis of the deltoid muscle can effectively reduce this phenomenon Figure 12.5.

M. pectoralis major

Often, especially with pronounced flexion spasticity of the upper arm, there is an increase in tonus in the pectoralis major muscle with a clear adduction of the upper arm, which can be treated with good results with an injection of the muscle. This significantly improves the extension of the upper arm and the mobility in the shoulder girdle, making it easier for the child to reach upwards.

12.4 Combination with Hand Orthoses

Treatment with botulinum toxin reduces spasticity, but paresis remains unaffected. Especially at the wrist, this often leads to an instability that is perceived as unpleasant. This can be effectively counteracted by adapting a silicone functional orthosis that guides the wrist. The silicone hand orthosis should support the hand function in such a way that the muscular imbalance of the hand muscles is balanced as much as possible. The correction of the wrist leads to a positive influence on the pathological activity of the wrist flex-

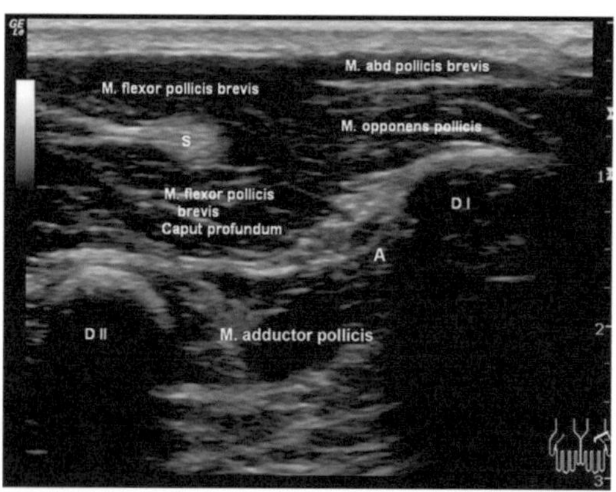

Fig. 12.4 Thenar eminence. (Courtesy of Ulf Hustedt)

Fig. 12.5 M. deltoideus. (Courtesy of Ulf Hustedt)

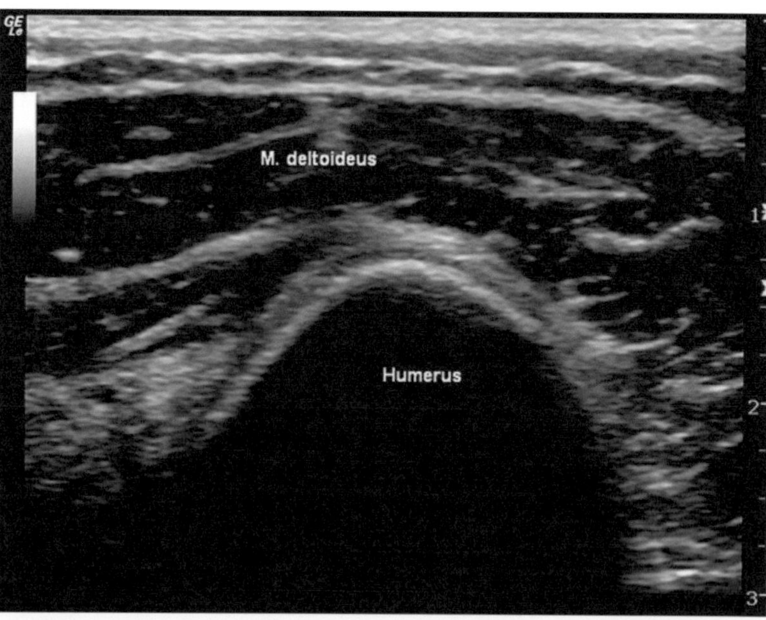

ors (especially flexor carpi ulnaris and radialis muscles) and to dynamic support of the extensors.

When correcting the wrist position, care should be taken to ensure that the child does not experience any significant restrictions on mobility as a result of the correction. If the finger flexors are already shortened, the wrist should not be raised too far. Taking away too much freedom of movement from the children can result in a restriction of function and activity and thus a rejection of the hand orthosis or at least significantly reduce the wearing time. Due to its unique properties, silicone is particularly suitable for hand orthosis construction and is being used more and more frequently. Silicone is breathable, dirt-repellent, anti-allergenic and 400% stretchable. For cleaning, it can simply be boiled out, and its durability is very high. To a certain extent, a silicone hand orthosis can grow with the child (depending on its age), due to the adjustable Velcro fastener [9].

12.5 Use of Botulinum Toxin in Flaccid Pareses

In the last 15 years, there have been several reports about the successful use of botulinum toxin in childhood plexus paresis in two situations [10].

– With **functionally interfering co-contractions between biceps and triceps** with active inhibition of elbow flexion: If a neuroma of the upper trunk does not allow a separate impulse conduction to both antagonists by the neuromatous mixed reinnervation, this leads to simultaneous control of the antagonists (well visible in the EMG surface) and thus to an impeding bending inhibition, which makes a hand-to-mouth movement impossible despite well-developed biceps. 100 units of botulinum toxin placed intramuscularly directly in the triceps allow a targeted, uninhibited exercise of the biceps for 6 months, whose control and strength increase during this time; after the expiration of the effective-

ness time of the Botox, the bicep often retains the functional upper hand.

– In the case of an **internal rotation malposition of the shoulder**, the essential pathophysiological element is clearly the subscapularis muscle, which is antagonised insufficiently or not at all. In a short mask anaesthesia, botulinum toxin can be applied directly intramuscularly in several places by dorsal-medial access directly under the raised scapula in the subscapularis of the sedated child; the stretching exercise of this muscle can be significantly facilitated for the parents and therapists, if necessary with a repetition after 6 months, which can then also lead to a permanent reduction in the strength of this muscle.

Due to its good success, this procedure has been firmly integrated into the incremental therapy strategy for internal rotation malposition of the shoulder in childhood plexus paresis in Aachen for 10 years—either as a single procedure or in combination with a selective nerve transfer to reactivate the external rotation of the shoulder (transfer of the distal branch of the accessory nerve to the suprascapular nerve via dorsal access).

References

1. Fehlings D, Novak I, Berweck S, et al. Botulinum toxin assessment, intervention and follow-up for paediatric upper limb hypertonicity: international consensus statement. Eur J Neurol. 2010;17: 38–56.
2. Hoare BJ, Wallen MA, Imms C, et al. Botulinum toxin a as an adjunct to treatment in the management of the upper limb in children with spastic cerebral palsy (Cochrane update 2010). Cochrane Database Syst Rev. 2010; https://doi.org/10.1002/14651858. CD003469.pub4.
3. Braendvik S, Elvrum AG, Vereijken B, et al. Relationship between neuromuscular body functions and upper extremity activity in children with cerebral palsy. Dev Med Child Neurol. 2009;52: e29–34.
4. Lidman G, Nachemson A, Peny-Dahlstrand M, et al. Botulinum toxin a injections and occupational therapy in children with unilateral spastic cerebral palsy: a randomized controlled trial. Dev Med Child Neurol. 2015;57:754–61.

5. Berweck S, Feldkamp A, Francke A, et al. Sonography-guided injection of botulinum toxin a in children with cerebral palsy. Neuropediatrics. 2002;33: 221–3.

6. Gesellschaft für Neuropädiatrie (GNP), Arbeitsgemeinschaft der niedergelassenen Neuropädiater (AG-NNP), Deutsche Gesellschaft für Sozialpädiatrie und Jugendmedizin (DGSPJ), Arbeitskreis Infantile Cerebralparesen der Deutschen Gesellschaft für Orthopädie und Orthopädische Chirurgie (DGOOC), Deutsche Gesellschaft für Neurologische Rehabilitation (DGNR), Deutschsprachige Vereinigung für Kinderorthopädie, et al. Botulinumtoxin für Kinder mit Zerebralparesen: 10-Punkte-Tabelle, 2007. Monatsschr Kinderheilkd. 2007;155:537–43.

7. Heinen F, et al. The updated European consensus 2009 on the use of botulinum toxin for children with cerebral palsy. Eur J Paediatr Neurol. 2010;14:45–66.

8. Schroeder AS, Berweck S, Fietzek UM et al. Munich Ultrasound Course. 2016. http://www.munichultrasoundcourse.com. Zugriff: Accessed 17 May 2016.

9. Becher T, Hägele A, Tenckhoff C. Interdisziplinäre Therapie der Handfunktion bei Kindern und Jugendlichen mit ICP-Schwerpunkt Handorthetik. Orthopädie Technik. 2016:18–21.

10. Bahm J, Becker M, Disselhorst-Klug C, Williams C, Meinecke L, Müller H, Sellhaus B, Schröder JM, Rau G. Surgical strategy in obstetric brachial plexus palsy—the Aachen experience. Semin Plast Surg. 2004;18:285–99.

Self-Concept

13

T. Becher

13.1 Introduction

A person's conception of their own competence, their confidence in their own actions, and the experience of self-efficacy are essential goals of successful therapy. In the ICF, these factors are reflected in the domain of "personal factors" and must be taken into account in the planning and implementation of therapy, in the therapeutic attitude, and in the therapy goals. If improved participation is the superior goal of therapeutic efforts, then positively influencing the self-concept must be an essential goal of all therapy.

13.2 Self-Concept: What Is it?

The "self-concept" construct describes a person's ideas about themselves.

Numerous definitions of the self-concept can be found in specialist literature. Other terms used are, for example, self-image, self-model, self-theory, and self-esteem. So far, there is no univocally accepted definition of the "self-concept" construct: "The continuous experiences with and concerning one's own person condense into the 'I', the 'self', the concept or pattern of one's own person, the self-concept. It is continuously altered and fed by experiences. (…) It is the summarised, concentrated, yet malleable sum of the thousand-fold experiences of a person with himself and about himself: What he is like, how he lives, what he can do and what he cannot do" [1].

According to Eggert et al. [2], individuals construct their own self-concept from the processed experiences and information about themselves; only those experiences that have emotional significance for the person are decisive (Fig. 13.1).

The basis of this view is a constructivist attitude, according to which our reality is a construction that is based on our experience. Constructivism is a scientific-theoretical approach that emphasises the part that the subject plays in cognitive achievements: Reality is regarded as being something that is generated by a person, and cognitive achievements are not seen as something that represents an apparently objective reality, but instead as an act of individual reality construction.

From this epistemological perspective, reality is an individually created concept, which necessarily differs from the reality of "the other", which eludes an external examination of its "validity". The decisive drivers of "construction" are the activities of the individual in the world: "Perceiving, thinking, acting, communicating" result in a reality of experience that can only be evaluated in terms of its viability [3]. Thus,

T. Becher (✉)
Kinderneurologisches Zentrum Gerresheim,
SANA Kliniken Düsseldorf, Duesseldorf, Germany
e-mail: thomas.becher@sana.de

© Springer Nature Switzerland AG 2021
J. Bahm (ed.), *Movement Disorders of the Upper Extremities in Children*,
https://doi.org/10.1007/978-3-030-53622-0_13

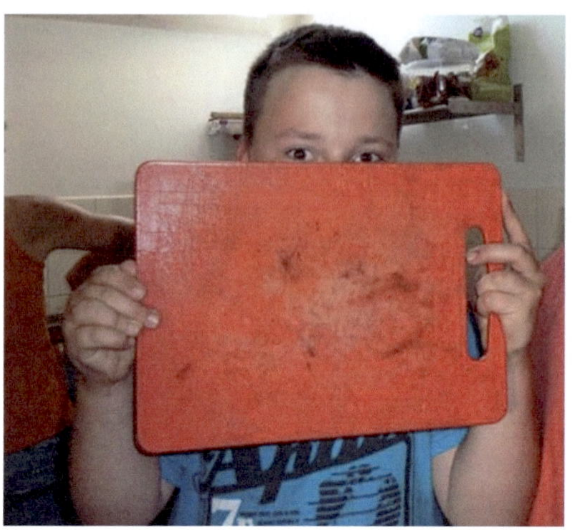

Fig. 13.1 The ongoing experiences with and about one's own person condense into the "I"

according to constructivist principles, knowledge is not passively absorbed, but actively built up by the thinking and acting subject; cognitive performances take place adaptively and aim at viability; they serve to organise the subject's world of experience.

This way, the self-concept also emerges unconsciously as the construction of an individual "self-reality".

There is a reciprocal relationship between self-concept and action, in which "the self-concept influences action, and conversely the individual learns something about itself in action situations". It is a living system consisting of various interconnected sub-areas [2].

> The self-concept also includes the future-oriented expectations of a person.

The self-concept of a child is fundamentally shaped by the experiences of the child in its family and close environment. For children with motor impairments, doctors and therapists are often part of the closer environment, and long-term relationships with regular contact often develop. Experts are the contact persons of the child and the parents concerning the disability, the resulting limitations, and overcoming these limitations. The attitude of therapists and doctors has a significant influence on the development of the child's self-concept – they can provide new

positive experiences and the experience of self-efficacy, but they can also effectively prevent this from happening.

13.3 Different Dimensions of the Self-Concept

In her papers, Saskia Schuppener worked out the various dimensions of the self-concept. She distinguishes between social, emotional, cognitive, performance-related, and physical self-concept, which she divides into two sub-dimensions each (Fig. 13.2).

Other authors make different classifications, but it is ultimately the consideration of different ideas from different areas that is essential. According to Eggert et al., for example, the self-concept consists of the dimensions "self-assessment", "body concept", "ability concept", and "self-image and self-assessment", which interact with each other (Eggert et al. [2], Table 13.1).

For therapeutic concerns, self-assessment, the body concept, and the ability concept are of particular importance. The expectation of success or failure as an expression of self-assessment has a lasting influence on the choice of and reaction to challenging life situations; the explanation of success as a result of one's actions or as a coincidental event depends above all on the self-assessment. With such a negative attitude without compensation in other areas, the experienced self-efficacy is further reduced, which in turn leads to the avoidance of potentially challenging situations, usually with social consequences.

The fact that one's own body plays a major role in the development of the self-concept is certainly logical. Especially the performance in sports is of great importance. Overall, young people of both genders who are active in sports seem to have a more positive body concept and self-concept than those who are not active [5]. Sonstroem and Morgan [6] assume that sports and exercise in the sense of bottom-up processes initially contribute to a higher physical self-efficacy. This experience of competence influences the perceived sports competence at a

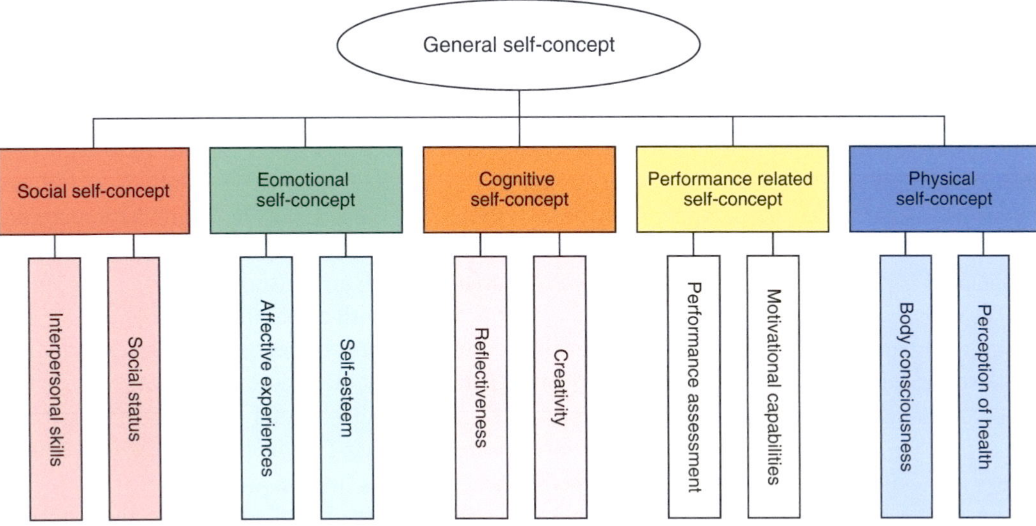

Fig. 13.2 Self-concept. (Modified acc. to [4])

Table 13.1 Self-concept according to Eggert

Self-assessment	Self-confidence (mental anticipation) Self-esteem (current component) Self-assessment (supersituative, generalised)	
Body concept	Body diagram	Body knowledge Body extension Body orientation Body in space and time
	Body sensation	Body attitude Body expression Physical exclusion Body awareness
Capability concept	Perception of one's own abilities Knowledge of one's own abilities Evaluation of own abilities	
Self-assessment	Emotional assessment of one's own actions Feelings regarding your own evaluations	
Self-image	Own "objective" assessments of own actions	

higher level, which further contributes to an increase in physical acceptance. Both—perceived sports competence and physical acceptance—influence the general self-esteem at the highest level [7].

The perception, knowledge, and evaluation of one's own abilities are further factors in the shaping of action and reaction in the world. A realistic assessment of one's own abilities is particularly important for people with a physical disability who have more difficulties comparing themselves to others.

It is an important task of all therapeutic efforts to contribute to a realistic assessment and expansion of one's own abilities through accompanied work at the limit of one's capacities.

13.4 Self-Concept in Children with Unilateral Motor Impairments

In 2011, a Norwegian working group with a very unusual composition of hand surgeons and psychiatrists for children and adolescents examined the self-concept and psychological well-being of children and adolescents with hand deformities and reduction defects of the arms. 92 children (53 boys, 9–11 years) were divided into two groups (severe vs. mild finger-hand-arm deformities) and examined with the Piers-Harris Children's Self-Concept Scale (PHCSCS). Overall, the PHCSCS values showed that the entire group of children with hand deformities had a "good" self-concept with values above 60 points, comparable to the values of a group of healthy children. Those with mild changes had lower values than those with severe deformities; boys had lower values than girls. The children with severe deformities had better values in the area of "intellectual and school status" and in the area of "popularity".

The authors conclude that children in this age group with hand deformities generally have the same self-esteem as children in the comparison group. Although these results may seem surprising at first, the clinical experience of the authors shows that children with severe changes experience a lot of empathy and understanding from the beginning. According to the authors, it is impossible to hide the disability and handicap, and it is obvious to the child and the environment. Other studies with children with different types of disability also showed equal or higher self-esteem among children receiving psychological support from a specialised team. Children with minor disabilities appear to be almost normal, and they—and their parents—may wish to hide them. Both the lack of special support and sympathy and the attempts to hide the disability could contribute to the inferior self-concept [8].

A Swedish working group reports on aspects of activities and participation in daily life resulting from body structures and functions in adolescents with plexus palsy (OBPP). Adolescents with OBPP reported interests, activities, and a social life similar to those of the adolescents in the comparison group. Differences were found in self-esteem for sport/motor activities; the self-esteem was lowest in the group of adolescents with the most severe form. The young people were concerned about risks for their affected and unaffected arm. Adolescents with OBPP report a typical teenage life in this study, but the authors believe that indicators of stress and worry related to disability should still be considered [9].

"He does not see himself as different"—under this title, Schiariti and colleagues present the perspectives of children and caregivers on relevant areas of functional capacity in cerebral palsy. The children examined usually described the same areas of functional capacity as their caregivers, but the two groups each had their own perspectives. The children talked more often about their skills with cerebral palsy, while the parents and caregivers talked more about their concerns regarding their children's limitations and bigger problems. These results highlight the importance of assessing the perspectives of parents and children when characterising the profile of abilities of children with cerebral palsy [10].

In the course of another qualitative and quantitative study, 18 adolescents between 10 and 17 years with neonatal plexus brachialis palsy were examined. Factors identified as contributing to the quality of life were social impact, peer acceptance, emotional adjustment, aesthetic concerns and body image, functional limitations, physiotherapy and occupational therapy, finance, pain, and family dynamics. Most adolescents and parents reported a good quality of life; adolescents reported a slightly higher quality of life than their parents [11].

In a systematic review of the self-concept of children with CP and the parents' point of view, it became clear that parents were not able to accurately assess the child's self-concept. There was no connection between the child's and parental assessments in all five dimensions of the self-concept. According to the authors, "health professionals" should obtain this information from the child itself [12].

In a comparison of the self-concept of 47 children with cerebral palsy with that of children without disabilities, no differences were found in the areas of global self-esteem, physical appearance, and social behaviour. Lower values were found in school competence (boys), social acceptance (girls), and athletic competence (girls and boys). According to the authors, children with cerebral palsy do not generally have lower self-esteem, even if they experience themselves to be less competent in certain aspects of the self-concept. Therapists should take this into account when making decisions on therapy management and should inform parents, caregivers, and health professionals that the diagnosis of cerebral palsy is not necessarily accompanied by a low self-concept.

13.5 Self-Concept and ICF

There are direct and indirect connections between the self-concept of a child and the components activities and participation of the ICF-CY. Christine Imms and an international working group [13] illustrated this impressively: They developed a conceptual approach to the concept of participation that contains a "family of participation-related constructs" (fPRC). They describe the relationship between intrinsic factors and participation: "Intrinsic person-related concepts that are related to participation in the fPRC, but are not the same as participation, include activity competence, sense of self, and preferences. These intrinsic factors influence future participation and are influenced by past and present participation". The working group reflects on the relationship between self-perception and participation and highlights the importance of having options to choose from: "The interaction between participation and sense of self involves the processes of engaging and perceiving. The sense of self evolves as a result of participation, and perceptions of self can predict future participation. Engaging can be seen as an internal state, and perceiving involves imagining one's ability or opportunity to participate. The relationship between participation and preference is expressed through choosing and complying. The importance of having the opportunity (or not) for choice and control over participation has been highlighted by many authors. Children choose what they will participate in (e.g., a preferred sport), or they comply (or cope) with choices made by others (e.g., reading at school), based on prior participation experiences and expectations of/for future participation".

Here, too, it becomes clear how important the active participation of the child is in the therapeutic process.

13.6 What Does the Self-Concept Theory Mean for Therapy?

These results have a concrete relation to therapy and its orientation. The support of children and adolescents with unilateral motor disorders in the testing of everyday, self-determined, and relevant actions for their own environment can lead to improvements in the self-efficacy experience if adequately accompanied. Children and adolescents should co-determine their therapy goals according to their age; respective agreements are possible from pre-school age onwards.

Self-efficacy is defined as the conviction that one's own competencies enable one to perform desired actions successfully or to provide appropriate performance in a certain situation [14]. According to Bandura, essential sources of self-efficacy are one's own active action and mastering a difficult task (direct experience), the observation of a model person during an action (representative experience), self-instruction such as "I can do it!" (linguistic conviction), and physiological reactions as a basis for the assessment of our situation and self-efficacy (e.g., increased heart rate when facing a task). Therapists should know and observe these principles of self-efficacious action. If a child, unlike in everyday life, learns that his assisting hand can play an essential role in his actions, and new actions become possible, he will use this hand first consciously and then later more and more automatically; if he expects positive self-efficacy, he will dare to approach new tasks, achieve successes, and be able to deal with failures more easily.

The agreement of the child on (co-)determined therapy goals relevant to everyday life is the ideal basis for direct experiences and for transferring new motor skills into everyday life. Thereby, approaches to motor learning are equivalent to active modifications of the environment: "A therapeutic approach that focuses more on changing the task and the environment than on the impairment of the child can be a viable treatment strategy" [15] and "child- and context-focused therapeutic approaches are equally effective" [16].

The change in self-concept is sometimes also evident in drawn self-images. Before and after hemi-intensive therapy, a 14-year-old girl drew a picture of herself (Fig. 13.3). The affected right arm is drawn much larger, the body tension is increased, the shoulders are wider, and growth has taken place!

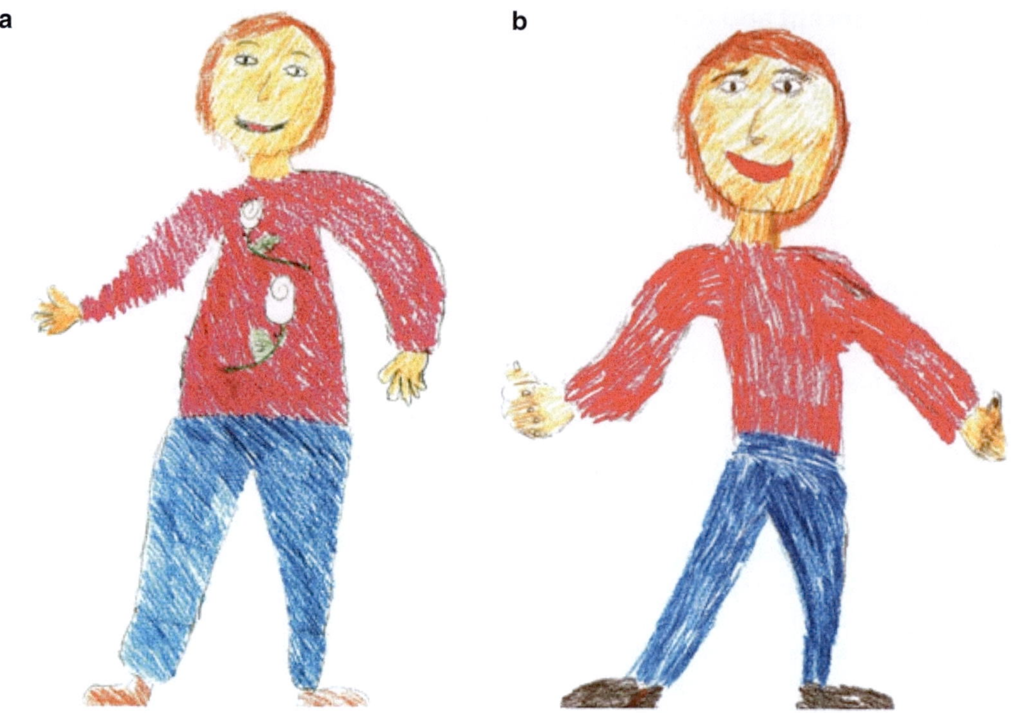

Fig. 13.3 (**a, b**) A 14-year-old girl with unilateral cerebral palsy. (**a**) Self-image before therapy. (**b**) Self-image after therapy

References

1. Tausch R, Tausch AM. Erziehungspsychologie: Begegnung von Person zu Person. Göttingen: Hogrefe; 1998.
2. Eggert D, Reichenbach C, Bode S. Das Selbstkonzept Inventar (SKI) für Kinder im Vorschul- und Grundschulalter. Dortmund: Borgmann; 2014.
3. Schmidt SJ. Kognitive Autonomie und soziale Orientierung. Konstruktivistische Bemerkungen zum Zusammenhang von Kognition, Kommunikation, Medien und Kultur. Frankfurt a.M: Suhrkamp; 1996.
4. Schuppener S. Selbstkonzept und Kreativität von Menschen mit geistiger Behinderung. Bad Heilbrunn: Klinkhardt; 2005.
5. Alfermann D. Selbstkonzept und Körperkonzept In Boes, K, Brehm, W (ed), Gesundheitssport. Ein Handbuch. Schorndorf: Hofmann. 1998;214–20.
6. Sonstroem RJ, Morgan WP. Exercise and self esteem: rationale and model. Med Sci Sports Exerc. 1989;21:329–37.
7. Stiller J, Alfermann D. Selbstkonzept im Sport. Z Sportpsychol. 2005;12:119–26.
8. Andersson GB, et al. Children with surgically corrected hand deformities and upper limb deficiencies: self-concept and psychological Well-being. J Hand Surg Eur. 2011;36:795–801.
9. Strömbeck C, Fernell E. Aspects of activities and participation in daily life related to body structure and function in adolescents with obstetrical brachial plexus palsy: a descriptive follow-up study. Acta Paediatr. 2003;92:740–6.
10. Schiariti V, et al. "He does not see himself as being different": the perspectives of children and caregivers on relevant areas of functioning in cerebral palsy. Dev Med Child Neurol. 2014;56:853–61.
11. Squitieri L, et al. Understanding quality of life and patient expectations among adolescents with neonatal brachial plexus palsy: a qualitative and quantitative pilot study. J Hand Surg [Am]. 2013;38:2387.e2–97.e2.
12. Dunn N, et al. Comparing the self concept of children with cerebral palsy to the perceptions of their parents. Disabil Rehabil. 2009;31:387–93.
13. Imms C, et al. Participation, both a means and an end: a conceptual analysis of processes and outcomes in childhood disability. Dev Med Child Neurol. 2017;59:16–25. http://doi.org/10.1111/dmcn.13237.
14. Bandura A. Self-efficacy: the exercise of control. New York: Freeman; 1997.
15. Darrah J, et al. Context therapy: a new intervention approach for children with cerebral palsy. Dev Med Child Neurol. 2011;53:615–20.
16. Law MC, et al. Focus on function: a cluster, randomized controlled trial comparing child- versus context-focused intervention for young children with cerebral palsy. Dev Med Child Neurol. 2011;53:621–9.

Inclusion

14

M. Mahler

14.1 Accommodation for Disadvantages at School

The purpose of accommodation measures at school is to compensate for the disadvantages caused to students by a disability through technical, educational, and other appropriate measures, thereby creating equal opportunities.

How and by what measure the compensation for disadvantages is granted must always be decided individually. A meaningful medical certificate, possibly supplemented by further expert opinions and examinations, is indispensable for this process.

The school examines and decides, ideally in collaboration with the parents, how the compensation for disadvantages can be implemented and achieved. The teacher conference decides on and documents the compensation for disadvantages, which is then binding. Disadvantage compensation is not noted in the grade report. The compensation for disadvantages must be regularly reviewed and adapted to the general conditions, the technical requirements of the student, and his or her needs.

> It is very helpful if the affected children, supported by their parents, openly communicate their limitations and needs and formulate their support needs as concretely as possible.

The affected children are experts in their impairment and are usually best able to explain what they can and cannot do. The parents know the strengths and weaknesses of their child and can describe the type and extent of the movement restriction as well as possible aids, measures and tools.

For many children it is unpleasant to talk about their special needs and to demand compensatory measures. They want to participate as normally as possible in everyday school life. Teachers and parents are therefore particularly called upon to find appropriate measures that reduce the inequality of opportunity and that are acceptable to the child concerned, the teachers, and the classmates. Openness and transparency help to improve acceptance and avoid conflicts.

Teachers and classmates need to be educated to understand the impairment and its consequences. The expectations of the affected child must be based on its capabilities. Where necessary, support must be offered.

The author is the mother of a son with an obstetrical brachial plexus injury. She is the chairperson of Plexuskinder e.V., a German self-help association that provides information, advice and support to affected children and adults and their families.

This chapter describes the situation in Germany at the time of the publication of the first German edition and might not apply elsewhere or at a different point in time.

M. Mahler (✉)
Plexuskinder e.V., Ulm, Germany
e-mail: info@plexuskinder.de

© Springer Nature Switzerland AG 2021
J. Bahm (ed.), *Movement Disorders of the Upper Extremities in Children*,
https://doi.org/10.1007/978-3-030-53622-0_14

Students and parents can obtain advice and support from the school office, a support center, a counseling center for integrating disabled children, or a support group for disabled children. Parents should submit their request for compensation for disadvantages in writing to the school and also have the school or the school office explain the regulations applicable in their location in writing.

In Germany the legal basis is the Grundgesetz, the Disabled Persons Act, and various administrative regulations and decrees of the Ministries of Education and Cultural Affairs of the Länder. The regulations and procedures in the federal states and also from school district to school district partly differ.

14.2　The Medical Certificate

The medical certificate for the application for compensation for disadvantages should describe not only the functional impairment but also the consequences for all movements in everyday school life in a detailed and concrete manner.

In the case of a brachial plexus injury, for example, the affected arm cannot be used for a throwing movement. Throwing with the unaffected side is also more difficult, as the entire movement sequence is impaired. When drawing with a ruler, it cannot be held straight and fixed; when measuring an angle, the ruler slips. Even the correct insertion of sheets into the hole punch is difficult. The handwriting is usually worse; the affected children can often not write as fast and enduringly as other children. All actions that require both hands, from putting the books in the bag to opening the correct page of a book to sharpening the pencil, take more time, are inaccurate, or sometimes are even impossible without outside help.

It is helpful for the application for compensation for disadvantages to document the additional time required for some concrete actions from everyday school life in comparison to peers of the same age, for example, writing a dictation, the packing and unpacking of the school bag, opening several pages in a book, changing clothes for sports lessons, and much more.

Examples of Compensation for Disadvantages with Limited Hand or Arm Function

- More time for written work.
- Shortened tasks.
- More frequent and longer breaks, even during a class test.
- Technical and other aids such as dictation devices, laptops, tablets, desk pads, clipboards, larger desks or individual desks, rulers with handles, writing materials for left-handed people, one-handed keyboards, and notebooks with larger lines.
- Use of enlarged worksheets.
- Educational measures, e.g., oral tasks instead of written work, multiple-choice tasks, and gap texts.
- Greater accuracy tolerance for handwriting, drawing, and geometric tasks.
- No recording of blackboard texts, provision of texts, or transcript by classmates.
- Two sets of textbooks, one for home and one for school, locker, and shelf in the classroom.
- Different weighting of oral grades in relation to written grades and different weighting of the keeping of notebooks.
- If the students do craft work, for example, in art lessons or in an experiment: grading of group work instead of individual performance.
- Only as an exception modified tasks.
- Exemption from grading or assignment of different tasks where the task cannot be completed due to the impairment and group work is not possible, for example, in sports, crafts, and shopwork. However, many of the affected children are proud of their achievements despite their impairment and participate as best they can.
- More time for changing clothes during physical education.
- More time for toilet visits.
- Sponsorship among classmates who, for example, can help with dressing or carrying school books and creating and duplicating blackboard scripts.
- Adaptation of the timetable, e.g., exemption from afternoon activities offers to attend therapy appointments.

- Special sports and exercise offers and relaxation techniques.
- Reduction of requirements in more practical subjects.

14.3 A Glimpse into the Everyday Life of Affected Children

Anton has a brachial plexus injury. In kindergarten Anton's impairment was hardly noticed. Many children could only dress themselves slowly and needed help with crafts and going to the toilet.

Anton has practiced diligently tying his shoes and cutting with scissors with his therapist. Often he was even faster than his friends. Anton did not experience himself as injured or disabled during his kindergarten years. In the mixed-age group, his abilities were not directly compared with those of other children or perhaps did not attract further attention. The many hours of therapy have greatly supported his development, Anton's somersaults were a bit crooked, but that was fine for everyone.

With the switch to primary school, Anton was confronted for the first time with the consequences of his injury. The teacher had no time to close his zipper after gym class or to help him put on his gloves.

In school it was no longer irrelevant that he sometimes needed a little longer to cut something out or just to open his lunch box.

At the sports festival, all students had to show their skills at different stations. Anton is a good athlete; he swims, plays soccer, and does martial arts; but he could not keep up in direct competition in disciplines such as jumping rope, bowling, long jump, and basketball. The other children in his group complained about him, because due to his impairment the group result was clearly worse.

Lisa also has a brachial plexus injury and is in the seventh grade. She can't write as fast as her classmates. Lisa sometimes can't complete the tests in the time allotted and often can't copy everything from the blackboard. Not all teachers are aware of her impairment or remember it. Every school year her mother has to inform all her teachers anew.

Anton and Lisa are sometimes sad, angry, and disappointed. In everyday life they experience themselves as different and disadvantaged. Coping with the injury and its consequences can lead to problems again and again.

14.4 A Primary School Student Tells His Classmates About His Disability

My right arm is paralyzed since birth. When I was born, the nerves in my neck were very stretched. Some were torn. That's how the injury happened. If the nerves are injured, as with me, the muscles are also weaker, and the messages from the brain are not so well received.

My right arm has less strength than my left arm. I can't move it that well, and I can't feel that well with it. It's a little shorter, too. Some movements are difficult for me. Some things I can't do or I do them differently from you.

I'm good at that:

- Math
- Playing soccer
- Inventing stories

I'll do it differently:

I write in block letters and use erasable pens, not a fountain pen. I cannot write so beautifully and not so fast, although I practice a lot.

I need more time for these things:

- Handwriting.
- Changing clothes simply takes longer, and if the zipper gets stuck, I need help.
- Packing and unpacking my school bag.

I need help or tools that help me:

- Tying my shoelaces – but now I have rubber shoelaces, so I don't need any help any more.
- A clipboard and desk pad to prevent the sheets from slipping away when writing.
- A big table or my pencil case will fall down all the time.

This isn't going well:

- Crafts, such as knitting and weaving, are not possible and not fun at all, but instead I can model with clay and draw but I cannot carry a heavy tray.

I need some help with sports, but most of the time, I find my own way of doing different things. This sometimes looks a little different or takes longer than with the other children. I always try everything, even if it's hard for me sometimes.

14.5 Conclusion

The affected children, their parents, and the school are called upon to work together to find suitable measures that create equal opportunities and are acceptable to the students, parents, teachers, and fellow students.

In an open dialogue, a solution should be sought which allows the student to make the most of his or her opportunities and at the same time compensates as far as possible for the disadvantages associated with the disability.

Part IV

Primary Reconstructive Interventions

Reconstruction of Traumatized Nerves

Jörg Bahm

15.1 Peripheral Nerve Surgery

Surgery on structures of the peripheral nervous system, especially on the extremities, is not the sole responsibility of one specialist group (neurosurgery), since it is a question not only of knowing the nerves alone and restoring them but also of other function-improving procedures and special surgical techniques such as microsurgery. Accordingly, plastic surgeons, hand surgeons and overall orthopaedic surgeons, who invented that discipline, are concerned with this topic, which also enables a rounded consideration of all facets again and again.

Peripheral nerve surgery "stricto sensu" is performed according to a fixed schedule: searching for the nerve path through a gentle (tissue-sparing) approach; visualization of the injured area, which often has to be prepared from a scarred soft tissue mantle (sometimes referred to as "external" neurolysis); and then intraoperative analysis (including direct electrical nerve stimulation) and nerve continuity restoration by neurolysis, suture, insertion of an interposition graft and/or various accompanying nerve transfers [1, 2].

J. Bahm (✉)
Department of Plastic, Hand and Burn Surgery,
Section for Plexus Surgery, University Hospital,
Aachen, Germany
e-mail: jbahm@ukaachen.de,
jorg.bahm@belgacom.net

In the following, we describe the individual surgical steps, which should always be performed under optical magnification (magnifying glasses or microscope) and with the provision of microsurgical instruments.

15.2 Exploration

In order to reach the affected nerve structure, it requires a *gentle soft tissue access*. It is especially important not to damage the musculature in the long term and to protect important vessels and also to maintain a good gliding bed for the repaired nerve.

The brachial plexus is approached by a straight *supraclavicular access* after reflection of the adipo-lymphatic soft tissue cushion at the level of the interscalene triangle (anterior gap between the scalenus anterior and medius muscles) (Bahm [3]; Fig. 15.1). From here, the retro- and somewhat also the infraclavicular space (by lifting the clavicle with a sling) can also be prepared. For the display of divisions, cords and main nerves, a combined *deltopectoral access* is required (Fig. 15.2).

In the case of children, no interventions are performed directly on the spinal cord through a dorsal laminotomy for the procedures described by us.

© Springer Nature Switzerland AG 2021
J. Bahm (ed.), *Movement Disorders of the Upper Extremities in Children*,
https://doi.org/10.1007/978-3-030-53622-0_15

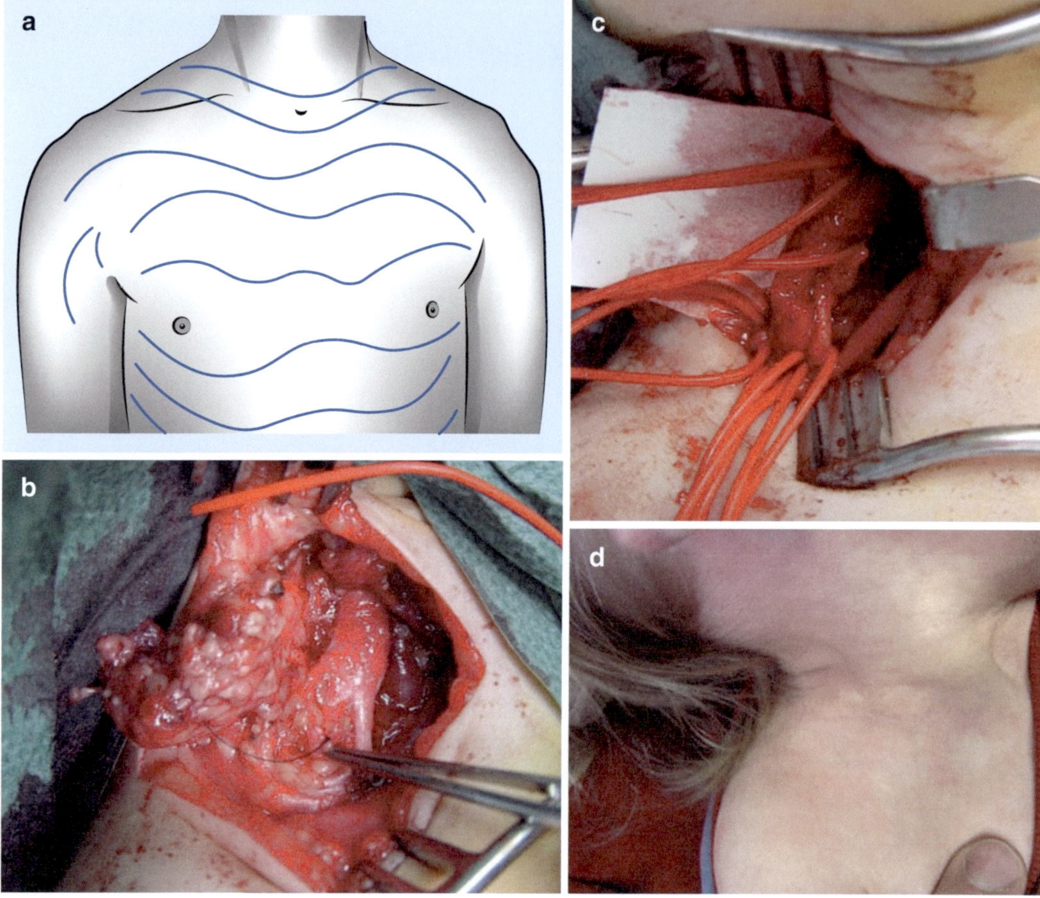

Fig. 15.1 (**a–d**) Supraclavicular access. (**a**) The access lies in a skin fold line. (**b**) After severing the subcutaneous tissue and keeping the adipo-lymphatic soft tissue away, the view of the scalenus triangle is clear. (**c**) Subsequently, a subtle preparation of the individual nerve strands is possible. (**d**) The remaining skin scar is always inconspicuous

The nerves located in the arm or leg are usually accessed through an access through the skin area, which lies directly above the injury site [4].

15.3 Neurolysis

Once the nerve structure has been found and separated from the surrounding soft tissue (possible post-traumatic adhesions to muscle and fat gliding tissue have been cleared), the lesion site can usually be delimited and by an access from the healthy nerve parts both proximal and distal.

Now the question arises to what extent fibrosis/scar tissue has spread into and around the nerves and thus impedes, restricts or cancels restoration of function by reinnervation. This is where the intraoperative electrodiagnosis (Fig. 15.3) by means of a stimulation catheter is applied, as used by the anaesthetists when performing a peripheral nerve blockade: A low stimulation current is applied above and below the injury zone; this current is constantly reduced in intensity, and the electrical conductivity of the injured segment is tested. If no muscle response can be triggered from above the lesion, this proves a conduction blockage; if more or less current stimulation is transmitted, there is a *conductive neuroma* or "conducting neuroma in continuity".

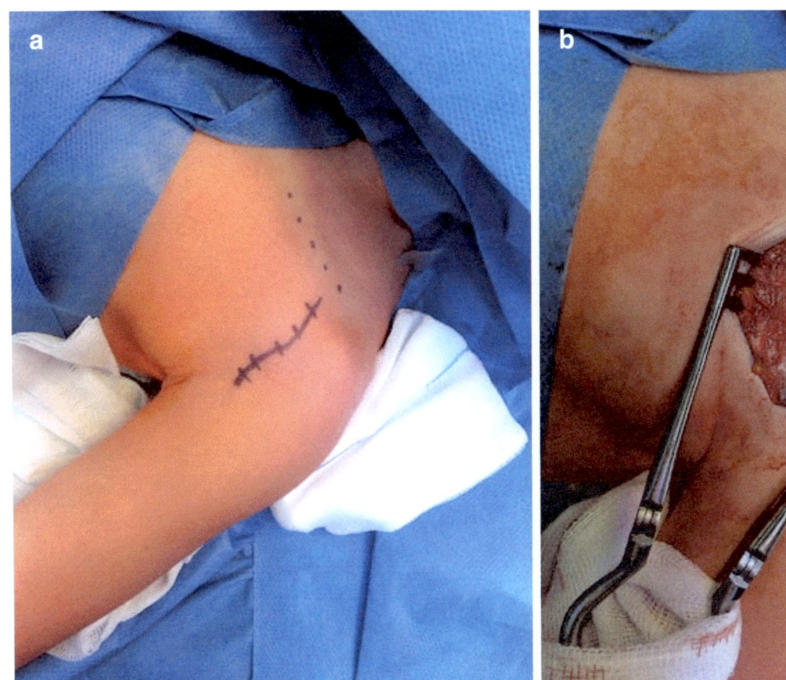

Fig. 15.2 (**a**, **b**) Deltopectoral access

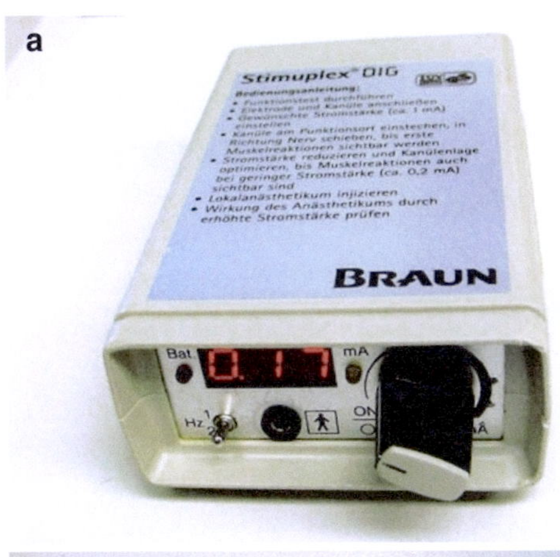

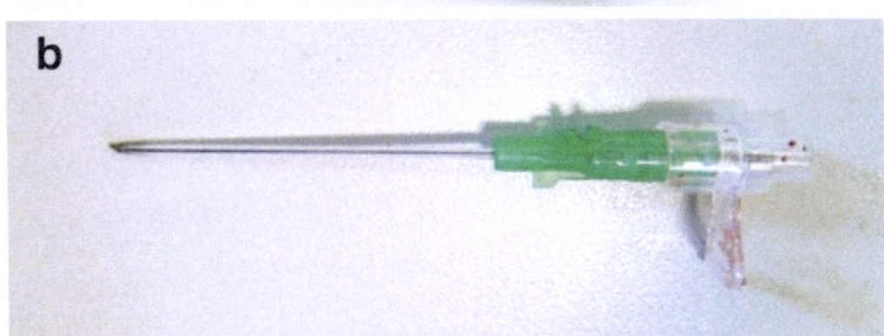

Fig. 15.3 (**a**, **b**) Intraoperative electrostimulation

The nerve conductivity should be improved as much as possible, through subtle scar tissue removal in the epineurium and eventually within the perineurium between the fascicular groups; here, the staged rules and empirical values described by Millesi are generally applied (Fig. 15.4; Millesi [5]). A clinical example can be found in Figs. 15.5 and 15.6.

If the internal anatomy of the nerve is destroyed or largely fibrosed, the injured segment must be excised, and the two ends must be connected again by a direct suture (avoiding excessive tension) or otherwise by bridging using a graft.

About the question on *tension on the nerve suture*, there are several investigations which show how, on the one hand, the blood flow to the nerve endings is reduced more and more with increasing tension on the nerve endings and, on the other hand, depending on the filament thickness used, the tear strength is no longer given. Here it is empirically valid that with small nerves, tensions should be supported by a 10/0 filament (if it breaks, a graft must be inserted); with thicker nerves up to 8/0 or 7/0 filament can be used.

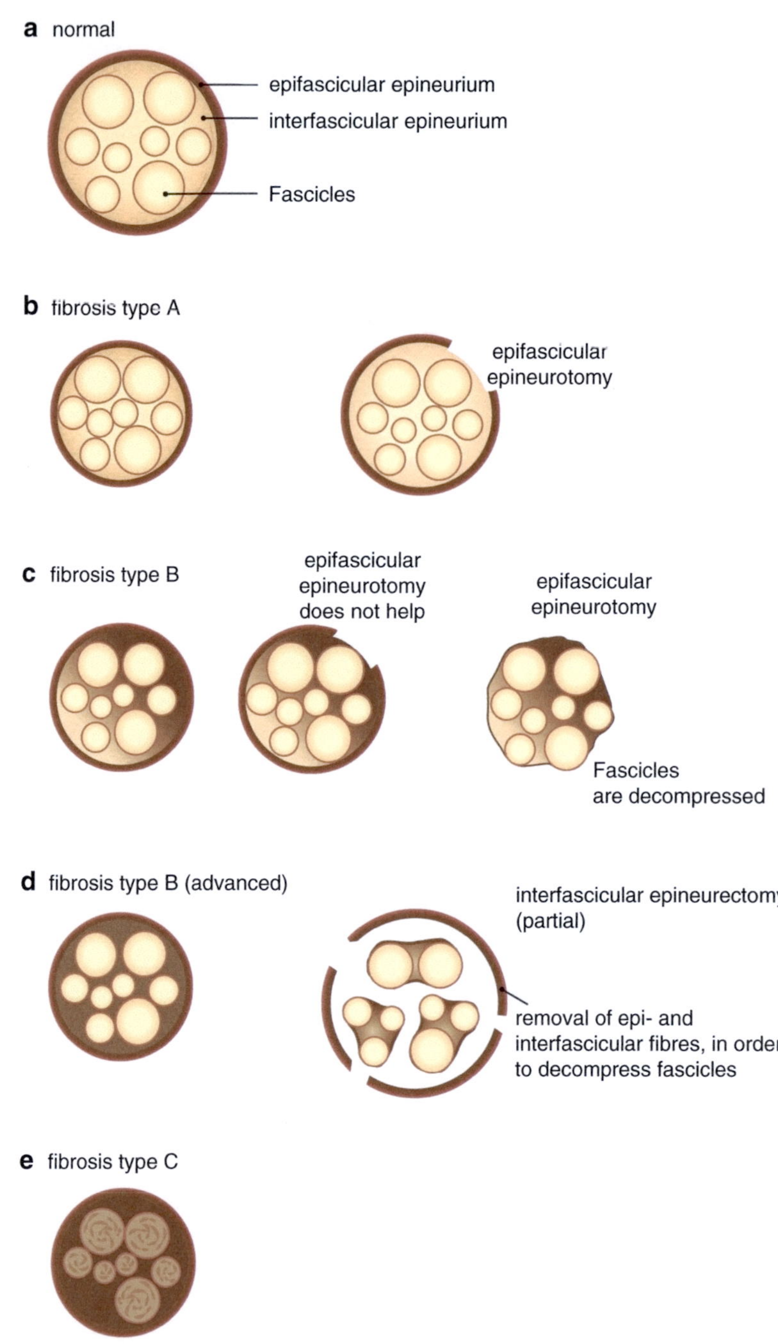

Fig. 15.4 Stages of neurolysis according to Millesi

Any existing anatomical variation of root and trunk branches or post-traumatic functional nerve connections must be carefully identified, checked and, if necessary, preserved (Fig. 15.7).

15.4 Direct Sutures

Here we perform in common microsurgical technique the so-called epiperineural end-to-end sutures which grip both the usually thin

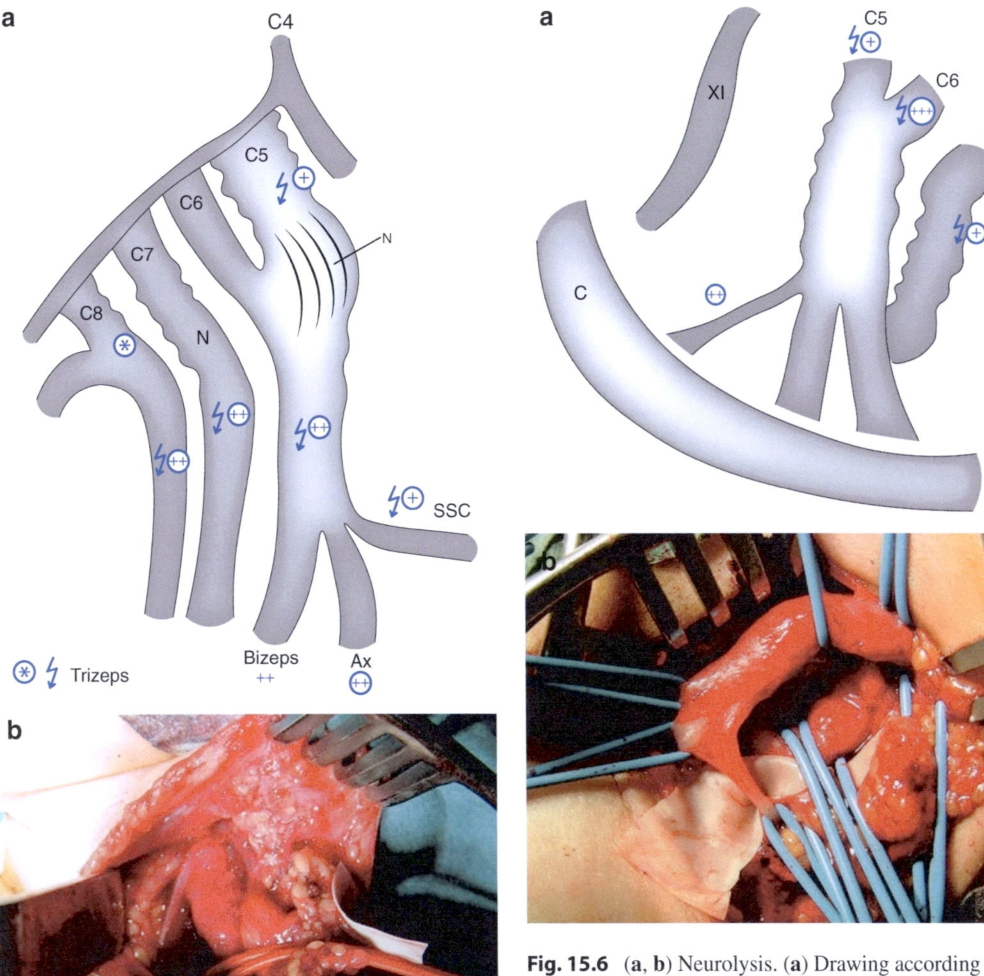

Fig. 15.5 (**a**, **b**) Neurolysis. (**a**) Drawing according to an operation sketch by Dr. Bahm (appendix). (**b**) Photo documentation

Fig. 15.6 (**a**, **b**) Neurolysis. (**a**) Drawing according to an operation sketch by Dr. Bahm (appendix). (**b**) Photo documentation

epineurium and the peripheral perineurium (Fig. 15.8). The suture material is not resorbable and therefore remains as foreign material on and within the nerve, but without any significant inflammatory reaction, as is usual with resorbable sutures. We assume that the coaptation is loadable after 2 weeks.

15.5 Interposition Grafts

If a direct suture is not possible or not advisable due to the length of the gap or the suture tension, a fascicular bridging is performed with autologous material, in the case of a short distance as a "cable interposition" (Fig. 15.9), in the case of a longer defect distance as an interfascicular interposition. The strands of graft are spread out across the bed of tissues the best possible way, so to promote revascularization (Fig. 15.10).

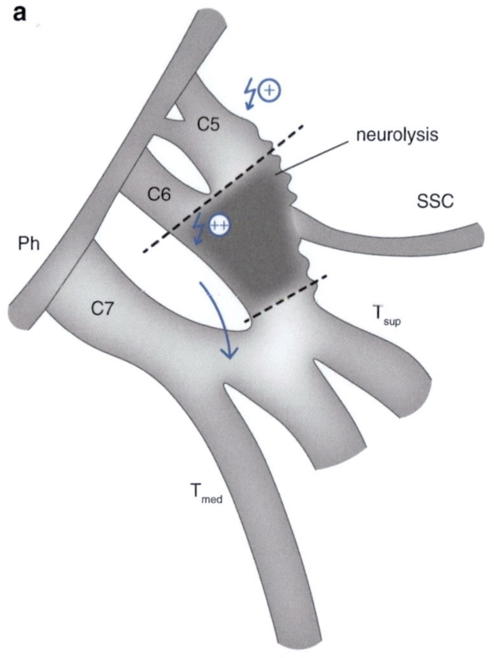

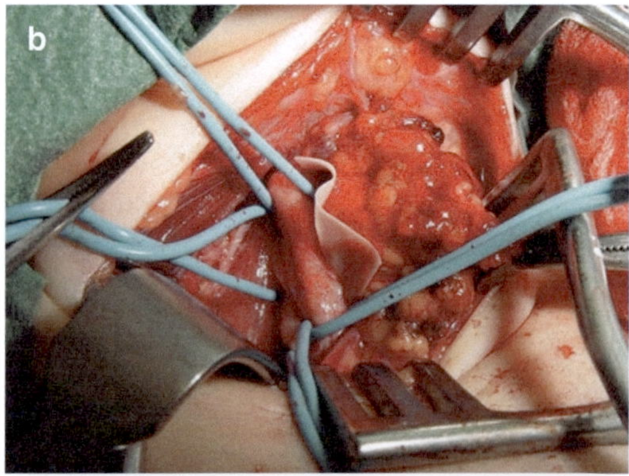

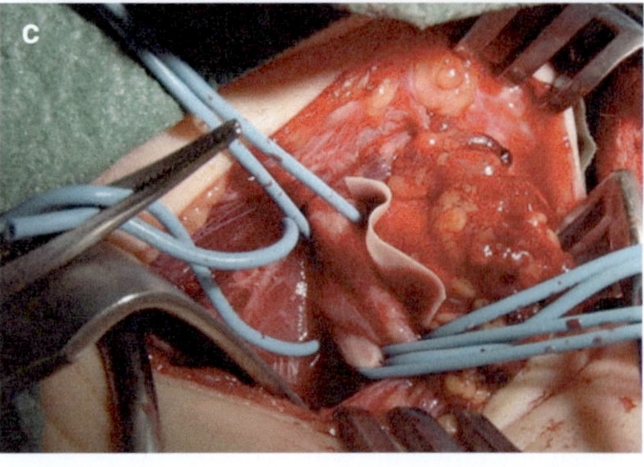

Fig. 15.7 (**a–c**) The root C7 contributes to the superior trunk. (**a**) Drawing according to an operation sketch by Dr. Bahm (appendix). (**b**, **c**) Intraoperative view ((**a**) Neurolyse = neurolysis)

15.5.1 Graft Donors and Harvesting Defect

Only dispensable autologous sensible nerves can be considered as graft donors, *N. suralis* on the lower leg or a sensible nerve branch on the forearm, such as the cutaneous divisions of the musculocutaneous nerve or the radial nerve. In the case of extensive defects, we may also harvest at the level of the upper thigh the *N. saphenus* along the medial vascular-nerve road. In addition to the unavoidable formation of scars on the skin, the loss of sensibility in the corresponding dermatome must always be considered. In small children, there is evidence showing that the deficit is compensated over time by the surrounding sensible nerves through overlap.

Of course, only nerves of cutaneous sensation are removed; they degenerate as a result of the removal and essentially serve as a guide rail for the regeneration cones.

15.5.2 Conduits and Tubes

Due to the limited number of autologous nerve donors, "artificial" nerves have been researched for several decades (Chap. 25).

Various hollow tubes or conduits are propagated today—from allogenic nerve cables to so-called bioartificial conduits, the individual components of which are of either synthetic or animal origin or are cultivated in the laboratory from human stem cells.

Some are now also available in clinical practice such as allogeneic nerve fascicles like Axogen® and chitin tubes like Reaxon®. However, they are preferred in adults and short defects and give better results in purely sensible or motor nerves. Here even more clinical experience is required before they can be used freely and in place of autologous transplants in small children. It is important to think about the immune reaction and its effect on a nerve regeneration process; it is also important to find out more about what kind of regeneration the bridging cables are made

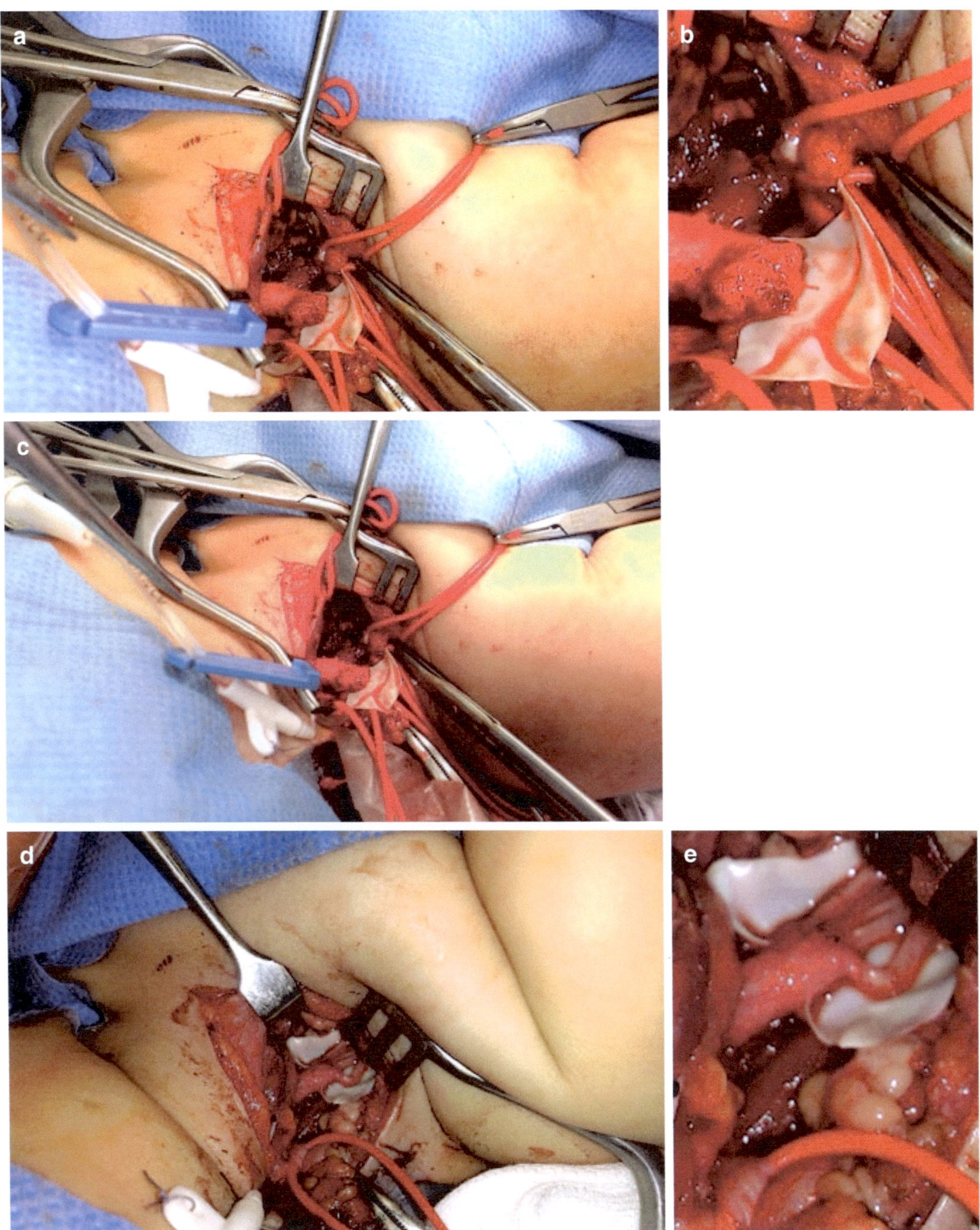

Fig. 15.8 (a–e) Direct suture of the upper trunk

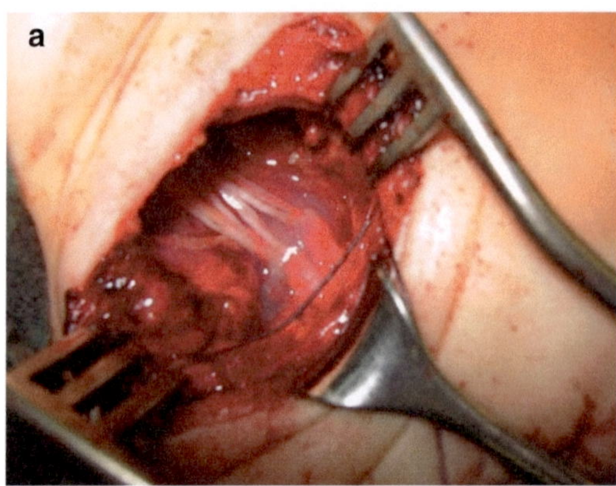

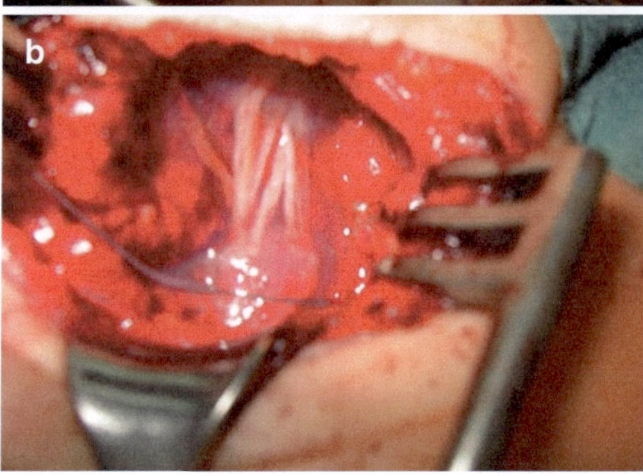

Fig. 15.9 (**a**, **b**) Interposition grafts. View after proximal and distal graft apposition and fixation with fibrin adhesive (milky zone)

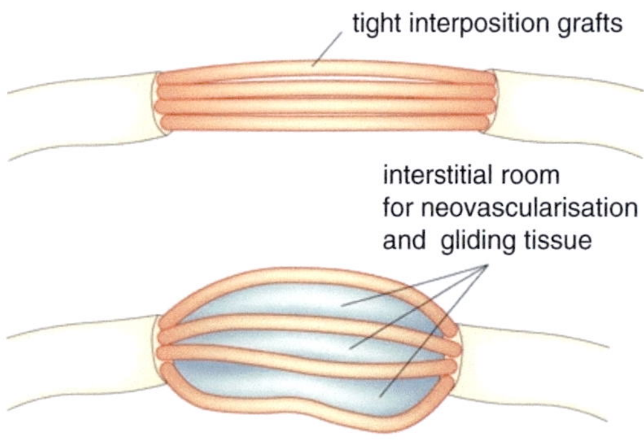

Fig. 15.10 Cable arrangement

of. Do they contain only unorganized minifascicles as in a neuroma, which lose their reinnervation potential after a short distance, or is it possible to organize them into real fascicle structures with the assignment of specific sensible and motor functions? (Fig. 15.11).

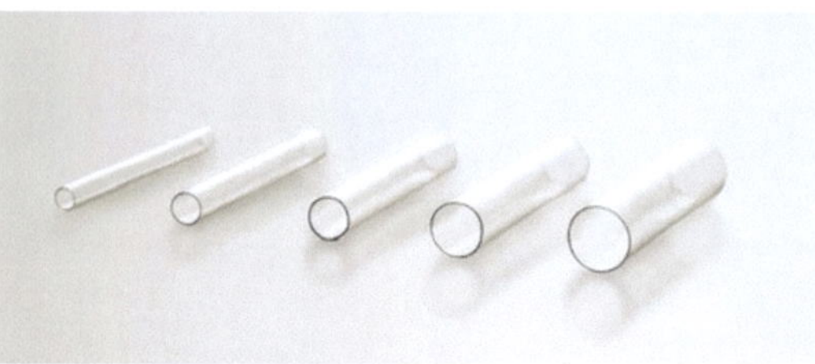

Fig. 15.11 Reaxon® tubes

15.6 Nerve Transfers

In a nerve transfer, a dispensable sensible or motor donor is coapted to a monofunctional target nerve, if a direct coaptation of the proximal and distal nerve ends is not (no longer) possible.

This is the case, for example, after a nerve root avulsion in the case of plexus damage (the "power socket" is no longer available and a replacement donor must therefore be redirected to the important—usually motor—target function) or in the case of injuries in which the proximal nerve end is difficult to reach (e.g., reconstruction of the axillary nerve after its crushing in the quadrangular space within the axilla, by transferring the first motor radial branch for the triceps muscle to the motor part of the axillary nerve; Fig. 15.13).

Table 15.1 gives an overview [6] of the donors and recipients currently available in peripheral nerve surgery who have more or less made their way into reconstruction strategies in children. Figs. 15.12, 15.13, 15.14 and 15.15 show intraoperative images of frequently used nerve transfers.

Today, a nerve transfer using the whole phrenic nerve as a donor is no longer accepted, as the vital respiratory function may be compromised early or over time, which is unacceptable in the reconstruction of a non-vital limb motor function. Its description figures in Table 15.1 only for complete listing and consideration for a partial or side to end transfer.

15.6.1 Nerve Versus Musculo-Tendinous Transfer

Sometimes in a long-standing peripheral nerve injury such as radial nerve palsy after humeral

Table 15.1 Nerve transfers: donor and recipient

Donor	Receivers	Author
XI	Suprascapularis (Mm. spinati)	Malessy et al. [11]; Bahm et al. [12]
XI	Musculocutaneous (M. biceps)	Narakas [13]
Intercostal nerves	Musculocutaneous (M. biceps)	Malessy et al. [14]
Intercostal nerves	Axillary nerve (M. deltoid)	Malungpaishrope et al. [15]
Ulnar	Musculocutaneous (M. biceps or brachialis)	Oberlin et al. [7]; Liverneaux et al. [16]
Ulnar	Radial (M. triceps)	Pet et al. [17]
Median	Musculocutaneous (M. biceps or brachialis)	Oberlin et al. [8]
Median	Radial (N. interosseus posterior)	Mackinnon et al. [18]; Bertelli and Ghizoni [19]
Radial	Axillar (M. deltoid)	Leechavengvongs et al. [9, 10]; Colbert and Mackinnon [20]; Bertelli et al. [21]
Musculocutaneous (branch for M. brachialis)	Median (finger flexion)	Palazzi et al. [22]
Thoracodorsalis	Thoracicus longus (M. serratus anterior)	Uerpairojkit et al. [23]
Phrenic	Musculocutaneous	Gu et al. [24, 25]; Siqueira and Martins [26]
Phrenic	Suprascapularis	Sinis et al. [27]
Contralateral C7	Numerous receivers	Gu et al. [28]; Terzis and Kokkalis [29]

shaft fracture, the question raises whether proximal primary reconstruction with end-to-end coaptation should be preferred, (with uncertain prognosis in the case of a longer defect in a mixed nerve, due to uncertain sensible and motor assignment of the corresponding proximal and distal fascicles) to a classical musculotendinous transfer of redundant donors or should we perform as an alternative elective distal nerve transfers.

Musculo-tendinous transfers have a reliable tradition and show actually predictable results after 6–8 weeks; distal selective nerve transfers have a failure rate and are not "reversible"; however, in the case of partial damage and the failure of only one specific muscle, they may well become a good alternative in the future, especially since local nerve transfer requires only a single, limited, anatomical approach. Also may a reinnervated extensor communis muscle provide again independent long finger extension, very interesting for piano players, what a tendon transfer definitely will not offer.

15.7 Intra- and Extraplexual Reconstruction

In cases of severe or extensive damage to the brachial plexus, not always enough roots are available for a complete intraplexual reconstruction (three roots are a minimum for the three trunks). That is why sometimes we have to add so-called extraplexual neurotization to compensate for the lack of proximal stumps.

These neurotizations consist of nerve transfers (usually without grafts) of available extraplexual nerve donors in the vicinity of the cervical plexus, i.e. of the 11th cranial nerve (accessorius XI nerve), the intercostal nerves, the phrenic nerve (only as end-to-side coaptation due to its high functional value) and, in the case of the most severe injuries, parts of the healthy contralateral root C7 (Table 15.1).

A detailed analysis of this selection exceeds the scope of this chapter; interested readers should consult specific surgical literature (in appendix) and also study the viewpoint of a neurosurgical colleague (Chap. 17) in parallel in this book.

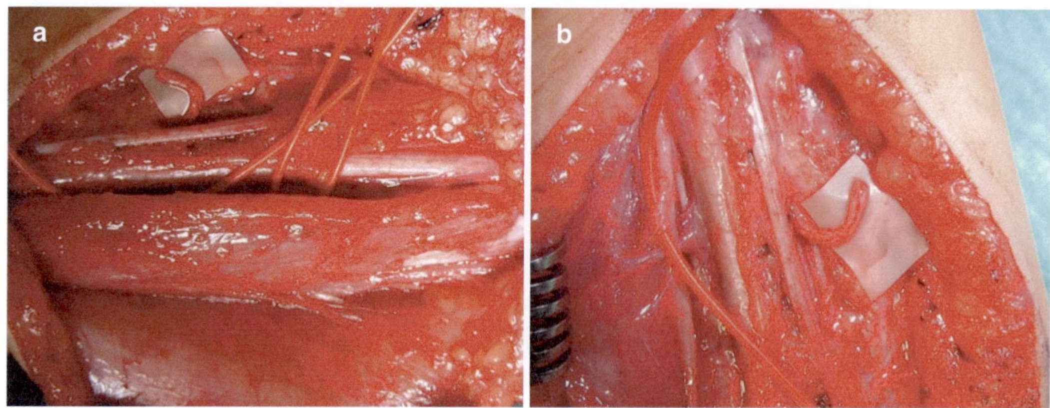

Fig. 15.12 (**a, b**) Example of a nerve transfer according to Oberlin with donor and recipient fascicles [7, 8]

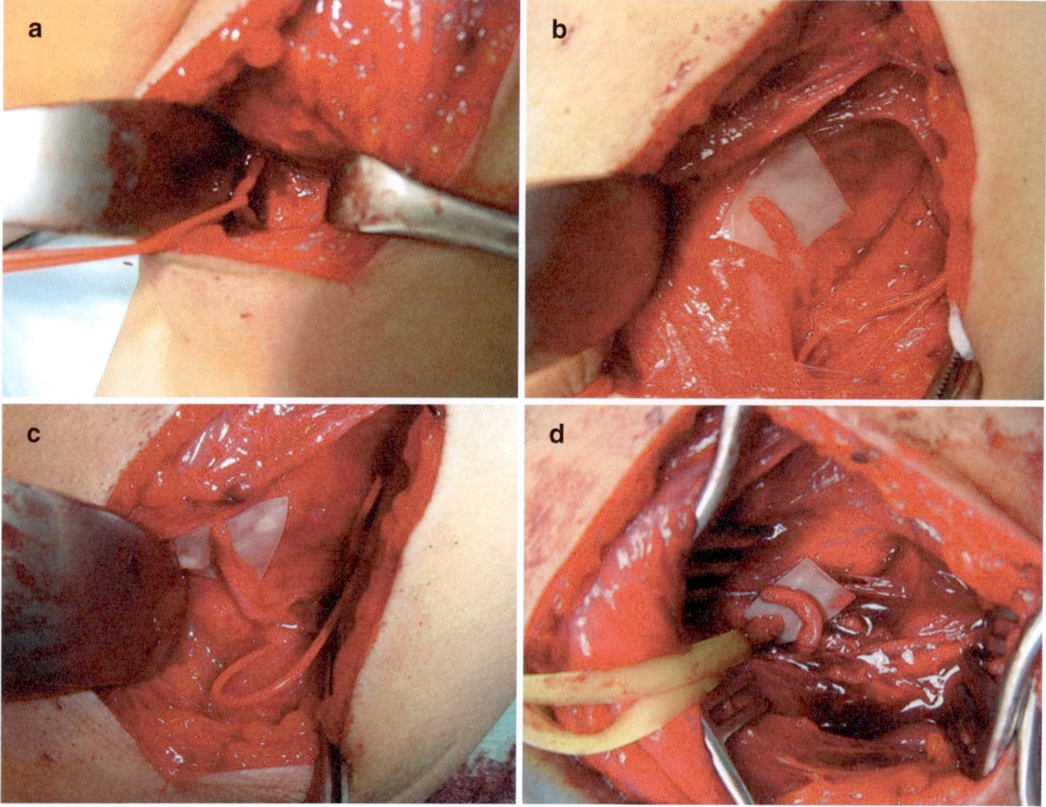

Fig. 15.13 (**a–d**) Nerve transfer according to Somsack with donor and recipient fascicles [9, 10]

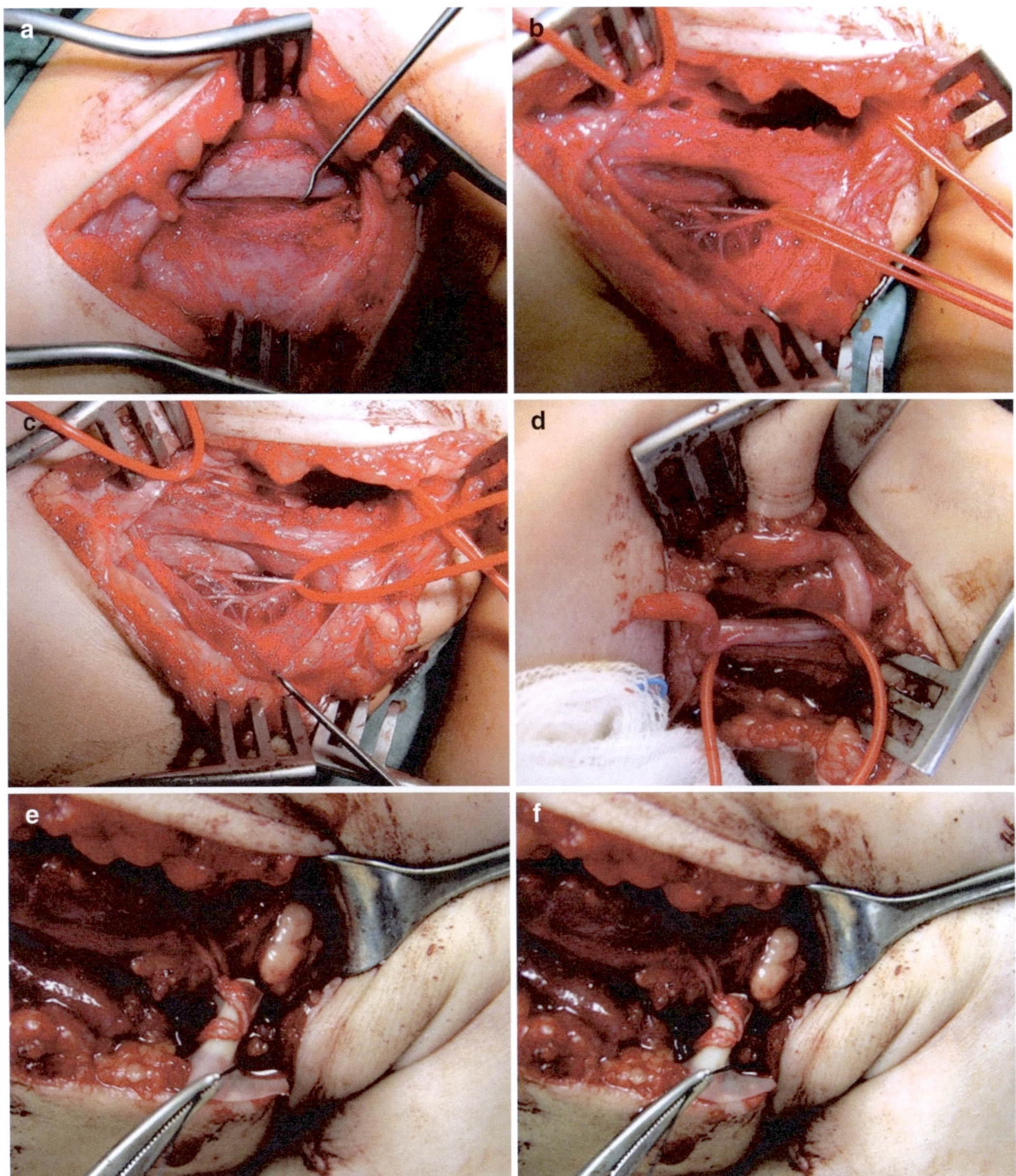

Fig. 15.14 (a–f) Transfer of intercostal nerves

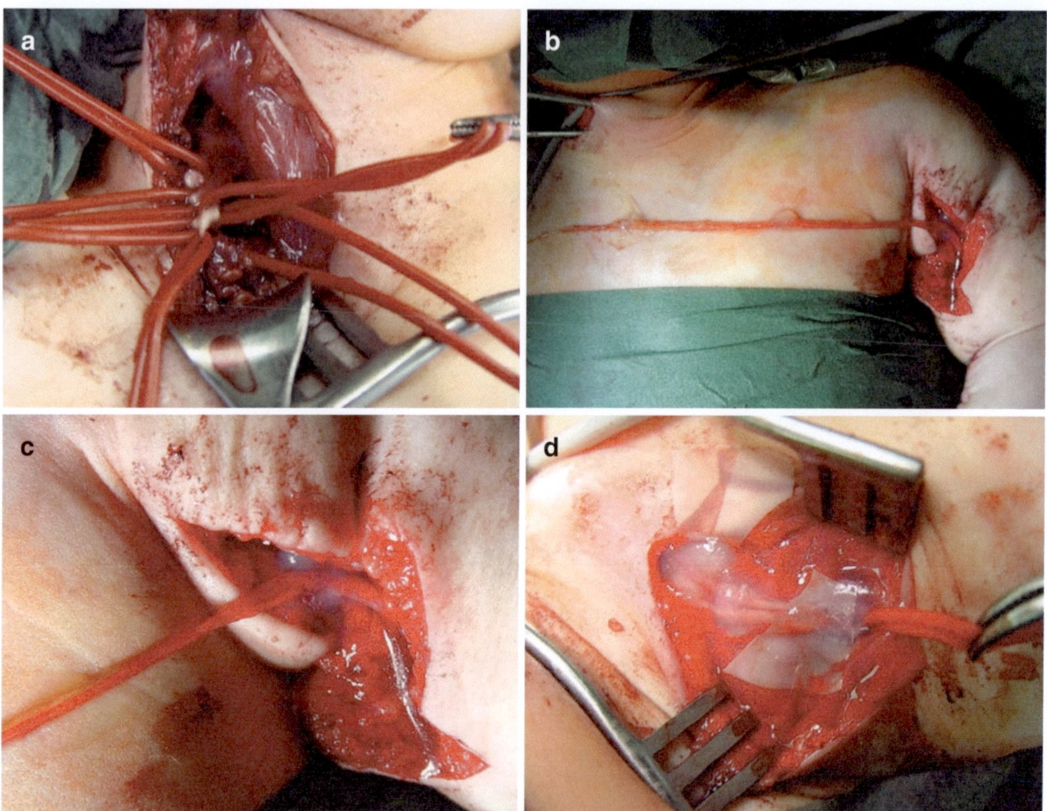

Fig. 15.15 (**a–d**) Transfer of the contralateral C7 root (partial)

15.8 Strategies and Examples

In the following, we present single examples of surgical strategies for different injury patterns, which illustrate the range of variation of plexus injuries on the one hand and of reconstruction possibilities at the upper extremity on the other hand.

Let us first consider the more frequent *upper lesions* which in the birth lesion usually have an in continuity neuroma (Figs. 15.16, 15.17 and 15.18).

If the root C7 and the middle trunk are also involved, we speak of an *extended upper lesion.* This often requires an accompanying reconstruction of the elbow and wrist extension (Figs. 15.19, 15.20, 15.21 and 15.22).

With a breech birth and otherwise only with maximum stretch forces, we may find *pregangli-onic lesions, with avulsion of the upper spinal nerves* (Figs. 15.23, 15.24, 15.25, 15.26 and 15.27).

Root avulsions also may occur in the severe extended upper lesions according to the same mechanism, whereby C5 is usually spared or rup-tured (Figs. 15.28, 15.29, 15.30, 15.31, 15.32 and 15.33).

In *subtotal lesions* only Th1 is intact (Figs. 15.34, 15.35 and 15.36).

Complete lesions are rare, but show severe traction damage, especially in the lower parts (Figs. 15.37, 15.38, 15.39 and 15.40).

An accessory, *cervical rib*, can increase the extent of injury to the middle plexus elements by acting as a lever or hypomochlion on the middle trunk (Figs. 15.41 and 15.42) [30].

The isolated reconstruction of the active exter-nal rotation of the shoulder can be performed via a ventral supraclavicular or a dorsal approach (Figs. 15.43 and 15.44).

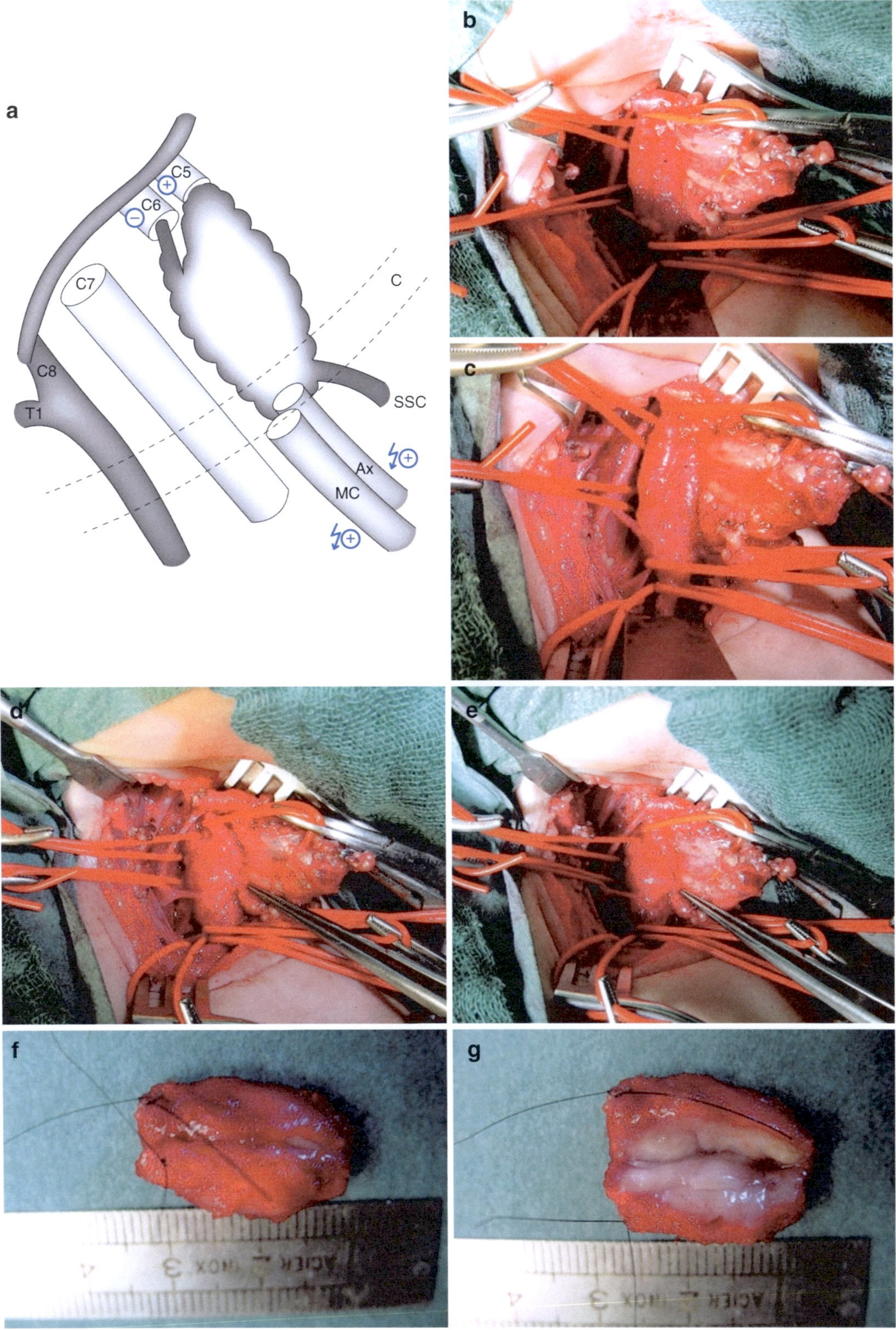

Fig. 15.16 (**a–g**) Obstetric plexus, lesion C5–C6 with continuity neuroma of the upper trunk, first example. (**a**) Drawing according to an operation sketch by Dr. Bahm (appendix). (**b–e**) Preparing the neuroma. (**f, g**) Open neuroma in which one sees the inner scarring

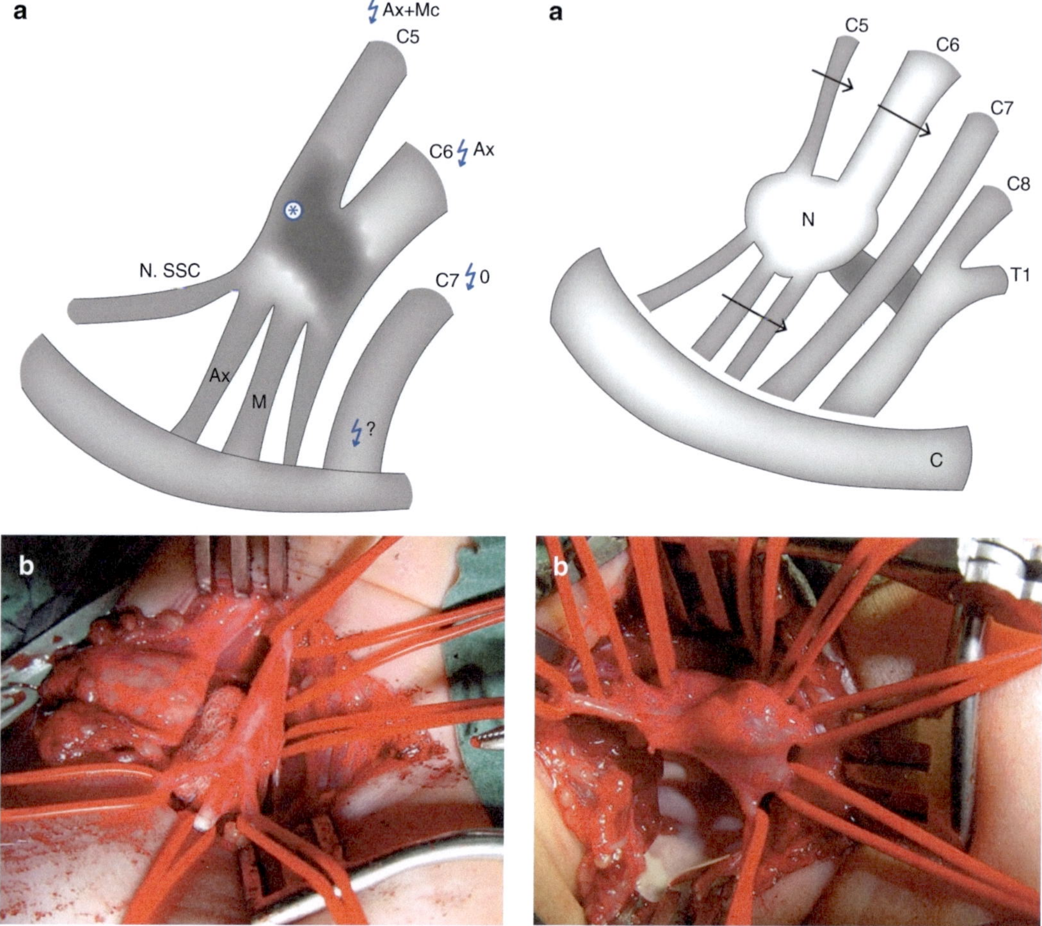

Fig. 15.17 (**a, b**) Obstetric plexus, lesion C5–C6 with continuity neuroma of the upper trunk, second example. (**a**) Drawing according to an operation sketch by Dr. Bahm (appendix). (**b**) Preparation of the neuroma

Fig. 15.18 (**a, b**) Obstetric plexus, lesion C5–C6 with continuity neuroma of the upper trunk, third example. (**a**) Drawing according to an operation sketch by Dr. Bahm (appendix). (**b**) Preparation of the neuroma

15.9 Time Schedule

Ideally, the children are presented at consultation in the first months of life, and one can then decide early (usually between 3 and 9 months of life) whether a primary nerve-repairing intervention is necessary. After that, it takes 12–18 months to allow sufficient time for the physiological regeneration of the peripheral nerves to rebuild the musculature accordingly, depending on the distance of the reinnervation target from the repair site. During this time, neurophysiologically based physiotherapy should continue. Apart from orthopaedic exceptions such as shoulder contrac-

ture, secondary surgery should not be indicated or performed.

Then comes the pre-school period between 3 and 5 years, in which period we frequently observe how variable and unreliable compliancy in the children can be: During this time it is therefore difficult to plan a secondary intervention that requires the postoperative cooperation of the small patient. On the other hand, it is preferable to complete surgical reconstruction before the children enter primary school. Muscle transfers on the shoulder and arm in particular benefit from the fact that the balance between arm weight and possible donor muscle strength has not yet

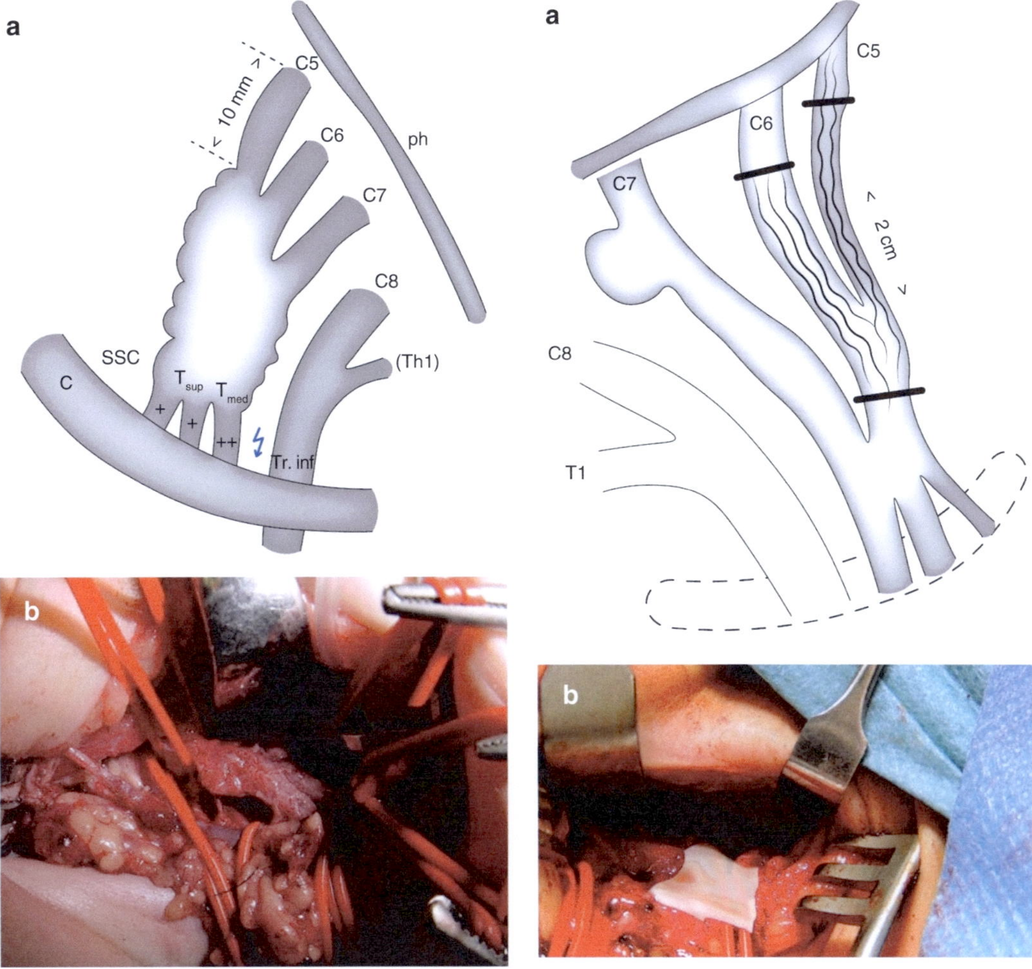

Fig. 15.19 (**a**, **b**) Extended upper lesion: involvement C5–C7, first example. (**a**) Drawing according to an operation sketch by Dr. Bahm (appendix). (**b**) Intraoperative view

Fig. 15.20 (**a**, **b**) Extended upper lesion: involvement C5–C7, second example. (**a**) Drawing according to an operation sketch by Dr. Bahm (appendix). (**b**) Intraoperative view

become too out of balance as a result of the pubertal growth spurt; therefore we usually recommend a period between 6 and 8 years of age.

The situation is different if the children are presented for the first time at an advanced age and have not been treated. Then, of course, one has to adapt to these conditions and tailor the treatment plan to what is still possible and, above all, functionally feasible. Bone corrections can also still be carried out without problems in adults, but experience has shown that muscle transfer at large, proximal joints such as the shoulder is no longer effective after puberty.

From school age on, it is also very important to involve the child in planning and decision-making, which not only values and motivates them but also relieves the parents of their sense of responsibility ("we don't want to be accused later of not having done everything").

An important time phase is puberty, when especially girls are confronted for the first time with aesthetic aspects concerning body image and arm position. This refers, for example, to the visibly "conspicuous" internal rotation malposition of the arm, the elbow contracture or a dropping hand.

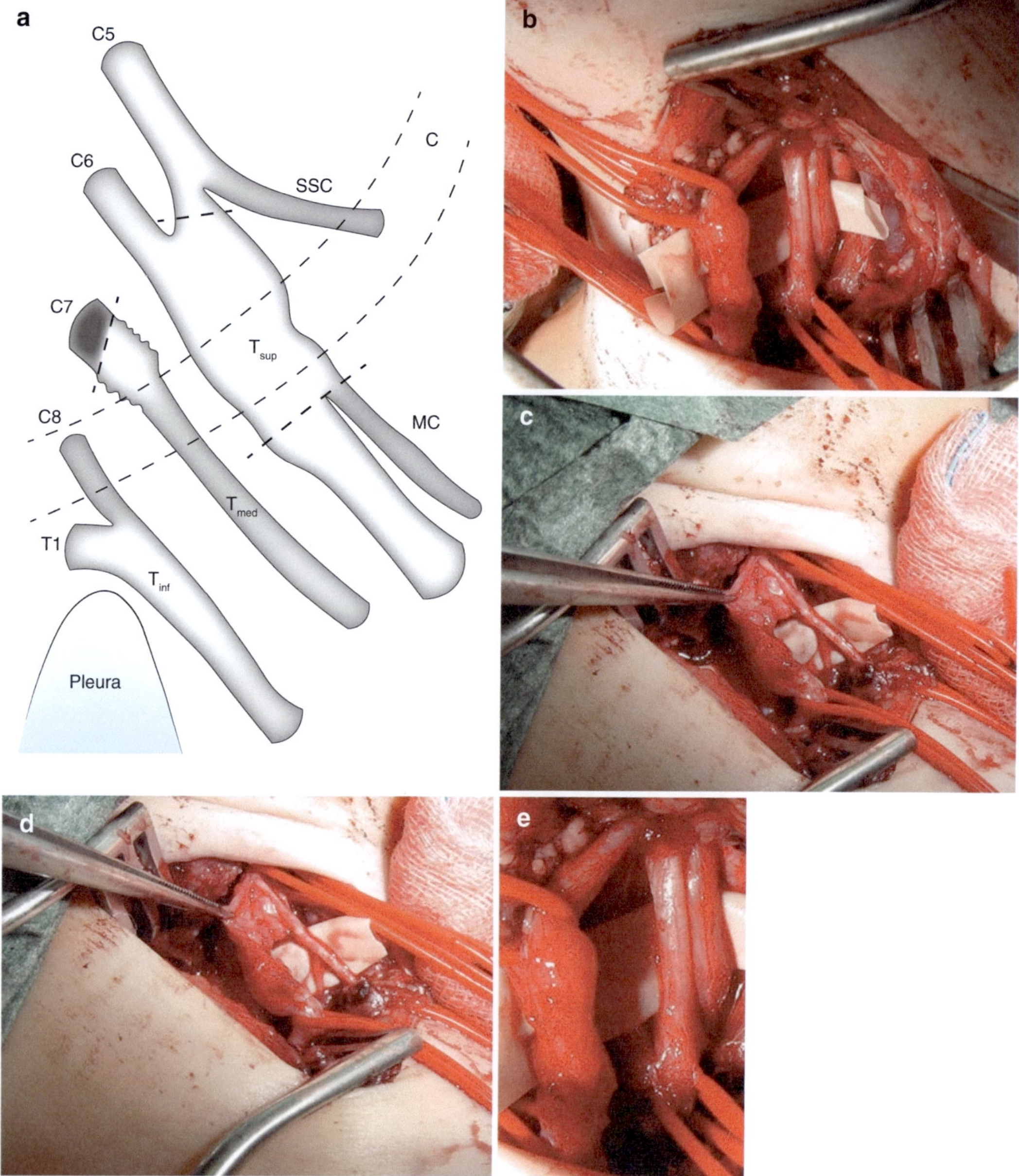

Fig. 15.21 (**a–e**) Extended upper lesion: involvement C5–C7, third example. (**a**) Drawing according to an operation sketch by Dr. Bahm (appendix). (**b–e**) Intraoperative view

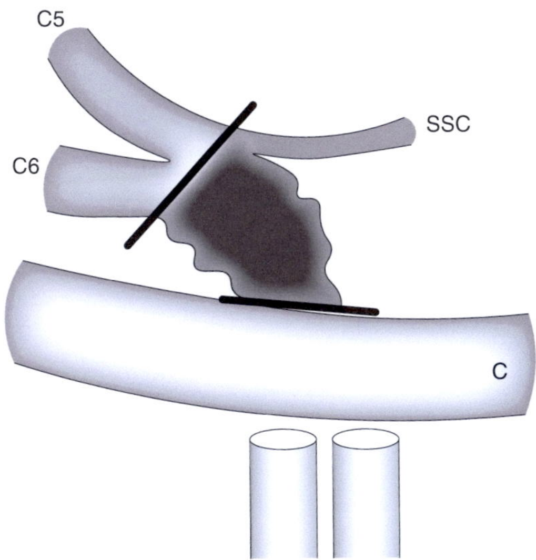

Fig. 15.22 Extended upper lesion: involvement C5–C7, fourth example. Drawing after an operation sketch by Dr. Bahm (appendix)

Young adults come to an initial presentation because they want to know what modern medicine and surgery can offer, or because the rotation deformity disturbs the motion sequences, or because the first load-dependent shoulder pain occurs. Consultation with an orthopaedic surgeon is helpful.

15.10 Results After Primary Nerve Reconstruction

Different centres have repeatedly reviewed retrospectively surgical procedures and functional results using different criteria (e.g., [31, 32]).

Ultimately, the reinnervation result for the arm depends on:

- Type and number of root injuries, especially number of avulsion lesions—with a special consideration of histological root quality [30]
- Density and quality of grafts and anastomoses
- Combination with selective (motor) nerve transfers, which show good reinnervation accuracy, but limited strength [33, 34]
- Quality of physiotherapeutic follow-up treatment
- Upgrading through well-chosen secondary procedures

Due to the almost intact hand function, upper lesions allow to re-integrate the upper extremity quite well; an active abduction of the shoulder of 90°–120°, a flexion of 90°, an active external rotation of about 40°–70° with abducted arm and of 30° with adducted arm, an active elbow flexion of 130° with force degree M3–M4 and a good triceps can be achieved.

Subtotal and complete lesions suffer from the reduced number of nerve root donors and in particular from the lost hand movement, which even with good neurotization of the inferior trunk clearly lags behind a normal hand (Fig. 15.34b–d). If contractures are rare in these arms, bone growth is affected, and many of the reinnervated muscles remain rather weak and limit the possibility of secondary muscle transfers. Usually the arm becomes a more or less usable auxiliary arm.

15.11 Secondary Nerve Surgery

The individual procedures are described in an anatomical-topographical manner in Chap. 21. They can generally be divided into two groups:

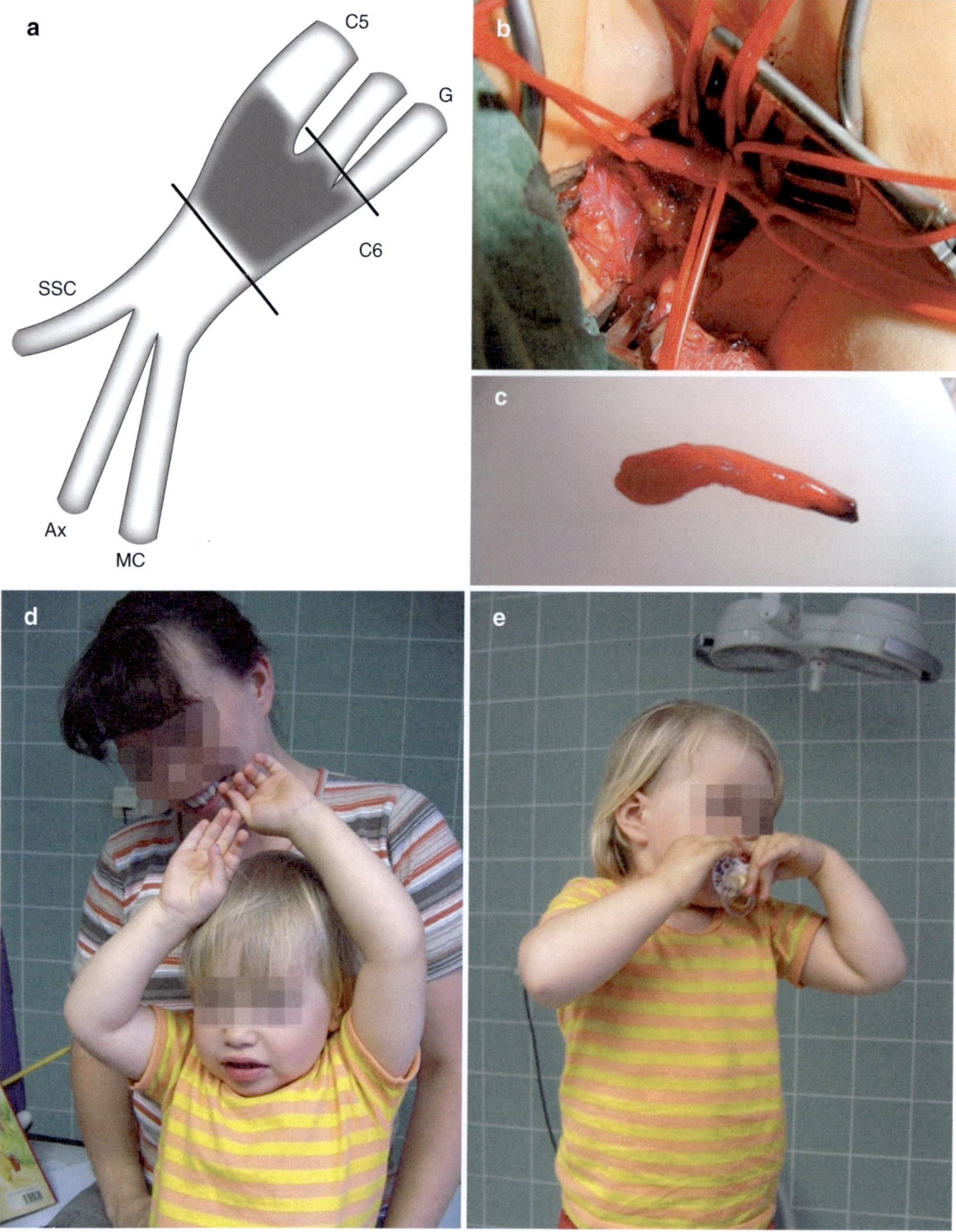

Fig. 15.23 (**a–e**) Upper lesion as in Fig. 15.16 with avulsion of root C6: reconstruction of C5, first example. (**a**) Drawing according to an operation sketch by Dr. Bahm (appendix). (**b**, **c**) Reconstruction of C5. (**d**, **e**) Postoperative function

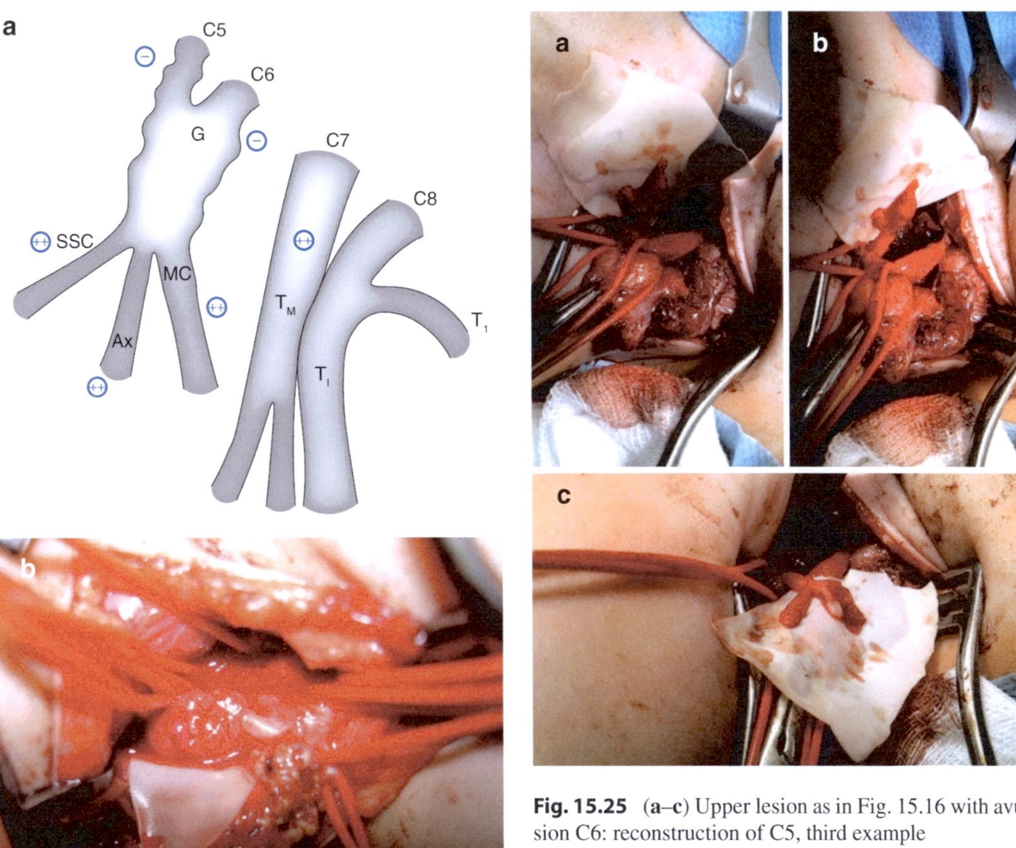

Fig. 15.24 (**a**, **b**) Upper lesion as in Fig. 15.16 with avulsion C6: reconstruction of C5, second example. (**a**) Drawing according to an operation sketch by Dr. Bahm (appendix). (**b**) Reconstruction of C5

Fig. 15.25 (**a–c**) Upper lesion as in Fig. 15.16 with avulsion C6: reconstruction of C5, third example

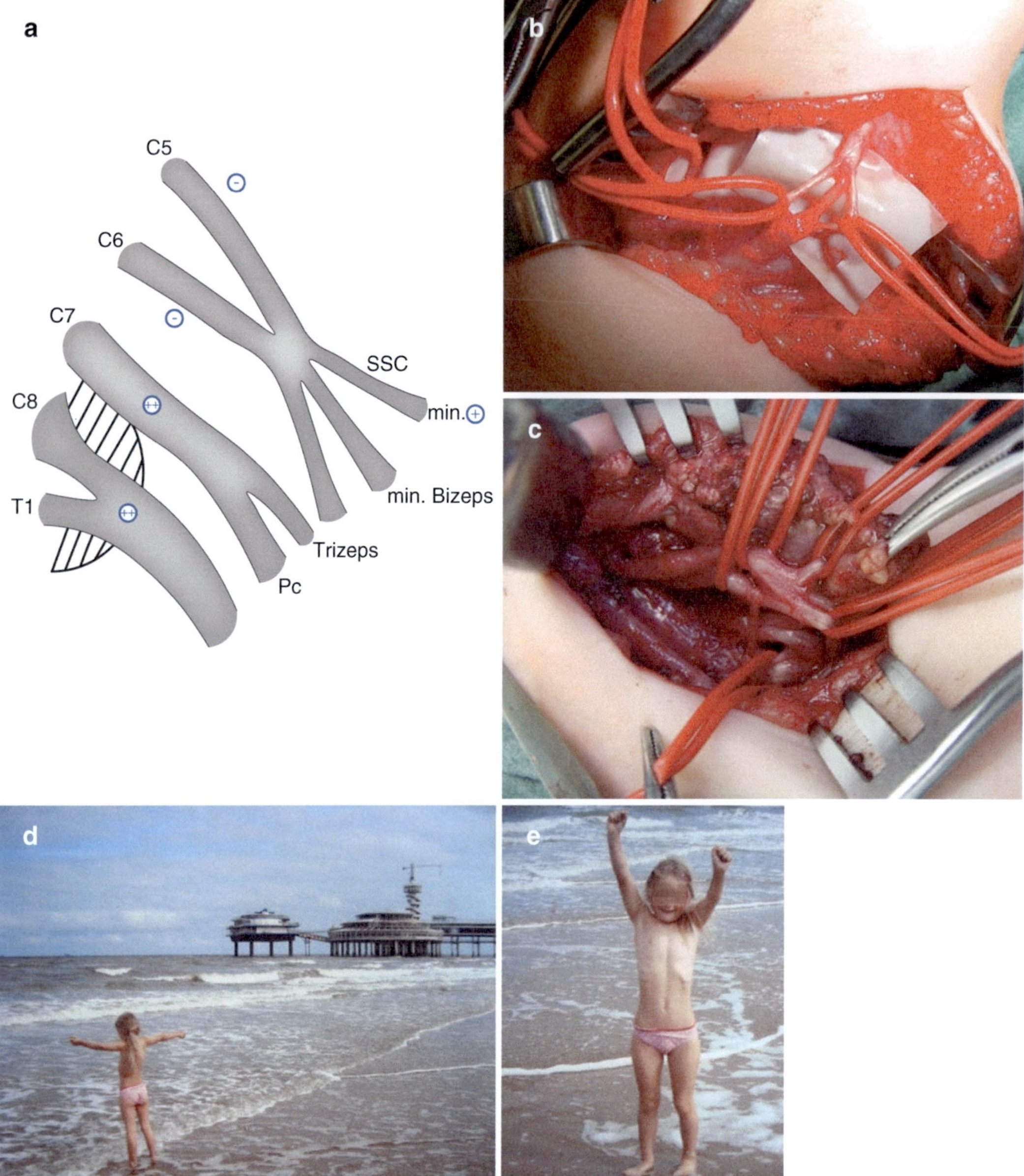

Fig. 15.26 (a–e) Upper lesion as in Fig. 15.16 after breech birth, avulsion of both C5 and C6 roots. (a) Drawing according to an operation sketch by Dr. Bahm (appendix). (b, c) Operative view. (d, e) Postoperative result after nerve transfers

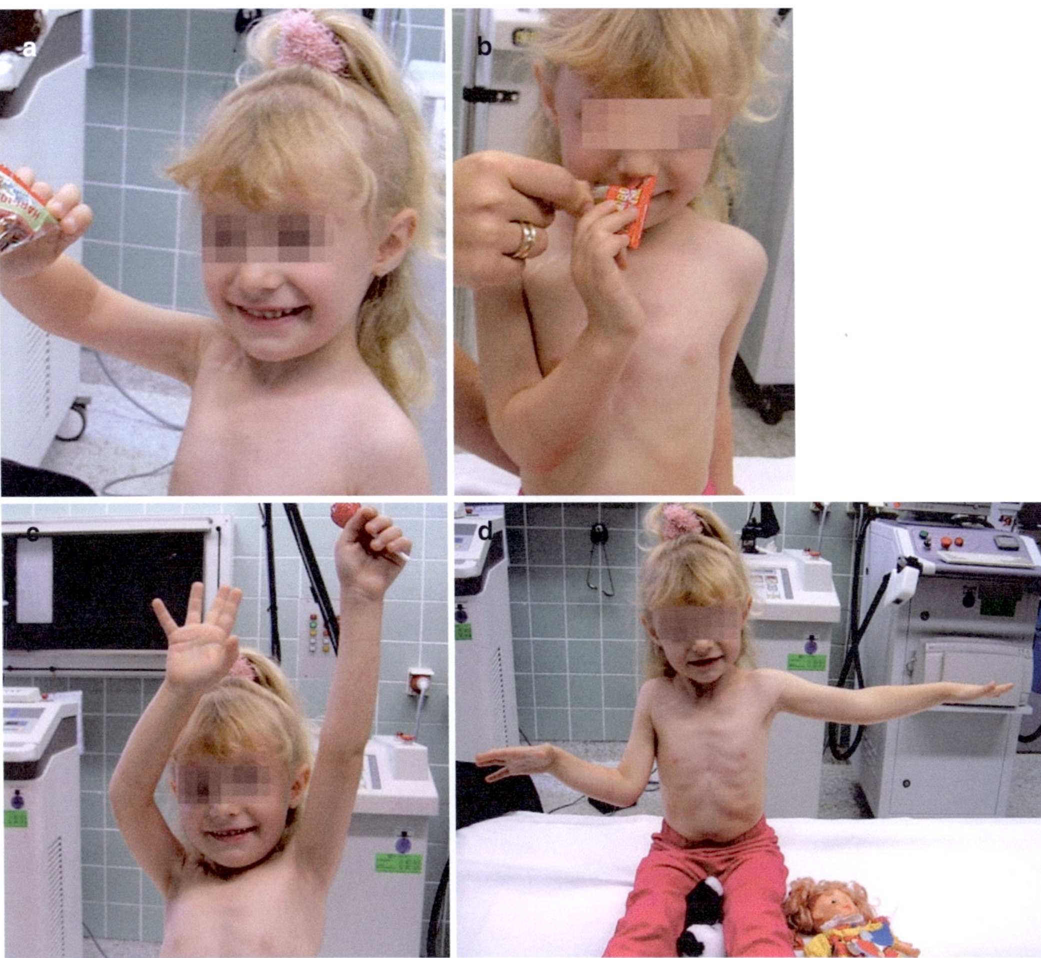

Fig. 15.27 (**a–d**) Postoperative condition in another child with avulsion of roots C5 and C6 as well as reconstruction with nerve transfers

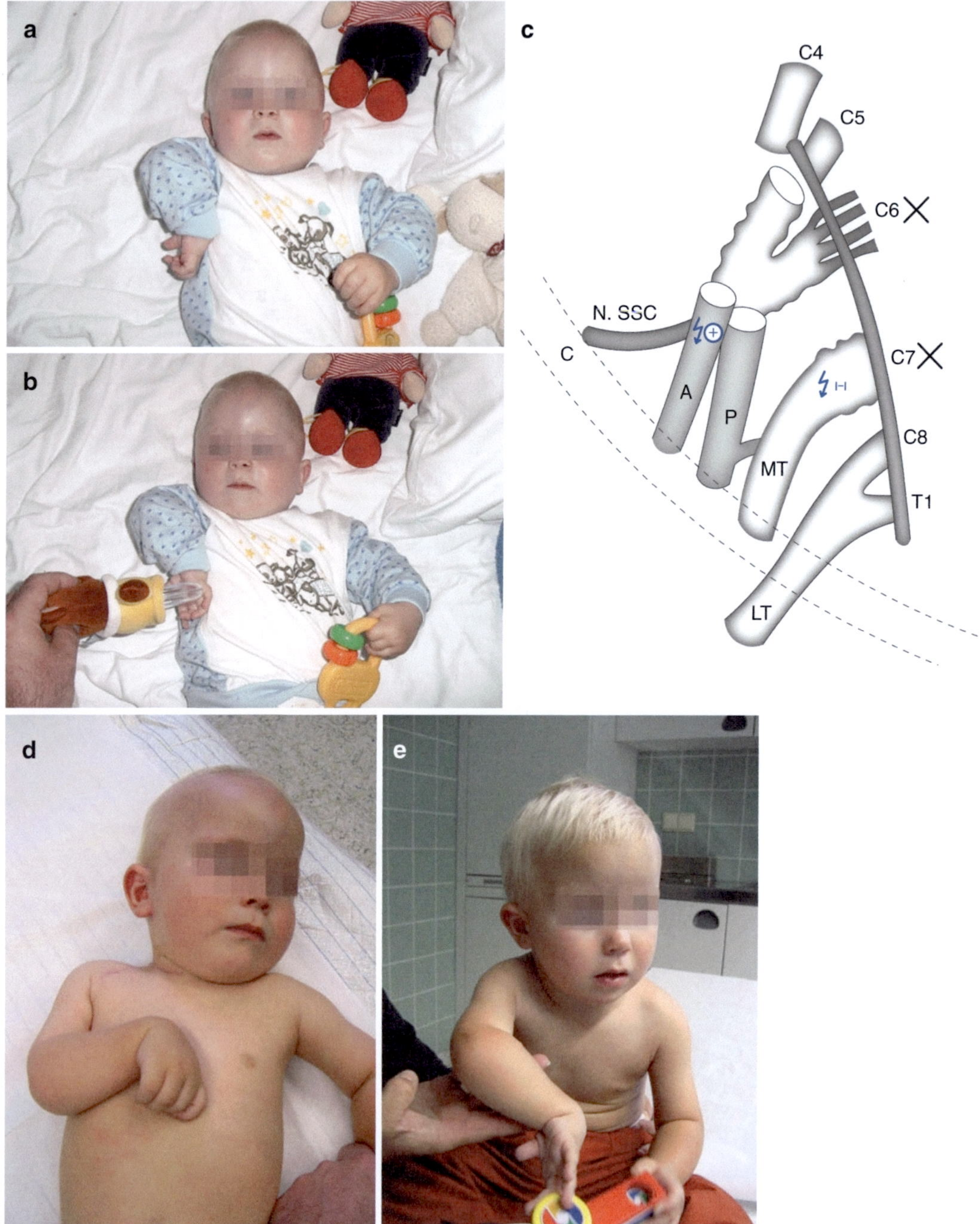

Fig. 15.28 (**a–e**) Avulsion of C6–C7, first example. (**a, b**) Preoperative findings. (**c**) Drawing according to an operation sketch by Dr. Bahm (appendix). (**d, e**) Postoperative findings

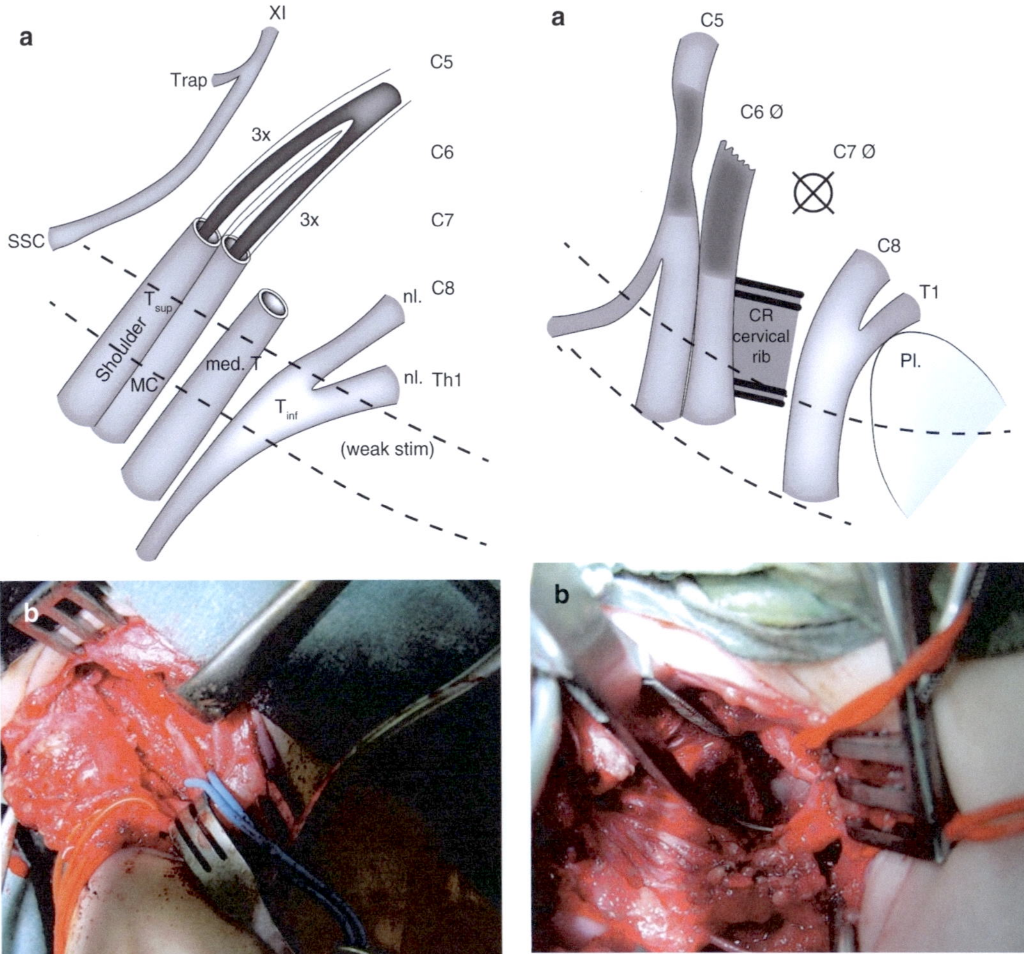

Fig. 15.29 (**a**, **b**) Avulsion C6–C7, second example. (**a**) Drawing according to an operation sketch by Dr. Bahm (appendix). (**b**) Intraoperative view ((**a**) Schulter = shoulder>; Stim.schwach = weak stim)

Fig. 15.30 (**a**, **b**) Avulsion C6–C7, third example, with a cervical rib. (**a**) Drawing according to an operation sketch by Dr. Bahm (appendix). (**b**) Intraoperative view

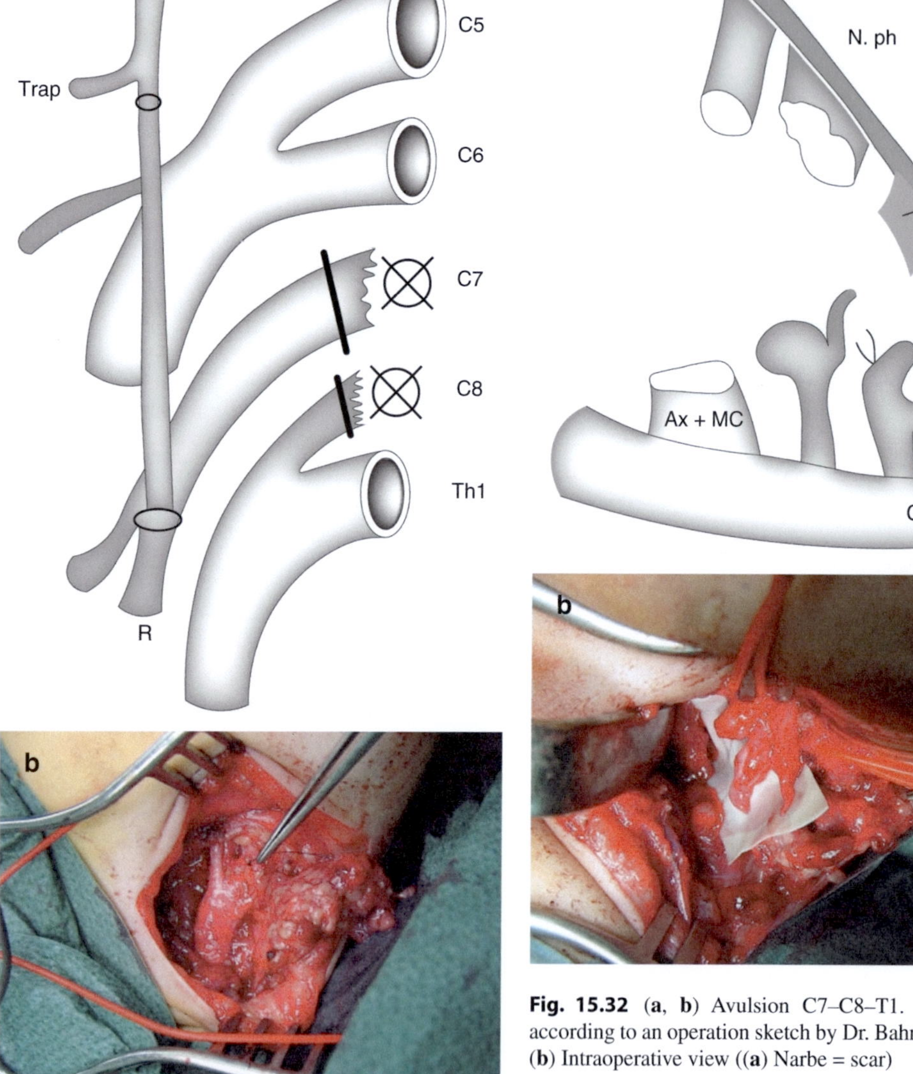

Fig. 15.31 (**a, b**) Avulsion C7–C8. (**a**) Drawing according to an operation sketch by Dr. Bahm (appendix). (**b**) Intraoperative view

Fig. 15.32 (**a, b**) Avulsion C7–C8–T1. (**a**) Drawing according to an operation sketch by Dr. Bahm (appendix). (**b**) Intraoperative view ((**a**) Narbe = scar)

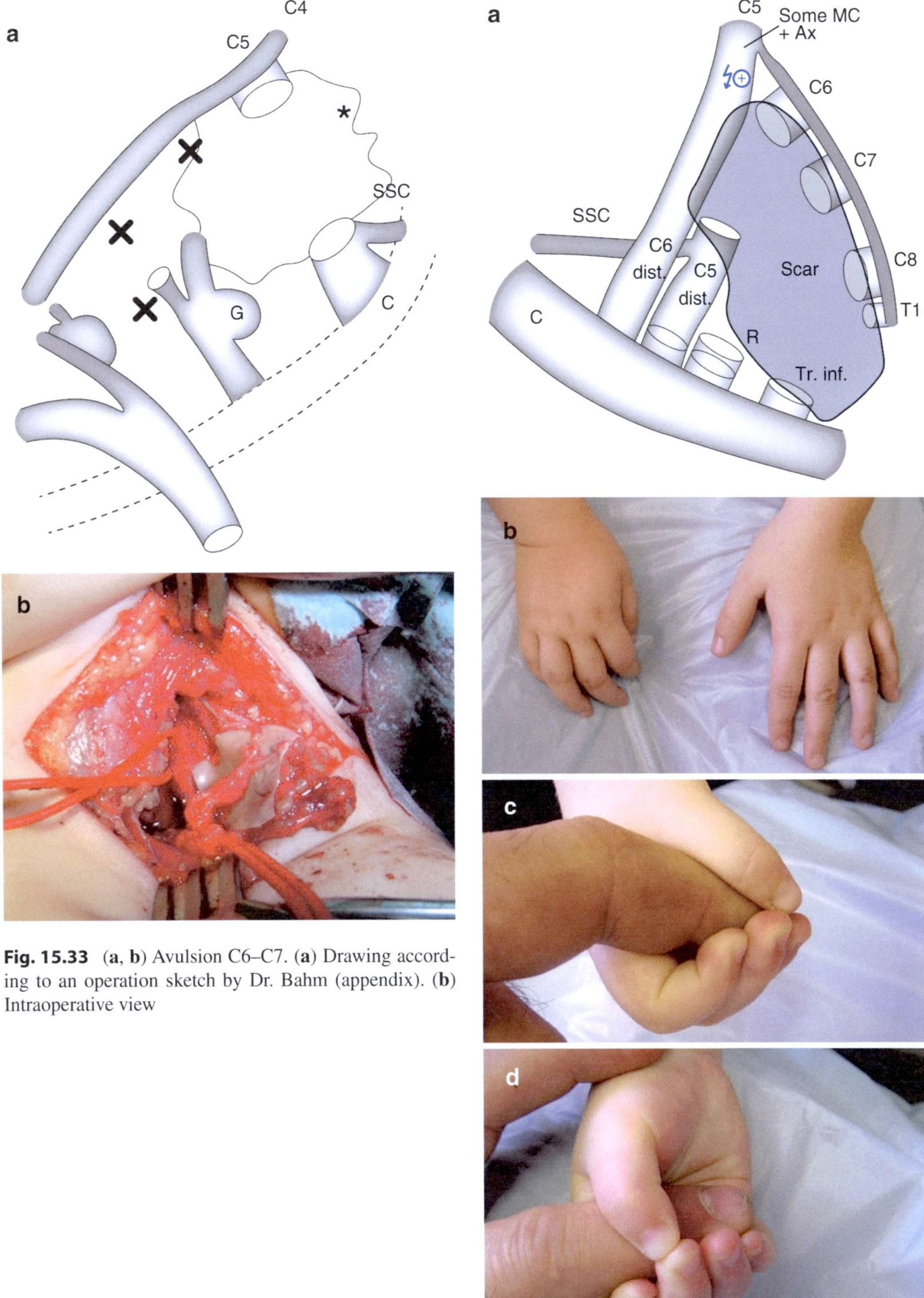

Fig. 15.33 (**a**, **b**) Avulsion C6–C7. (**a**) Drawing according to an operation sketch by Dr. Bahm (appendix). (**b**) Intraoperative view

Fig. 15.34 (**a–d**) Subtotal lesion C5–C8, T1 intact, first example. (**a**) Drawing according to an operation sketch by Dr. Bahm (appendix). (**b–d**) Postoperative hand function ((**a**) Etwas = some; Narbe = scar)

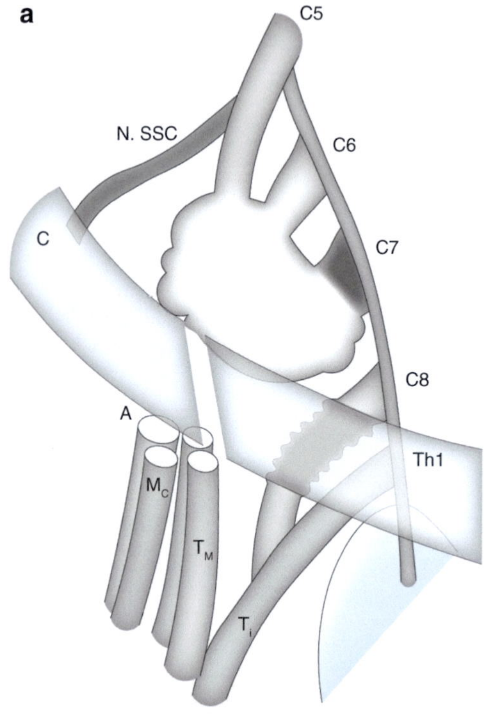

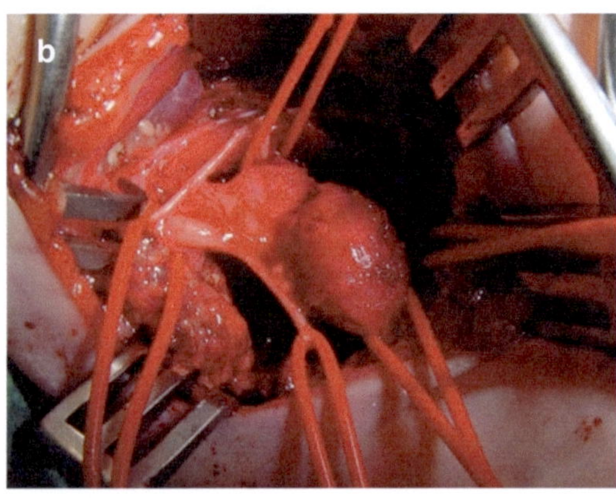

Fig. 15.35 (**a, b**) Subtotal lesion C5–C8, T1 intact, second example. (**a**) Drawing according to an operation sketch by Dr. Bahm (appendix). (**b**) Intraoperative view

– Interventions with predictable outcomes, having been well investigated. These include muscle transfer to enhance external rotation of the shoulder, correction of the drop hand or the supination malposition of the forearm.
– Experimental surgical solutions, with unpredictable results or technically difficult or impracticable: various manifestations of shoulder contracture with complex joint malformation, luxation of the radial head, pronounced flexion contracture of the elbow and ulnar deviation of the wrist. In particular, in severe complete paralysis, the weak distal reinnervation often makes it difficult to impossible to perform tendon transfers to improve hand function.

Current clinical research concentrates primarily on addressing these orphaned problems, preventing them and developing promising surgical techniques (see Chap. 21).

In general, it must be said about secondary surgery that it may be read like a recipe, but is by no means indispensable. It must be individually oriented to the needs and wishes of the growing child and should not be imposed by the parents: In a somewhat provocative manner, I always state to the parents that the child with plexus paresis will definitely be integrated and cope with our technical world—and therefore our "secondary plan" only represents an upgrading and balancing—provided that the patient can get a benefit in his everyday life (and accordingly participate postoperatively in the functional rehabilitation). At some point there comes the moment when a child who has undergone multiple previous operations should not be put back on the operating

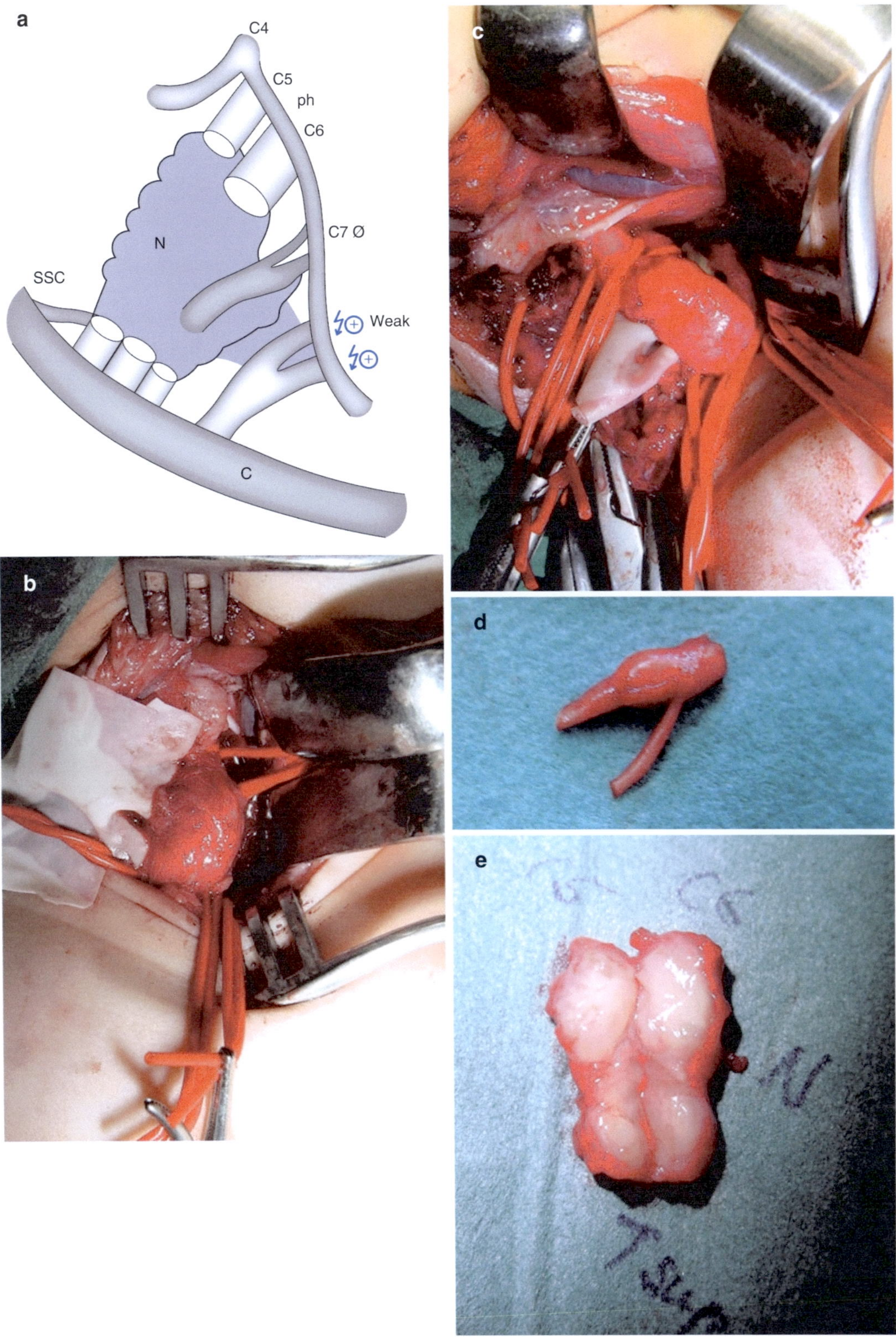

Fig. 15.36 (a–e) Subtotal lesion C5–C8, T1 intact, third example. (a) Drawing according to an operation sketch by Dr. Bahm (appendix). (b–e) Intraoperative view with avulsed root C7 (c) and neuroma C5–C6 (d, e) ((a) Schwach = weak)

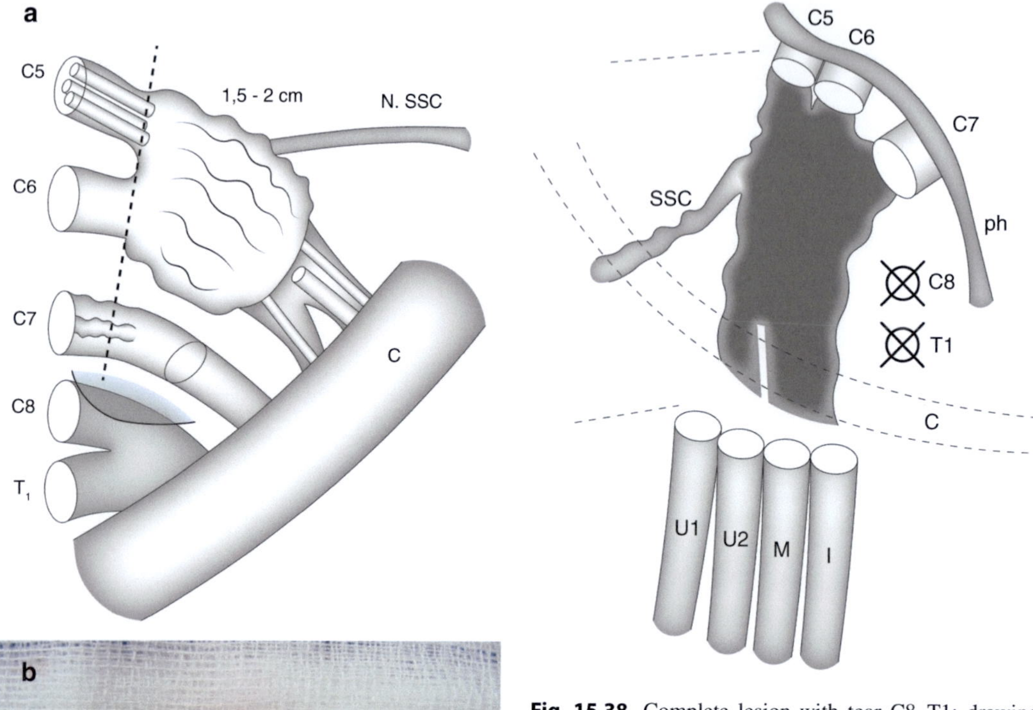

Fig. 15.38 Complete lesion with tear C8–T1; drawing after an operation sketch by Dr. Bahm (appendix)

Fig. 15.37 (**a**, **b**) Complete lesion with avulsion of root C8. (**a**) Drawing according to an operation sketch by Dr. Bahm (appendix). (**b**) Sliced

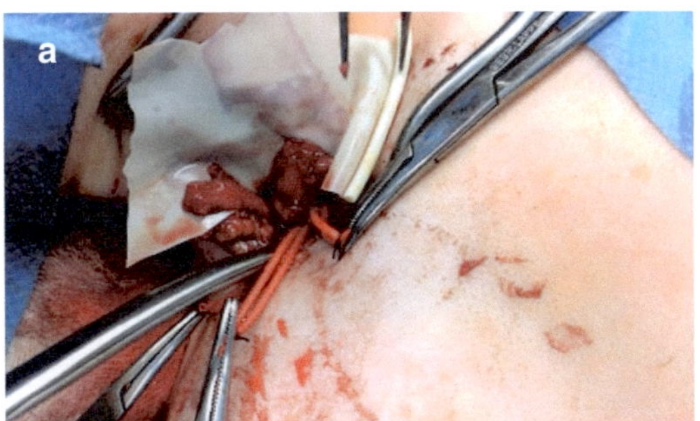

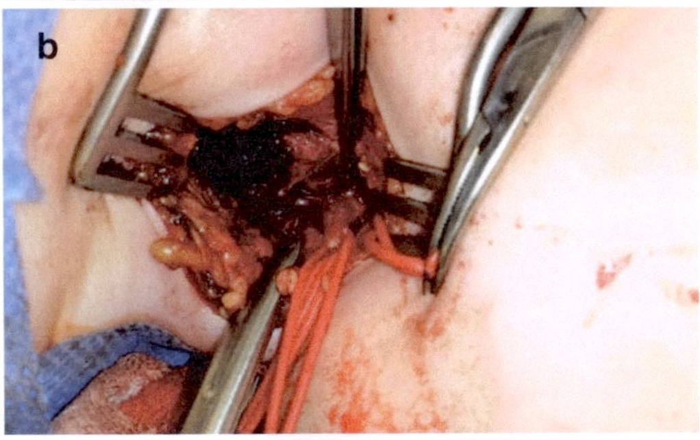

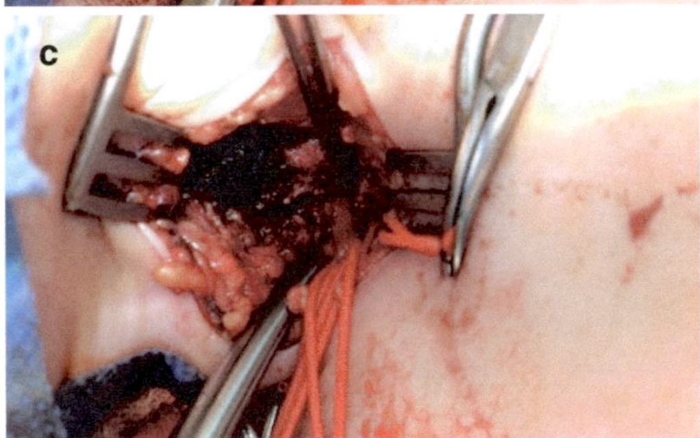

Fig. 15.39 (**a–c**) Complete lesion with three upper avulsions

table or when a functional status can only be minimally improved or when a patient temporarily or definitely withdraws from meaningful therapy or operation options. Here we may even encounter disease patterns of a serious nature, with somatic or psychological causes such as hyperactivity syndrome, borderline disorder and autism, which make a further intervention harmful or even impossible.

15.12 Late Nerve Surgery

Finally, some exceptional situations in the reconstruction plan that are somewhat outside the usual time schedule (so-called late nerve surgery) should be mentioned.

- Resensibilization of the insensible hand or presenting nail dystrophies (Fig. 15.45).
- Revision of previous primary interventions with little or no success (in which the failure to recover functions does not allow any alternative but delayed access to the original site of operation for revision and a new temptative of reconstruction).

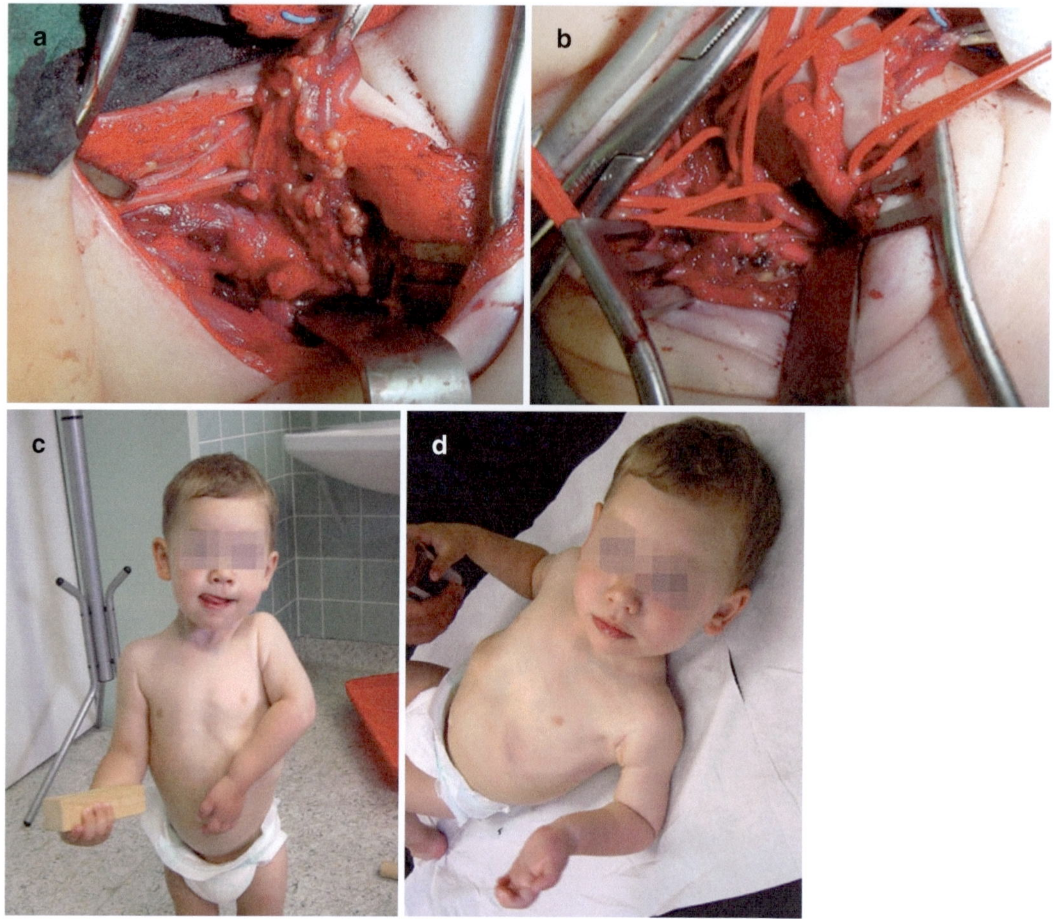

Fig. 15.40 (**a–d**) Complete lesion with four lower root avulsions. (**a**, **b**) Intraoperative view. (**c**, **d**) Postoperative result

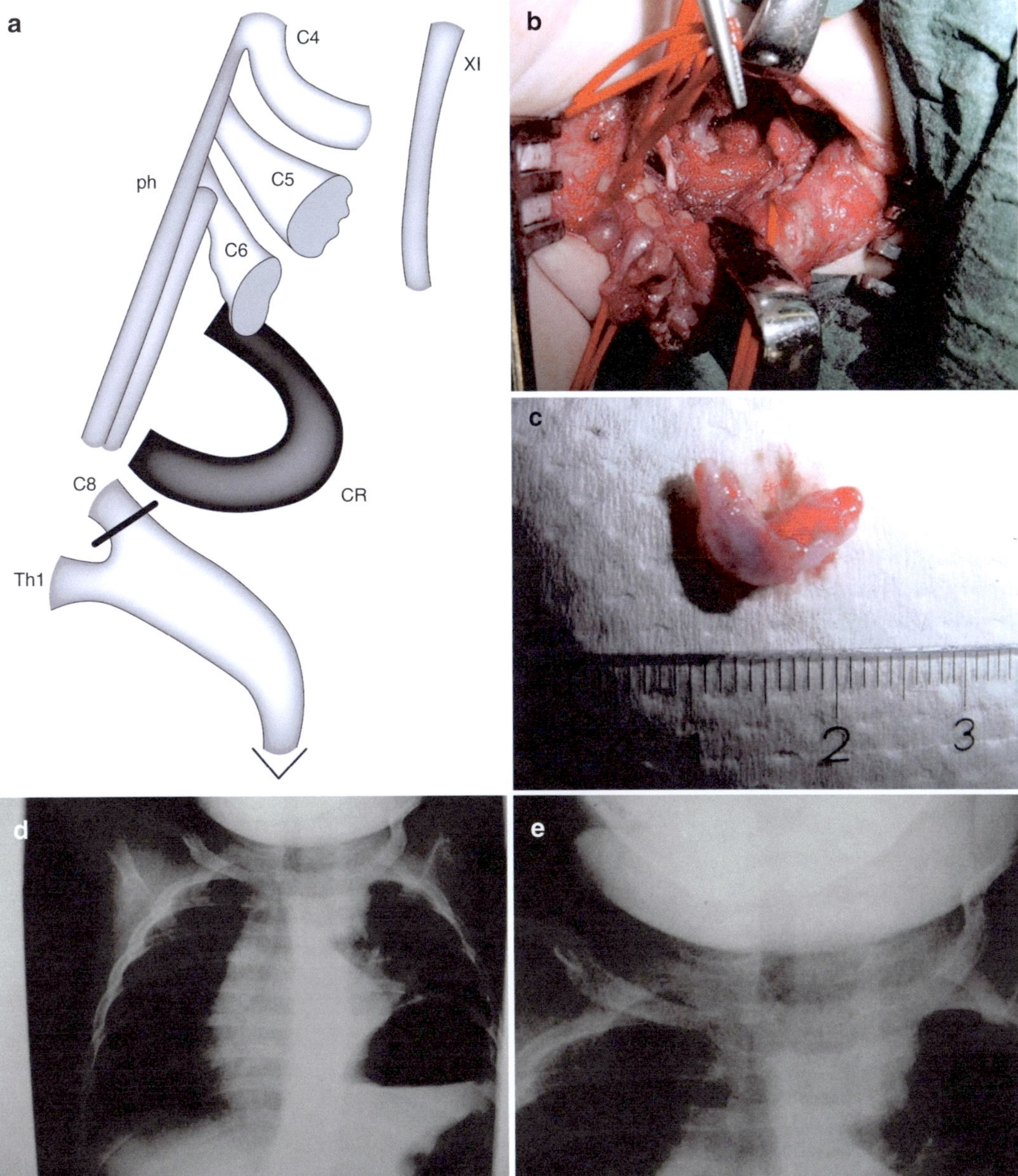

Fig. 15.41 (**a–e**) Cervical rib, first example. (**a**) Drawing according to an operation sketch by Dr. Bahm (appendix). (**b, c**) Intraoperative findings. (**d, e**) Radiological findings ((**a**) HR = CR)

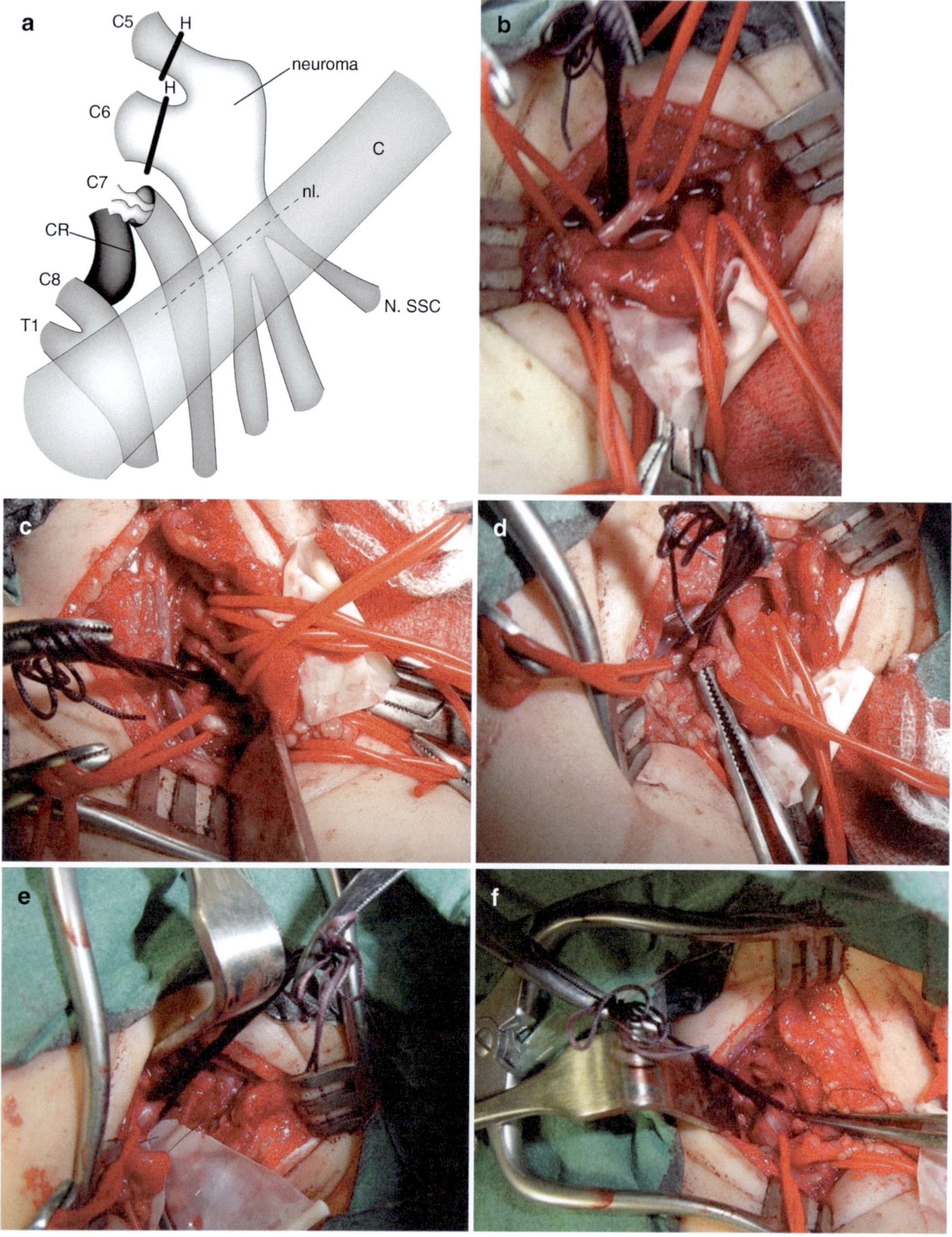

Fig. 15.42 (**a–f**) Cervical rib, second example. (**a**) Drawing according to an operation sketch by Dr. Bahm (appendix). (**b–f**) Intraoperative findings ((**a**) Neurom = neuroma)

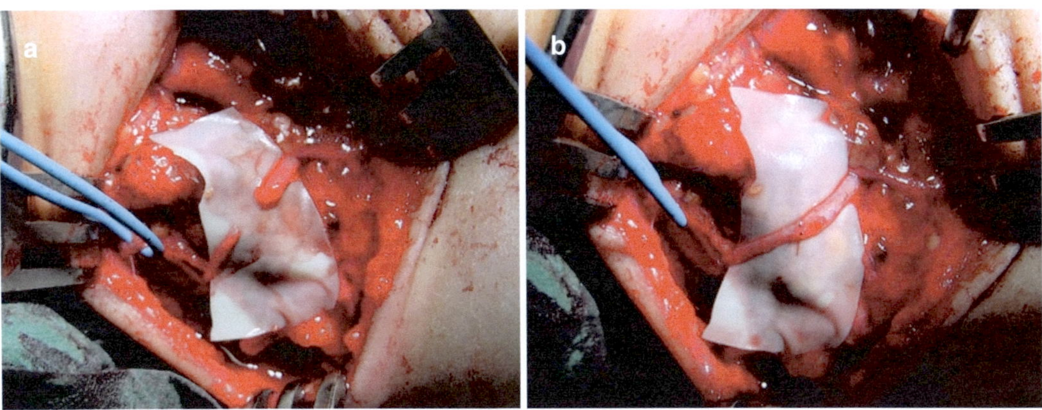

Fig. 15.43 (**a, b**) Reconstruction of the external rotation of the shoulder through supraclavicular incision

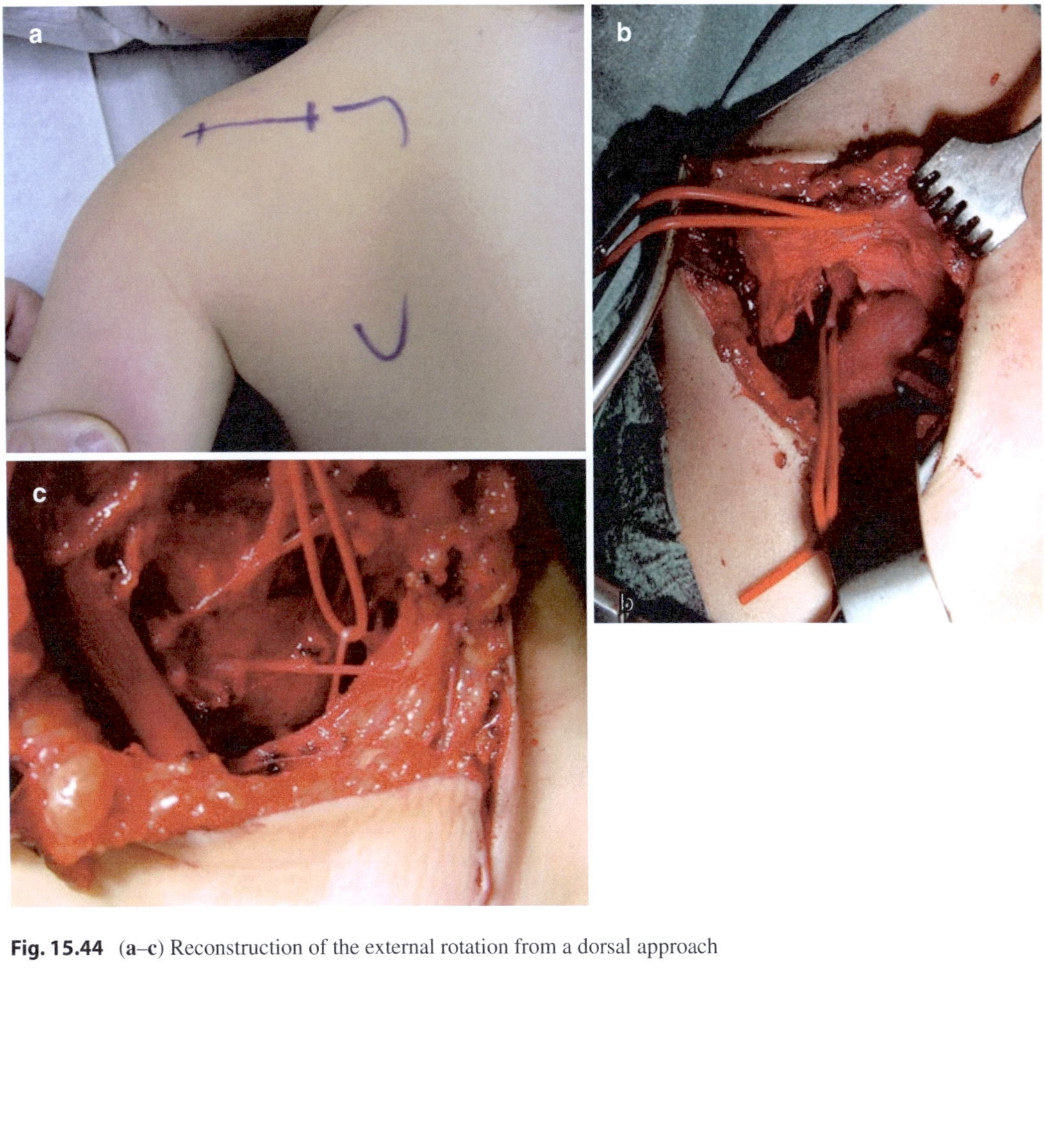

Fig. 15.44 (**a–c**) Reconstruction of the external rotation from a dorsal approach

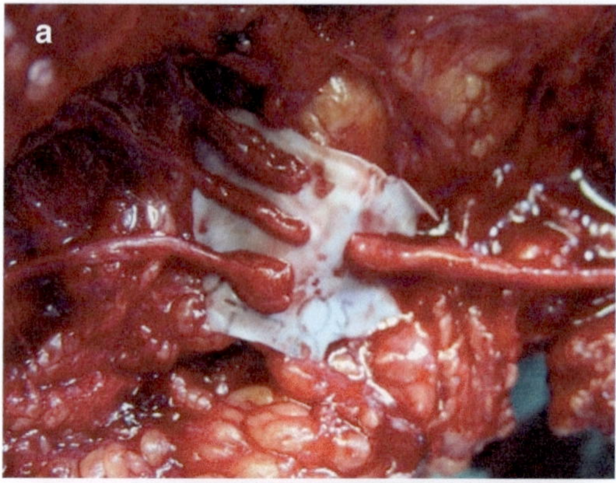

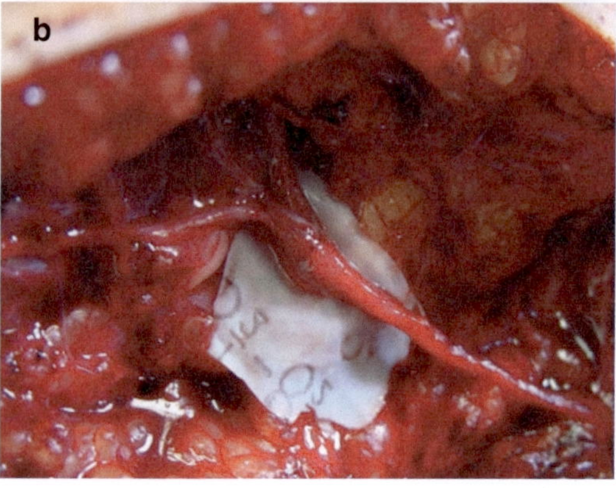

Fig. 15.45 (**a**, **b**) Resensibilization of the median nerve by transfer of the intercostobrachial nerve

References

1. Bahm J, Becker M, Disselhorst-Klug C, Williams C, Meinecke L, Müller H, Sellhaus B, Schröder JM, Rau G. Surgical strategy in obstetric brachial plexus palsy: the Aachen experience. Semin Plast Surg. 2004;18:285–99.

2. Blaauw G, Muhlig RS, Vredeveld JW. Management of brachial plexus injuries. In: Advances and technical standards in neurosurgery, vol 33. Berlin, Heidelberg/ New York: Springer; 2008. p. 201–31.

3. Bahm J. Die kindliche Armplexusparese-Übersicht zur Klinik, Pathophysiologie und chirurgischen Behandlungsstrategie. Handchir Mikrochir Plast Chir. 2003;35(2):83–97.

4. Kline DG, Hudson AR, Kim DH. Atlas of peripheral nerve surgery. Philadelphia: Saunders; 2001.

5. Millesi H. Neurolysis. In: Boome RS, editor. The brachial plexus. The hand and upper extremity, vol 14. Livingstone, New York: Churchill; 1997.

6. Bahm J, El Kazzi W, Schuind F. Nerve transfers. Rev Med Brux. 2011;32(6 Suppl):54–7.

7. Oberlin C, Ameur NE, Teboul F, Beaulieu JY, Vacher C. Restoration of elbow flexion in brachial plexus injury by transfer of ulnar nerve fascicles to the nerve to the biceps muscle. Tech Hand Up Extrem Surg. 2002;6:86–90.

8. Oberlin C, Durand S, Belheyar Z, Shafi M, David E, Asfazadourian H. Nerve transfers in brachial plexus palsies. Chir Main. 2008;25:S1297–302.

9. Leechavengvongs S, Witoonchart K, Uerpairojkit C, Thuvasethakul P. Nerve transfer to deltoid muscle using the nerve to the long head of the triceps. Part II a report of 7 cases. J Hand Surg [Am]. 2003;28:633–8.

10. Leechavengvongs S, Witoonchart K, Uerpairojkit C, Thuvasethakul P, Malungpaishrope K. Combined nerve transfers for C5 and C6 brachial plexus avulsion injury. J Hand Surg [Am]. 2006;31:183–9.

11. Malessy MJ, de Ruiter GC, de Boer KS, Thomeer RT. Evaluation of suprascapular nerve neurotisation after nerve graft or transfer in the treatment of brachial plexus traction lesions. J Neurosurg. 2004;101:377–89.

12. Bahm J, Noaman H, Becker M. The dorsal approach to the suprascapular nerve. Plast Reconstr Surg. 2005;115:240–4.

13. Narakas AO. Neurotization in the treatment of brachial plexus injuries. In: Gelberman RH, editor. Operative nerve repair and reconstruction. Philadelphia: Lippincott; 1991. p. 1329–58.

14. Malessy MJ, Thomeer RT, van Dijk JG. Changing central nervous system control following intercostals nerve transfer. J Neurosurg. 1998;89:568–74.

15. Malungpaishrope K, Leechavengvongs S, Uerpairojkit C, Witoonchart K, Jitprapaikulsarn S, Chongthammakun S. Nerve transfer to deltoid muscle using the intercostal nerves through the posterior approach: an anatomic study and two case reports. J Hand Surg [Am]. 2007;32:218–24.

16. Liverneaux PA, Diaz LC, Beaulieu JY, Durand S, Oberlin C. Preliminary results of double nerve transfer to restore elbow flexion in upper type brachial plexus palsies. Plast Reconstr Surg. 2006;117:915–9.

17. Pet MA, Ray WZ, Yee A, Mackinnon SE. Nerve transfer to the triceps after brachial plexus injury: report of four cases. J Hand Surg Am. 2011;36(3):398–405.

18. Mackinnon SE, Roque B, Tung TH. Median to radial nerve transfer for treatment of radial nerve palsy. Case report. J Neurosurg. 2007;107:666–71.

19. Bertelli JA, Ghizoni MF. Transfer of supinator motor branches to the posterior interosseous nerve in C7-T1 brachial plexus palsy. J Neurosurg. 2010;113:129–32.

20. Colbert SH, Mackinnon S. Posterior approach for double nerve transfer for restoration of shoulder function in upper brachial plexus palsy. Hand. 2006;1:71–7.

21. Bertelli JA, Santos MA, Kechele PR, Ghizoni MF, Duarte H. Triceps motor nerve branches as a donor or receiver in nerve transfers. Neurosurgery. 2007;61:333–8.

22. Palazzi S, Palazzi JL, Caceres JP. Neurotization with the brachialis muscle motor nerve. Microsurgery. 2006;26:330–3.

23. Uerpairojkit C, Leechavengvongs S, Witoonchart K, Malungpaishorpe K, Raksakulkiat R. Nerve transfer

to serratus anterior muscle using the thoracodorsal nerve for winged scapula in C5 and C6 brachial plexus root avulsions. J Hand Surg [Am]. 2009;34:74–8.

24. Gu YD, Wu MM, Zhen YL, et al. Phrenic nerve transfer for treatment of brachial plexus root avulsion. Lausanne: Report at Brachial Plexus Symposium; 1989.

25. Gu YD, Zhang GM, Chen DS, et al. Cervical nerve root transfer from healthy side for treatment of brachial plexus root avulsion. Lausanne: Report at Brachial Plexus Symposium; 1989.

26. Siqueira MG, Martins RS. Phrenic nerve transfer in the restoration of elbow flexion in brachial plexus avulsion injuries: how effective and safe is it? Neurosurgery. 2009;65:A125–31.

27. Sinis N, Boettcher M, Werdin F, Kraus A, Schaller HE. Restoration of shoulder abduction function by direct muscular neurotization with the phrenic nerve fascicles and nerve grafts: a case report. Microsurgery. 2009;29:552–5.

28. Gu YD, Wu MM, Zhen YL, et al. Microsurgical treatment for root avulsion of the brachial plexus. Chin Med J. 1987;100:519–22.

29. Terzis JK, Kokkalis ZT. Selective contralateral c7 transfer in posttraumatic brachial plexus injuries: a report of 56 cases. Plast Reconstr Surg. 2009;123:927–38.

30. Becker MHJ, Ingianni G, Lassner F, Atkins D, Schröder JM. Intraoperative Schnellschnittdiagnostik bei der geburtstraumatischen Plexusläsion-Gegenüberstellung von Makroskopie, HE-Schnellschnitten und Semidünnschnitten mit Toluidinblau-Färbung. Handchir Mikrochir Plast Chir. 2003;35:112–6.

31. Gilbert A, Hentz VR, Tassin FL. Brachial plexus reconstruction in obstetric palsy: operative indications and postoperative results. In: Urbaniak JR, editor. Microsurgery for major limb reconstruction. St Louis: Mosby; 1987.

32. Gilbert A, Pivato G, Kheiralla T. Long-term results of primary repair of brachial plexus lesions in children. Microsurgery. 2006;26(4):334–42.

33. Maricq C, Jeunehomme M, Mouraux D, Rémy P, Brassinne E, Bahm J, Schuind F. Objective evaluation of elbow flexion strength and fatigability after nerve transfer in adult traumatic upper brachial plexus injuries. Hand Surg. 2014;19(3):335–41.

34. Malessy MJ, Thomeer RT. Evaluation of intercostals to musculocutaneous nerve transfer in reconstructive brachial plexus surgery. J Neurosurg. 1998;88:266–71.

35. Merrell GA, Barrie KA, Katz DL, Wolfe SW. Results of nerve transfer techniques for restoration of shoulder and elbow function in the context of a meta-analysis of the English literature. J Hand Surg [Am]. 2001;26:303–14.

Neuro-Orthopaedic Management of Congenital Joint Stiffness and Muscle Spasticity

Leonhard Döderlein and Chakravarthy U. Dussa

16.1 Introduction and Definitions

The syndrome of congenital joint stiffness (incidence 1:3000 live births) is significantly less frequent than spastic disorders (incidence approx. 2–3:1000 live births). Patients with congenital joint stiffness (AMC) as well as children with spastic cerebral palsy (SCP) can easily be recognized by their characteristic joint deformities. Nevertheless both disorders differ substantially from each other.

AMC, also named amyoplasia because there is a definite lack of the formation of specific muscles or muscle groups, is the result of insufficient or absent formative joint movements [1]. Affected children are born with fully developed fixed malposition of a characteristic group of joints of both arms and hands and usually also of both legs. The deformities appear mostly in a symmetric manner and reflect a direct image of the absent muscles which are over-powered by the existing muscles and typical movement restrictions (Fig. 16.1) [2].

Congenital joint stiffness is a different designation for restriction of active and passive joint mobility as a result of lacking muscular and articular development. This is already present at birth with unmistakable typical symmetric malpositions.

The spasticity (spastic paresis; spastic cerebral palsy) is the peripheral manifestation of an acutely or chronically happening damage to the central upper motor neuron and/or central motor pathways in the brain and/or spinal cord.

Patients with spastic paresis of the upper extremity are usually born with normally developed and completely flexible extremities and have all muscles in place. The typical deformation pictures develop as a result of the centrally caused muscle imbalance and stereotyped movement patterns with further growth (Fig. 16.2).

Spastic paresis is the result of a damage to the upper motor neuron (UMN) and leads to characteristic and continuously changing posture and movement patterns due to inadequate central motor and proprioceptive control.

In contrast to congenital joint stiffness, in which the changes in shape and movement are already fully established at birth, the deformities in spastic disorders are subject to continuously acting dynamic influences.

L. Döderlein (✉)
Foot Surgery, Children's Orthop, Aukamm-klinik fur Orthopaedics, Wiesbaden, Germany

C. U. Dussa (✉)
Kinderorthopädie, Orthopädische Kinderklinik, Bernauerstrasse 18, Aschau, Deutschland
e-mail: c.dussa@bz-aschau.de

© Springer Nature Switzerland AG 2021
J. Bahm (ed.), *Movement Disorders of the Upper Extremities in Children*,
https://doi.org/10.1007/978-3-030-53622-0_16

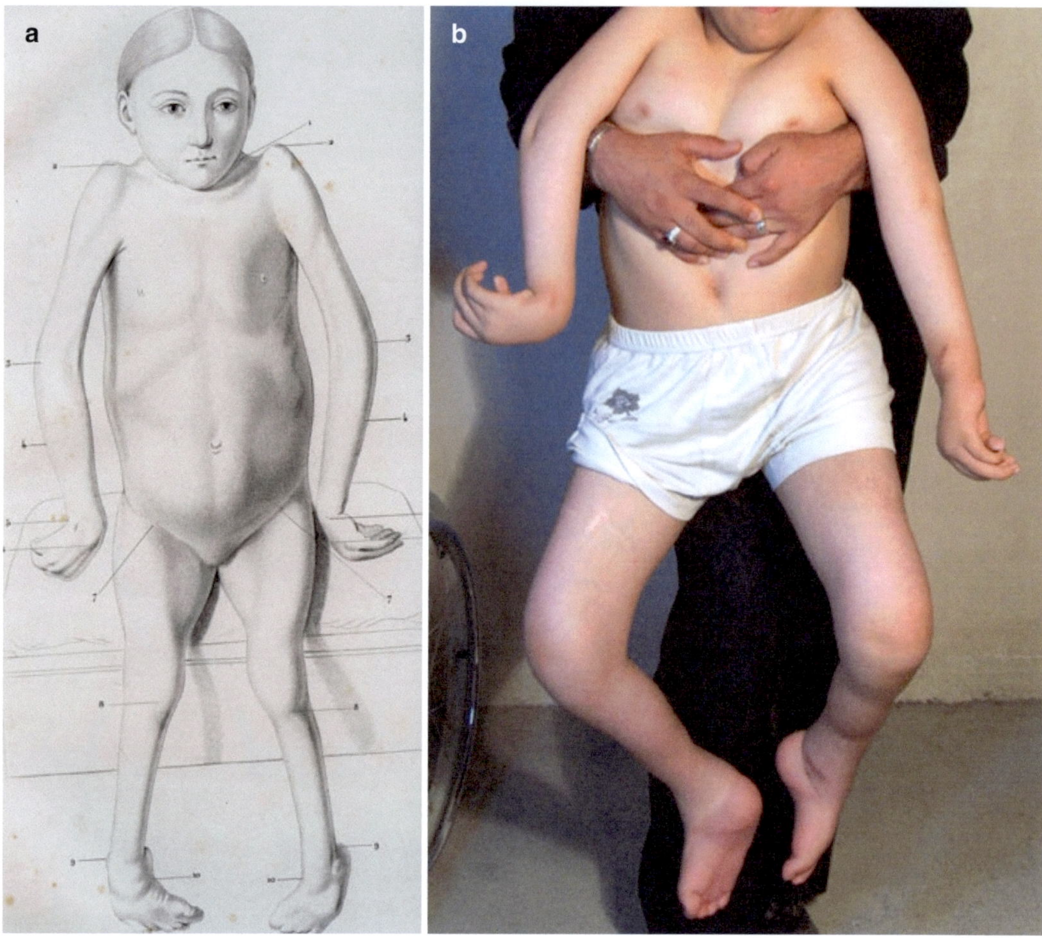

Fig. 16.1 (a, b) Typical examples of similar patients with fully established arthrogryposis and total body involvement, (a) historical picture from Guerin [3], (b): a 12-year-old boy with bilateral deformities of arms and legs

16.2 Causes and Development

In **congenital joint stiffness**, there are a hypo- or atrophy of the affected extremities and musculature and a deformity of the affected joints as a result of a lack of formation, insertion or/and innervation of single muscles or characteristic muscle groups. These muscle deficits cause joint contractures. For joints to normally shape and develop active movements and intact agonistic and antagonistic muscles as well as sufficient passive mobility are necessary. These prerequisites are only partially present or even completely absent. In addition to muscle deficits, connective tissue and neurogenic motor innervation deficits are causative factors [4]. Further accompanying

problems may be vascular disorders, chromosomal aberrations or maternal metabolic diseases. The characteristic joint postures result from gravity, muscular imbalances, activities, compensatory functional efforts and growth. The joint contractures are present from the very beginning. Sensitivity and proprioception as well as central motor programming remain always undisturbed.

In the **spastic paresis**, a variety of causative factors can be found, which include damages of the central sensorimotor centres and pathways. Distinctions can be made between oxygen deficits at birth, congenital brain malformations, CNS damages by infections or trauma, tumours or progressive neurodegenerative diseases.

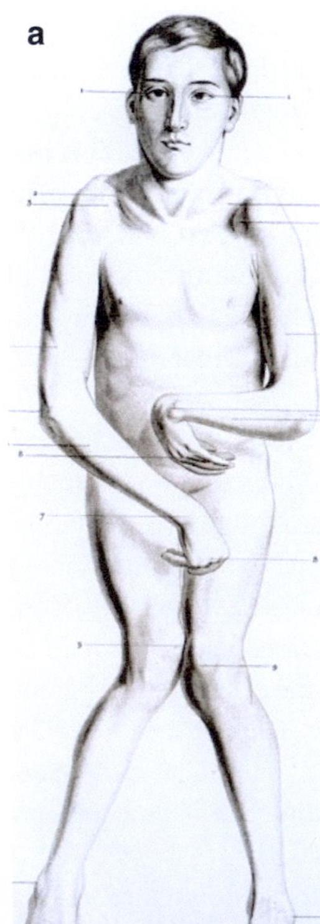

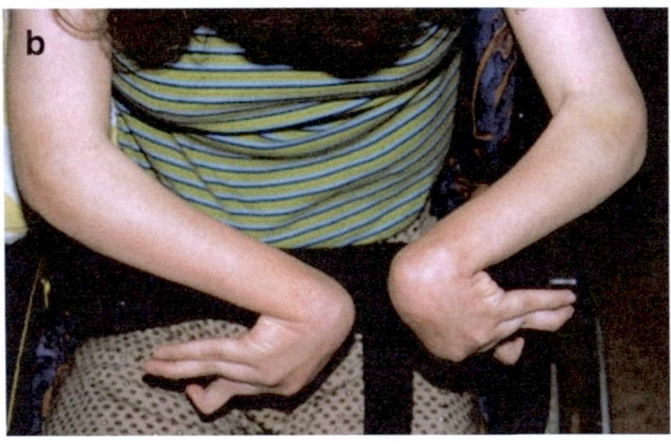

Fig. 16.2 (**a**, **b**) Characteristic pictures of two patients with bilateral spastic paresis, (**a**) historical depiction from Guerin [3], (**b**) a 14-year-old girl with bilateral spastic hemiplegia

Functional impairments of the upper extremity occur either in a unilateral or a bilateral distribution symmetric or asymmetric. The quality of the paresis can be described as spastic, dystonic, ataxic or mixed. The degree of functional impairment is usually graded with a variety of classifications, where the MACS scale (Manual Ability Classification System—[5]) is one of the most commonly used systems.

The main differences between congenital joint contractures (AMC) and spastic joint deformities are the normal central motor programming and the fixed deformities already at birth in congenital contractures in contrast to progressively evolving deformities with growth and disturbed central and proprioceptive motor functions in spastic disorders.

16.3 Functional Consequences

The functional consequences between both groups are fundamentally different. This fact must always be taken into account during diagnosis and treatment planning.

In **AMC** the central control and proprioceptive feedback are intact, but the motor implementation is disturbed. The affected joints are in characteristic malposition and are largely mobility restricted or stiff. The causes are muscle deficits, imbalances and weakness and also compensatory strategies in an attempt to overcome the restrictions. Shoulders, arms, hands and fingers are hypo- or atrophic, stiff and paralytic. Symmetric patterns largely overweigh. It is possible to distinguish predominantly distal distributions from affections of the whole extremity as well as flexion and extension types. The flexion type is a combination form of shoulder adduction and internal rotation, elbow flexion with a partial webbing and wrist and finger flexion and thumb adduction [6].

The extensor type shows similar shoulder, hand and wrist deformities but elbow extension stiffness. Interestingly in contrast to paralysed extrinsic hand and finger muscles, intrinsic function is mostly present but weak. The thumb is adducted because of a lack of active abductors and extensors. Ulnar deviation and interdigital web formation may occur. The fingers are usually contracted in extension or in slight flexion. Skin dimples overlying the affected joints are a characteristic sign (Fig. 16.3).

Proprioceptive function is always preserved as well as the central motor planning. So the affected patients have to develop their own compensatory

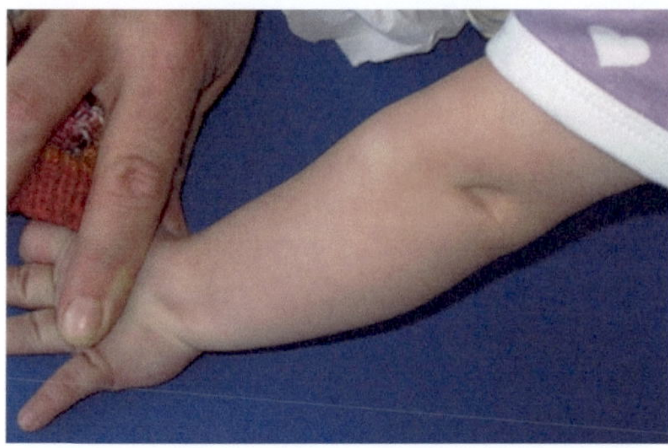

Fig. 16.3 The characteristic dimple sign over the elbow joint in a 2-year-old boy with congenital arthrogrypotic elbow extension stiffness

movement strategies and use the affected arms and hands individually or together like pincers and move them through the trunk activities. A slight flexion of the wrists is favourable for a combined use. In all cases with pronounced weakness and severe contractures, the trunk can be integrated into the motor patterns to compensate for the deficient arm and hand movements. The retained proprioceptive function allows for extremely complex tasks even in only minimal movement residues. This can make extremely deformed hands and stiff fingers still very valuable control instruments, often with computer assistance.

In the absence of active elbow flexion but retained passive excursion, the patient makes hand to mouth contact by throwing his arm up to the mouth or by creating a counter-support of the forearm through his bent leg or with the help of a table edge. Any additional flexion contracture of the wrist can be useful for this purpose as well.

The active innervation of retained muscles results in a constant tendency to worsen the contractures by the mechanism of muscular imbalance pull.

In the case of **spastic paresis**, there is a restriction or even a complete loss of the centrally controlled motor function, which is replaced by characteristic uniform movement patterns of muscles or muscle groups (Fig. 16.4). Spasticity is mostly accompanied by centrally and peripher-

ally mediated muscle weakness. This makes any measure to reduce increased muscle tone undesirable by its additionally weakening effects.

The central cause of muscle weakness is due to an insufficient activation of motor units. Its peripheral component has several components such as stiffening and shortening tendency of affected agonists, elongation of their antagonists, co-activation, joint instability and others.

In contrast to spastic paresis, dystonia is characterized by constantly alternating movements between the end positions of the affected joints. The fluctuating muscle activities represent a peculiar therapeutic challenge, because constantly changing muscle imbalances are hard to calculate and control. On the other hand, dystonic muscles have very little tendency to shorten. During sleep they are completely relaxed. Therefore nighttime splinting in dystonic patients is rarely necessary (Fig. 16.4).

In addition to the motor deficits, a reduction in proprioception but only rarely in sensation can be found. This can considerably restrict the voluntary and targeted use of the hand and arm in less affected patients. In severely impaired individuals, any useful movement of the extremity is impossible. Unilateral spastic paretic patients tend to use their involved extremity as a helping hand at best even if reconstructive surgery has been performed adequately. The more extended the central damage, the more the deformity, and the lesser the retained functional capacity.

Congenital joint stiffness on the other hand is a pure motor problem in which the affected person tries to use the remaining functions individually in the best possible way by use of his/her proprioceptive capabilities.

In spastic paresis on the other hand, there exists a combined problem of sensorimotor control and actuator function which allows the affected persons at best to perform gross motor tasks using few motor patterns. The central deficits are the key to understand the remaining motor capabilities.

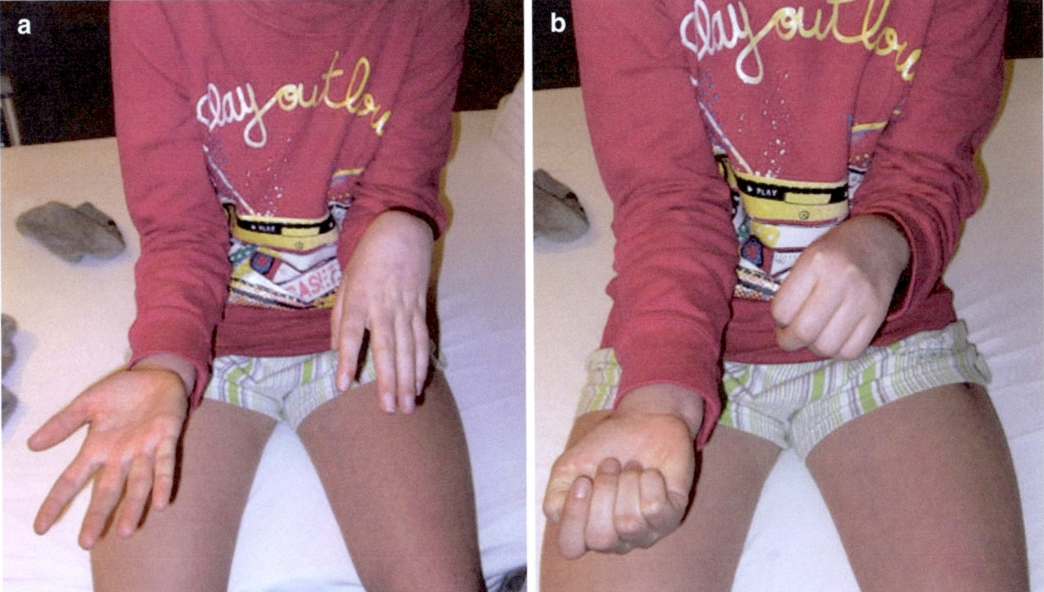

Fig. 16.4 (**a**, **b**) Unilateral spastic cerebral palsy left side with a typical combination deformity of elbow flexion, forearm pronation, wrist flexion and thumb adduction (11-year-old girl)

16.4 Differentiated Indications for Therapy

Every indication must start with a precise analysis of the existing deformities and functional limitations. The use of classification systems helps to define realistic treatment goals. After having set the diagnosis, the leading problems must be outlined, and an individual treatment program must be fixed. This has to be started by using appropriate methods in isolation or combined. Treatment alternatives must always be considered. The treatment program of paretic deformities should follow an integrated multidisciplinary approach. Bach et al. [7] have defined three therapeutic indication areas for the upper extremity in AMC patients:

- Creation of functional movement areas
- Improvement of hand use in everyday life
- Maximizing training and professional capacity

The results which can be achieved should be followed at regular intervals of 6–12 months and—depending on the findings and needs—may be complemented or replaced by new therapy goals as necessary.

In patients with congenital joint stiffness (AMC), treatment should be aimed at improving position, mobility and residual functions. The setting of an indication can be extremely complex in view of often very weak muscles and limited ranges of joint motion present. When there is almost no grip power, both arms and hands should be preserved symmetrically to function like a pair of tweezers (Fig. 16.5). The trunk functions as a moving element of the arms and hands unit. Creating one flexed and one extended arm has often been recommended in the past. The goal "one for the mouth and one for the toilet" could almost never be reached, and the loss of the tweezer function of both arms can thus be much worse than the preoperative situation. In every case of better muscle and movement functions, the main treatment focus should be given to improving functional joint excursion and restoring a grip function between thumb and fingers. In every case the entire upper extremity and the opposite arm must be included in the treatment

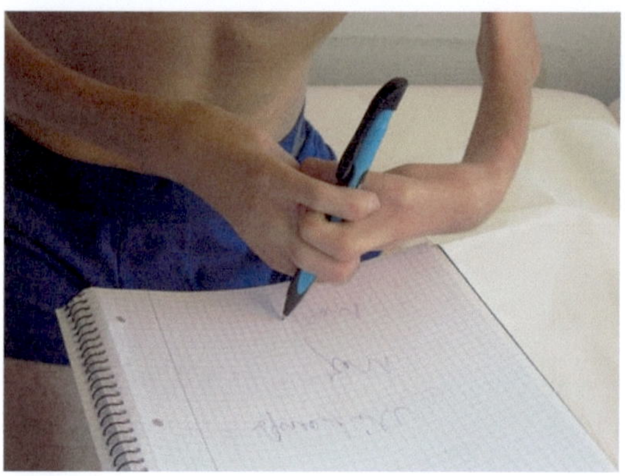

Fig. 16.5 This 5-year-old boy with bil. Congenital joint stiffness uses both hands like a pair of tweezers, which he manipulates by his trunk movements

plan before. Even small improvements in joint position (hand, fingers, wrist) can produce dramatic functional progress (Fig. 16.9).

In the spastic movement disorders, any treatment indication is based on an improvement of a restricted joint excursion and a simplification of complex movement strategies, e.g., gross grip and release hand function. The treatment goals have to be much more modest and depend on the preoperative hand function assessment. It should always consider the use of aids for daily living (grips, walking aids, computers, etc.) too. There are also examples where only hygienic indications are possible (Fig. 16.6).

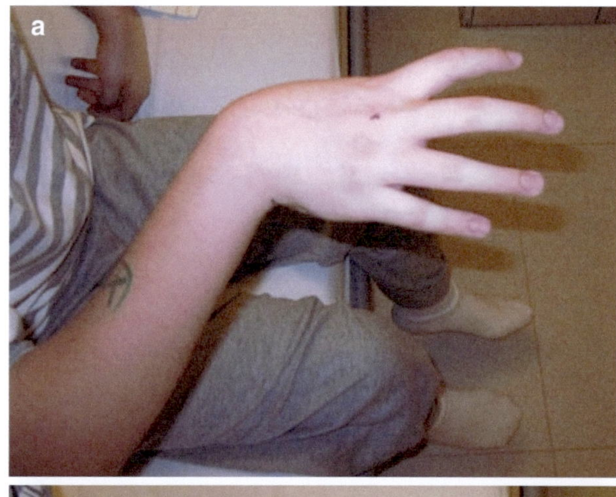

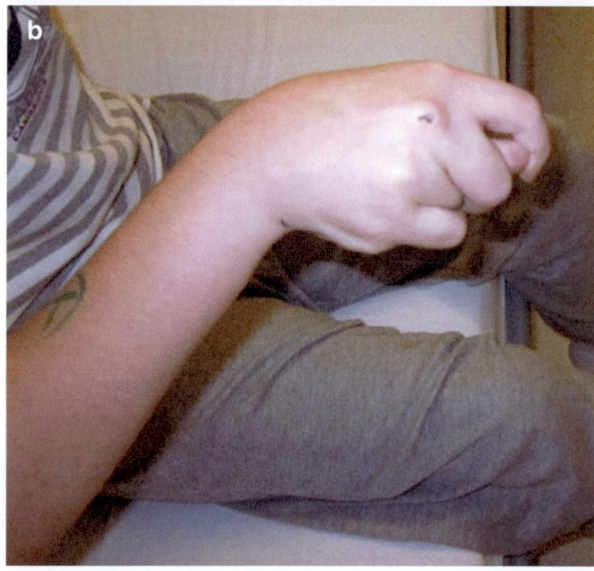

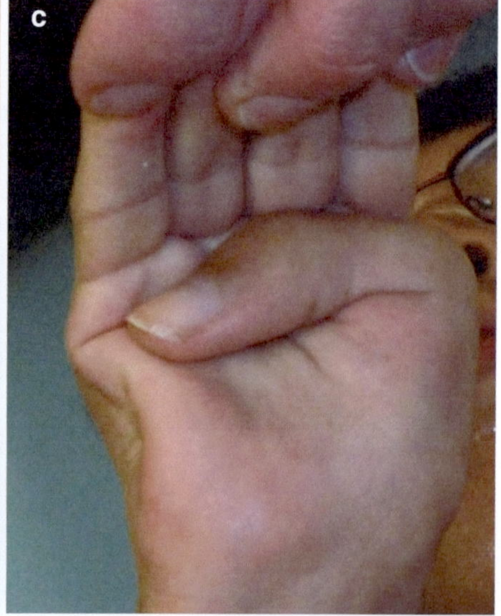

Fig. 16.6 (**a–c**) Palmar flexion spasticity. (**a, b**) Good surgical indication for functional improvement in a 12-year-old girl with unilateral spastic cerebral palsy (SCP), right side. (**c**) A palliative indication in a 13-year-old boy with severe SCP and fixed palmar flexion contractures

In spastic disorders as well as in AMC, the whole extremity must be incorporated in the treatment plan. An exception is cosmetic or hygienic indication. The functional improvements in spastic paretic disorders remain always limited and can only marginally be changed even with the best surgical technique.

16.5 Conservative Treatment

In congenital joint stiffness and in spastic paresis, conservative therapies play a permanent role starting from the beginning. But even after successful surgery, conservative therapies must be continued in most cases as the basic motor disorder with its long-lasting problems remains.

As with every conservative method, the art lies in the selection but also in the intensity of the best suited technique that has to be applied either in isolation or in combination. The effect of any conservative treatment should be checked similar to surgery.

The different conservative methods can be divided into orthotics, rehab technology, physiotherapy, occupational and hand therapy, physical treatments or injections (e.g., botulinum toxin into overactive muscles). These can be added as necessary. For an efficient use, it is of importance to know the basic working principle of each method in order to select the best suited treatment for each situation [8].

Orthotics work with exactly applied external corrective forces. It is necessary that each device has to be built individually for an exact fit. Corrective forces can be applied statically or dynamically by adjustable springs. Functional orthotics support inadequate muscle power and compensate for joint instabilities and deformities (Fig. 16.7). If joints are incorporated, their position must correspond with the anatomical joint axis. Postural orthotics is prescribed for nighttime use either to prevent further deformities or to protect operated joints from recurrent deformities.

In congenital joint contractures, orthoses are mainly prescribed for wrist, finger, and thumb joints. When evaluating an orthotic device, the following six points must be respected:

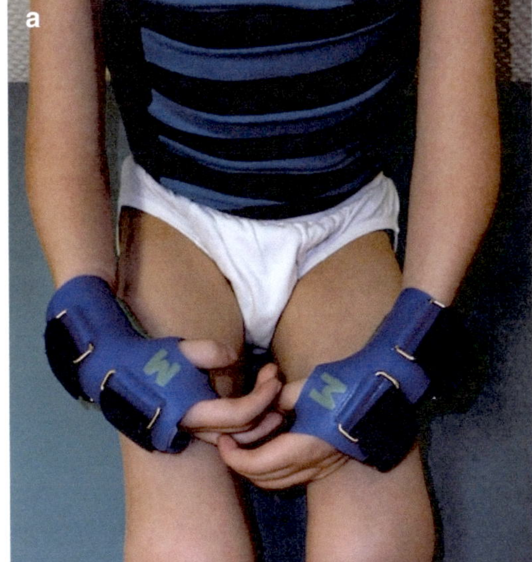

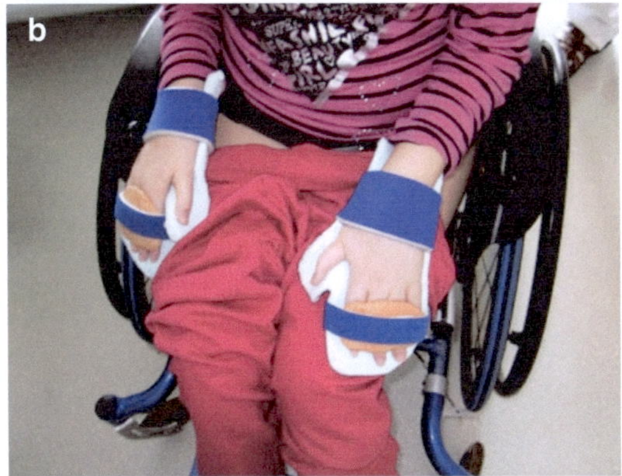

Fig. 16.7 (**a**, **b**) Orthotic management of deformities: (**a**) stable silicone wrist-hand orthoses in a 5-year-old boy with arthrogryposis and wrist flexion deformities. (**b**) Forearm-hand-finger braces to stretch spastic muscles (boy, 10 years old, bil. SCP)

– Is the indication correct?
– Are design and constructive properties correct?
– Is the choice of the materials correct?
– Does the orthosis fit snugly?
– Is the function fulfilled as desired?
– Is the acceptance of the device adequate?

If one or more of these points are not fulfilled, the orthosis must be reshaped or even newly constructed. An orthosis without a functional benefit does not make any sense.

In addition to orthotics, rehab technology takes care for wheeled and walking mobility and is also responsible for individual aids in everyday living situations.

Physiotherapy and occupational therapy including hand therapy: Their professionals are responsible for improvements of joint position, mobility, muscle power and self-care tasks.

They work closely together with orthotists and rehab technicians. Individual exercise procedures must be tailored to each patient and modified and adapted as patients grow. Furthermore the parents should always be instructed how to do specific exercises by themselves as they are members of the treatment team.

It should be pointed out that every treatment method be it conservative, surgical or both should be accompanied by a detailed analysis of functions and definition of treatment objectives. These have to be followed in regular intervals and adapted as necessary.

In the case of congenital joint stiffness, special custom-made positioning orthoses are used to prevent or correct deformities up to the degree which can be corrected manually. Functional orthoses are used to improve standing and walking functions by stabilizing unstable joints and supporting weak muscles. Orthoses for thumb opposition and wrist extension are the most frequent used constructions. Upper arm orthoses to correct elbow range of motion are prescribed postoperatively to stabilize the surgical corrections. These must always be constructed with static or (better) dynamic spring supports working in the desired direction.

Manual redressing joint mobilization techniques rank among the commonly used physiotherapeutic techniques. They are augmented by stretching and strengthening techniques. Hand and finger aids may also be used for improving the use of computers.

In the case of spastic paresis, specially designed exercise programs have been developed focusing towards a better use and recognition of the involved extremity in everyday tasks. These methods are named CIMT (constraint-induced movement therapy) where the less affected or better side is temporarily protected from its use in order to increase the use of the more affected

hand [9]. In the HABIT (hand and arm bimanual intensive training) program, both hands are similarly intensively activated. Injection treatment with botulinum toxin A is used as targeted injections into more spastic muscles. It can halp to better accept the other treatments but is almost never indicated in isolation.

Conservative treatment programs including physiotherapy, occupational therapy and orthotics arc also an important part of every surgical intervention [10]. These programs work best if offered in specialized centres by designated specialist staffs.

Every conservative treatment must be accompanied by individual treatment goals for the short, middle and long terms. These goals do not only consider functional aspects but must always also target towards social improvements of activity and participation International Classification of Functioning, Disability and Health (ICF) goals. The children should be regularly followed in special clinics at least until the end of their growth.

16.6 Surgical Treatment Procedures

Surgery plays an important additional role in both conditions of congenital joint stiffness and spastic paresis. It does however not work in isolation but is always a part of an integrated multidisciplinary treatment approach. Almost every operation should be seen only as a necessary temporary interruption of the long-term conservative treatment program. The only exceptions to this are cosmetic or hygienic indication.

Special surgical management can be offered in hospitals which have adequate facilities for preoperative evaluation and postoperative management programs. Specialists in reconstructive orthopaedics or hand surgery are the prerequisite for tailored approaches to the arms and hands of paralysed patients. The surgical indication setting on the upper extremity is fundamentally different among patients with congenital joint stiffness and patients suffering from spastic paresis.

16.6.1 Indications and Surgical Techniques for Congenital Joint Stiffness

All forms of this disorder have two characteristic features which remain permanent and must therefore be accepted as unchangeable. These consist of the permanent restriction of movement and the muscular imbalance and weakness.

The difficulty with indication lies in selecting the best possible compromise in terms of position, mobility and function.

In most cases, an attempt must be undertaken to shift the already existing limited range of motion to a more favourable range, for example, more towards the direction of extension or flexion depending on the presenting functional situation. According to Bach et al. [7], the indication for surgery in the upper extremity is only about 30%, while almost every patient with congenital joint stiffness (AMC) needs operations to his legs.

The following joint problems often constitute a surgical indication: They are dealt with subsequently pointing towards their indication, the operation principle, the surgical technique and possible problems.

16.6.1.1 Internal Rotation and Adduction Contracture of the Shoulder

Indication

Limited or completely absent passive external rotation and abduction of the shoulder joint complex with corresponding functional limitations (e.g. bimanual tasks, hand to mouth contact but also hygiene problems).

Operation Principle

Restoration or creation of a passive external rotation and abduction position.

Surgical Technique

Correction via a delto-pectoral approach with release of the surrounding contracted muscular and capsular structures (pectoralis major, subscapularis, latissimus dorsi) plus antero-inferior capsulotomy and possible addition of a sub-capital external rotation osteotomy fixed with a stabile locking plate if soft tissue release is not sufficient.

Problems

Insufficient primary correction (less than 30°–40° of abduction, less than 20°–30° of external rotation), recurrent deformity after adequate postoperative mobility due to insufficient postoperative splinting and mobilization and failure of osteosynthesis due to vigorous postoperative treatment.

16.6.1.2 Elbow Joint Extension Contracture

Indication

Insufficient passive flexion of the elbow with functional limitations (no hand to mouth contact), usually significantly less than 90° of passive flexion, but with adequate active distal hand and finger function. In bilateral weak hand and finger muscles, a bilateral extension position of both arms to function as a pair of tweezers is preferable.

Operation Principle

There is usually an aplasia of the elbow flexor muscles with preserved triceps brachii. So restoring passive elbow flexion by lengthening of the triceps tendon and dorsal elbow capsulotomy is performed so that passive support at the forearm enables hand to mouth contact. Adequate active extension function of the triceps should be preserved.

The creation of a sufficiently strong active elbow flexion although wishful thinking often fails because of lacking or weak donor muscles. Several muscles have been reported for this purpose (m. latissimus dorsi, pectoralis major, half of the triceps, sternocleido-mastoideus or a proximal transfer of the common wrist flexor origins). Furthermore the cosmetic appearance of these techniques is besides the small gains in active flexion often less favourable.

Surgical Technique

Access to the triceps tendon via a straight dorsal incision and Z-shaped division of the tendinous part. Access to the dorsal elbow joint is accomplished via visualization and protection of the ulnar nerve at the sulcus. The tendon halves are securely sutured in a position of about 90° of flexion with stable sutures for early mobilization purposes.

Problems

Undercorrection or recurrence of the extension contracture. Both are due to insufficient aftercare. An overcorrection with subsequent elbow flexion contracture and loss of extension power is due to generous and insufficient surgical technique. If an active flexion is planned, it should always be performed as a second step when passive flexion and active extension power have been preserved [11].

16.6.1.3 Elbow Joint Flexion Contracture

Indication

Insufficient or functionally disabling flexion contracture. However every possible hand to mouth contact is much more important and must therefore be preserved. In the absence of an active elbow extension, the risk of recurrence after surgery is extremely high.

Operation Principle

Restoration or improvement of passive elbow extension by lengthening the shortened elbow flexor muscles and anterior capsulotomy of the elbow joint; the intraoperatively gained degree of extension must be further improved by successive splinting. If adequate and functionally favourable extension could be reached, a second step extensor muscle augmentation may be performed provided strong donor muscles are present (e.g. deltoideus). This is however rarely the case.

Surgical Technique

Approach to the anterior elbow region via a lazy S-incision, visualization, dissection and protection of all neurovascular structures, also to check their stretch intraoperatively, lengthening or recession of all shortened flexors (biceps, brachialis, brachioradialis, common flexor pronator muscle origin), anterior transverse capsulotomy of elbow joint, checking of maximum extension possible without undue stretching of the neurovascular structures and plastering in this position.

Drop-out long arm casts with posterior opening of the dorsal upper part are a very efficient way to improve passive extension. Neural function must however continuously be checked. After having reached the best possible extension, long arm (dynamic) splinting is strongly recommended to prevent recurrent deformity.

Problems

Difficult indication, recurrence and neurovascular damage due to stretch.

16.6.1.4 Hyperpronation Contracture of the Forearm

Indication

A lack or a complete restriction of passive supination with consecutive loss of (bimanual) function, no finger to mouth contact possible despite theoretically possible and restriction of eye-hand functional tasks (Fig. 16.8).

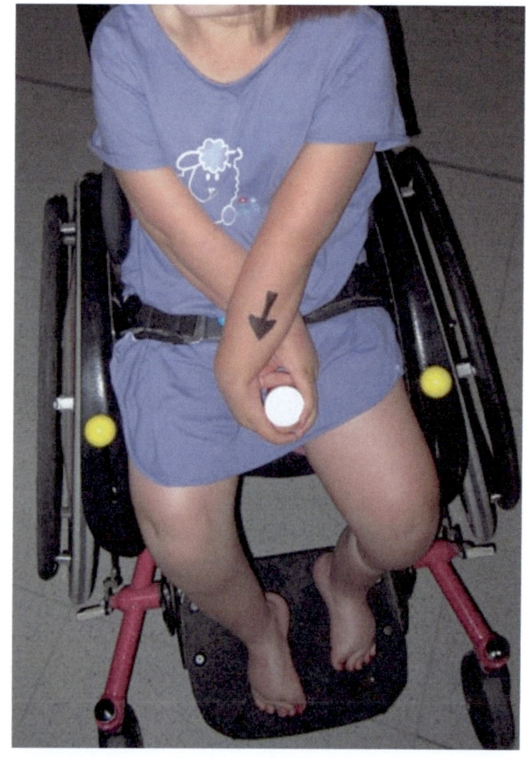

Fig. 16.8 Bilateral forearm pronation and wrist flexion contractures necessitate an adaptive crossing of both forearms for every active use (girl, 6 years old, AMC)

Operation Principle

Creation of a functionally adequate supination position of the forearm, by muscle and if necessary also by bony surgery.

Surgical Technique

Recession and removal of the contracted pronator teres tendon and muscle via a volar approach in the proximal radius; the creation of an active function as a supinator is only successful, if a passively adequate supination could be achieved and an active pronator muscle with sufficient excursion and strength is present. This scenario happens only very rarely in slight disorder types.

After having recessed the contracted pronator teres, another incision at the distal volar ulna is used to release the contracted pronator quadratus muscle as well, and through both approaches (anterior elbow and distal ulna), the interosseous membrane can be stripped off, which gives further freedom for passive supination. If this is still not adequate, a radius supination osteotomy can be performed and fixed with a 4–6-hole plate. The position of the forearm should be in the middle between supination and pronation.

Problems

Recurrence and overcorrection (only rarely, but need revision).

16.6.1.5 Wrist Flexion Contracture

Indication

Functional restriction of grip by significant wrist flexion contracture; additional ulnar deviation may occur. If the patient uses the back of his hand(s) for passive support, this function should be preserved after surgery by an adequate volar support. If the patient uses both hands as a pair of tweezers, the flexed wrist position may be preferable. Similarly the wrist flexion may help the hand to mouth contact, and any correction may make this worse.

Operation Principle

Achievement of a functionally more appropriate mid-position of the hand through a combination of soft tissue (tendons, capsules) and bony corrections; soft tissue corrections are adequate only for mild deviations.

Surgical Technique

The first step is volar ulnar incision and recession of the volar wrist flexors together with a volar transverse capsulotomy. If there are functionally intact flexor muscles with a sufficient excursion, they may be used to augment insufficient or lacking dorsal muscles. Any lengthening of already weak finger flexors should be done very cautiously in order not to worsen grip strength.

Correction is achieved by resecting a carpal dorsally/dorso-radially based wedge from the intercarpal bone row. Any ulnar deviation can be corrected as necessary. A wrist fusion may be an alternative, but wedge resection retains some degree of passive mobility at the wrist which is functionally superior. Any remaining active wrist flexor muscles may be additionally transferred do the dorsal side via the interosseous route. Intraoperative K-wires are used in open growth plates. Otherwise also plate or staple fixations are also an option (Fig. 16.9a, b).

Problems

Overcorrections and permanent loss of grip function (almost not curable). Undercorrection or loss of correction is also possible if volar flexor muscles are not detached before the wedge resection step; nerve stretch due to inadequate surgical accuracy.

16.6.1.6 Thumb Adduction Contracture

Indication

Any functionally disabling thumb adduction contracture with an insufficient or impossible grip; musculo-cutaneous shortening of the first intermetacarpal web space.

Operation Principle

Achievement of adequate abduction by release of short muscles combined with cutaneous enlarging of the web space; if possible also creation of an active abduction if donor muscles are available (Fig. 16.10).

Surgical Technique

Recession of all contracted adductors and short flexors in the first intermetacarpal space

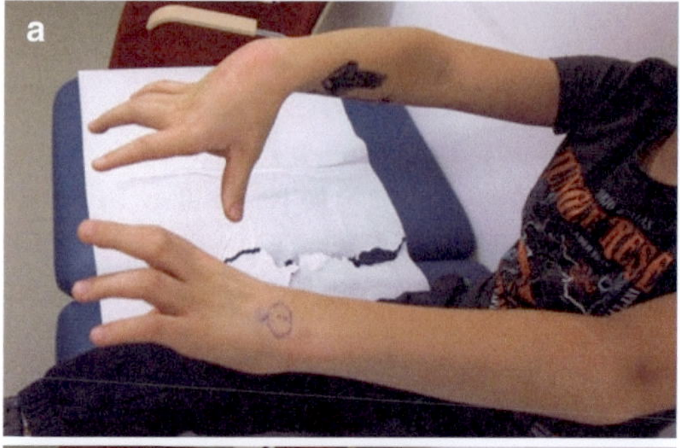

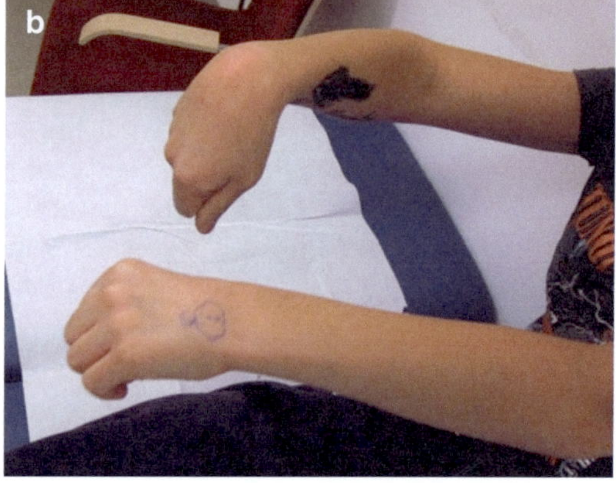

Fig. 16.9 (a, b) Surgical result of a wrist flexion and thumb adduction deformity on the left hand in comparison with the not yet corrected right side (boy, 8 years old, AMC, status after carpal wedge resection, flexor release and thumb abduction reconstruction left)

and enlargement of the first intermetacarpal distance by a proximally based long autologous skin graft from the radial side of the index finger possibly further augmented by a free flap skin graft. Additional MCP fusion or metacarpal corrective osteotomy, restoration of an active abduction and extension by augmentation and relocation of the intact EPL if an active donor muscle and tendon exist. The corrected position is temporarily fixed by an intermetacarpal K-wire between MC I and II.

Problems

Permanent weakness of the ab- or adduction, recurrence of adduction contracture especially if inadequate orthotic corrective spreading of the first intermetacarpal space had been used, scar formation with re-contracture.

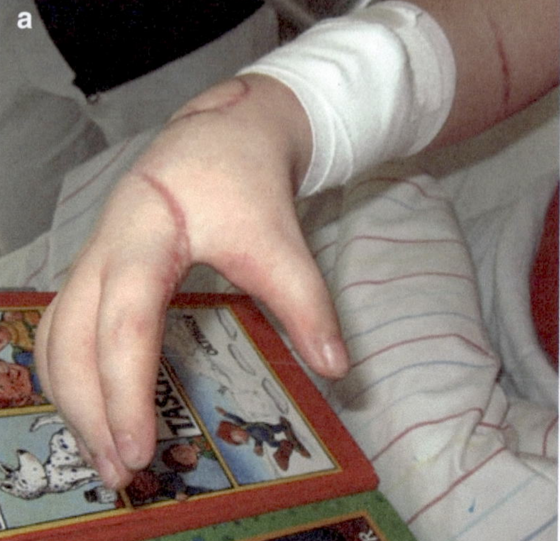

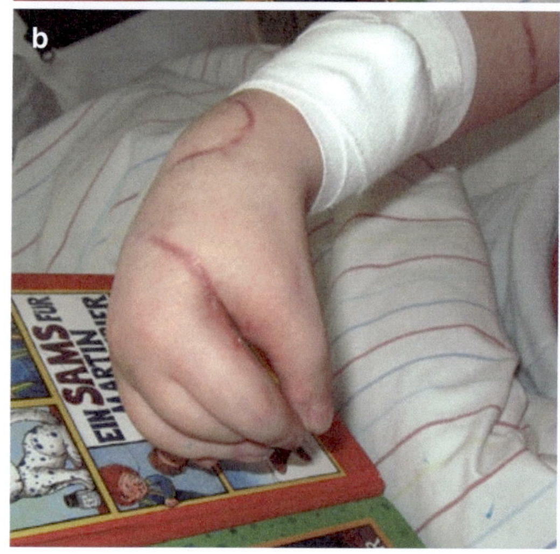

Fig. 16.10 (a, b) Another example of a combined correction of wrist flexion and thumb adduction contractures: active opposition requires muscle releases and plastic reconstruction of the web space as well as active donor tendons

16.6.2 Indications and Surgical Techniques in Spastic Paresis

In spastic disorders it is always important to distinguish functional and cosmetic issues, although both may often be present together. Any function-improvement operation will also have a positive effect on cosmetic appearance but hardly vice versa.

In the cases of spastic paresis, we are confronted with a central motor disorder of movement planning, execution and control, which never can be eliminated by surgery. JL Goldner simply stated: "The problem is in the brain and not in the arm" [12]. In analogy to the procedures for AMC, proper function and deformity analysis is of major importance before. An exact and detailed examination of the entire upper extremity allows for the selection of suitable surgical measures.

During any surgery a distinction must be made between spastic overactivity and structural muscle shortening. Although both are managed by similar techniques, the decisive factor is the dosage of muscle-tendon lengthenings or transfers.

The following deformities occur particularly frequent in the spastic arm and hand often in combination and are to be presented in the same sequence as above: indication, operation principle, surgical technique and problems. In almost every case, a combination of different procedures at different levels is entertained (multi-level correction). Soft tissue interventions in dystonia patients are extremely problematic due to the constant risks of overcorrection. Therefore arthrodesis should be taken into consideration in this patient group.

16.6.2.1 Internal Rotation and Adduction Contracture of the Shoulder Joint

Indication

Pain or/and restriction of function or care by a structural contracture of offending muscles.

Operation Principle

Correction of limited range of motion through elongation or release of shortened muscles and tendons (pectoralis major, subscapularis, latissimus dorsi); in difficult cases, additional correction at the bony level.

Surgical Technique

Delto-pectoral approach to the internally rotation and adducting muscle insertions at the proximal humerus, starting with the tendinous attachment of the pectoralis major and then correcting shortness of the subscapularis tendon without opening the joint capsule. If necessary

also elongation of the latissimus dorsi; muscular insertions should be retained and tendinous insertions lengthened or recessed.

If an external rotation of more than the midposition and abduction to approximately 90° cannot be achieved, a derotational osteotomy at the proximal humerus level can be discussed, although this is only seldom necessary in very severe long-standing cases.

Problems

Recurrence, especially after insufficient postop management without adequate physiotherapy and corrective positioning devices, overcorrection if too much weakening of the elongated muscles allows the antagonists to gradually overpower the agonists; in these cases re-intervention should be considered. In dystonic malpositioning, soft tissue corrections are fraught with complications. Therefore in these difficult cases, a primary shoulder joint fusion is best.

16.6.2.2 Elbow Flexion Contracture

Indication

Functional or cosmetic deficits through severe dynamic and/or static contractures of elbow flexor muscles and in severe cases also of the anterior joint capsule.

Operation Principle

Elongation of the offending shortened muscles, starting with the biceps brachii and brachialis muscles; in more severe cases, also detachment of the origin of the brachioradialis muscle and of the common flexor-pronator origin at the medial condyle of the humerus; in severe cases also transverse capsulotomy of the anterior elbow joint.

Surgical Technique

Lazy S-incision ventrally over the elbow region, starting lateral proximally and ending medial distally, and dissection of biceps tendon and Z-plasty and then aponeurotic intramuscular recession of the underlying brachialis muscle; when considering release of the brachioradialis muscle, the radial nerve must be dissected carefully and protected. The common flexor-pronator origin is released from the medial humerus condyle by simultaneously protecting the neurovascular structures. The anterior elbow joint capsule can be approached easily by blunt longitudinal splitting of the brachialis muscle fibres.

Postoperatively a drop-out long arm cast is preferable to further stretch the contracture. Nerve function must be monitored.

Problems

Undercorrection or recurrence of the deformity is not rare; overcorrections occur only in dystonic patients and are extremely difficult to manage.

16.6.2.3 Pronation Contracture of the Forearm

Indication

Every severe contracture of the forearm in pronation direction in severely handicapped patients; dynamic pronation spasticity in functional patients.

Principle of Operation

Complete release of the musculotendinous insertion of the pronator teres muscle at the proximal radius or preferably: rerouting of the insertion of the pronator teres tendon around the radius and changing its action from a pronator into a supinator (Tubby procedure).

Surgical Technique

Approach to the proximal insertion of the pronator teres tendon through a 6 cm longitudinal incision volarly over the proximal third of the radius; dissection of the superficial branch of the radial nerve and complete dissection of the pronator teres tendon down to its insertion. The tendon together with its tendo-muscular insertion is either completely released or preferably Z-lengthened as far as possible upwards and securely tied with non-absorbable sutures. With a curved clamp, which is put through the interosseous membrane from volar around the radios laterally, the distally based and tagged part of the pronator teres tendon is grasped, and after spreading the hole in the membrane generously, the tendon is pulled through this hole anteriorly into the interosseous space. Now it is possible to suture both tendon ends during passive supination of the forearm. By this way, the pronator muscle changes its action into a supinator.

In case if adequate passive supination cannot be achieved, the interosseous membrane may be stripped partially. In severely contracted cases, a radial supination osteotomy to the mid-position is the only solution. Release of the pronator quadratus together with the pronator teres is not recommended because of a higher risk of overcorrection into a supination deformity.

Problems

Recurrence, especially after simple pronator teres release operation; nerve damage to the superficial or/and deep radial nerve.

16.6.2.4 Wrist Flexion and Ulnar Deviation Contracture or Spasticity

Indication

Classical component of the multi-joint spastic flexor movement pattern; every higher degree of deformity or contracture; very severe stiff flexion deformities must be treated by wrist fusion.

Principle of Operation

Release of the common flexor-pronator origin at the medial epicondyle and the proximal ulna (Max Page operation). As this procedure causes unsightly scars and weakness, a distal release or better a transfer is preferable.

The tendons of the flexor carpi ulnaris (FCU) and if necessary also the extensor carpi ulnaris (ECU) are detached and tagged distally at the ulnar wrist insertion and then mobilized proximally and transferred either around the ulna or preferably through the interosseous membrane at the ulnar border to the extensor carpi radialis brevis tendon dorsally or if both are transferred also to the common extensor tendons of the fingers (EDC).

Any additional shortening of the FCR or superficial digital flexor tendons should be lengthened intramuscularly, but always very cautiously because of an overcorrection risk.

Severe wrist flexion contractures must be treated by wrist fusion and proximal row carpectomy following adequate soft tissue releases.

Surgical Technique

Distal volar approach at the distal ulna, 8 cm long, and dissection of the FCU tendon up to its insertion at the pisiform bone. Take care of the ulnaris nerve and its superficial branch. Mobilize the tendon proximally generously, and dissect the ECRB tendon through another incision dorsally at the wrist. The FCU tendon should be pulled through the interosseous membrane along the ulnar border and directed dorsally. Then, but only in severe contracted cases, intramuscular cautious lengthening of the FCR—if necessary—may be done. If ulnar deviation is strong, the ECU tendon is detached distally as well and mobilized proximally. The FCU tendon is fixed to the ECRB tendon by interweaving sutures and the ECU to the EDC tendons. We recommend always a temporary K-wire transfixation of the wrist but in only neutral position before suturing the tendons in order not to overtighten the sutures.

Wrist fusion in severe cases is done after surgical flexor tendon lengthenings through a dorsal approach. We remove the cartilage of all joints and put an inlay graft from the iliac crest under an 8-holed mini-fragment stable dynamic compression plate. Additional K-wires may be used in weak bone situations.

Problems

Overcorrection into extension deformity of the wrist only if tension is too high and the FCR had been lengthened concomitantly. Loss of correction, if no temporary orthotic protection had been used postoperatively. After generous lengthening of finger extrinsic flexors, an intrinsic plus deformity of the fingers develops which is also disabling (Fig. 16.11).

16.6.2.5 Weakness of Finger Opening

The FCU tendon can be rerouted through the interosseous membrane and sutured under slight tension into all long finger extensor tendons. Any weakness of finger opening needs the flexibility of the wrist to enable the tenodesis effect for opening. Wrist fusion is contraindicated in this problem.

16.6.2.6 Adduction Contracture of the Thumb (Different Types)

Indication

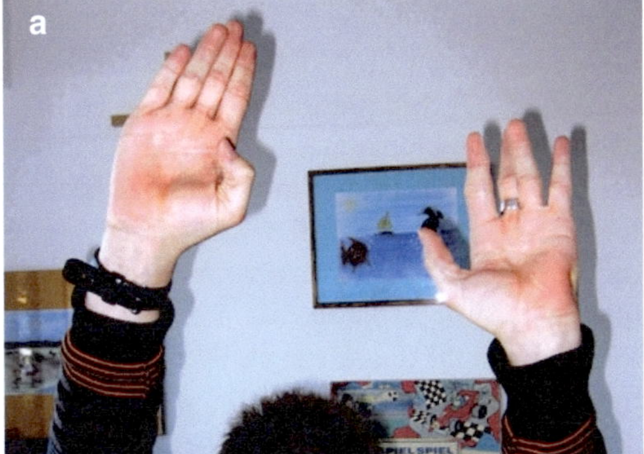
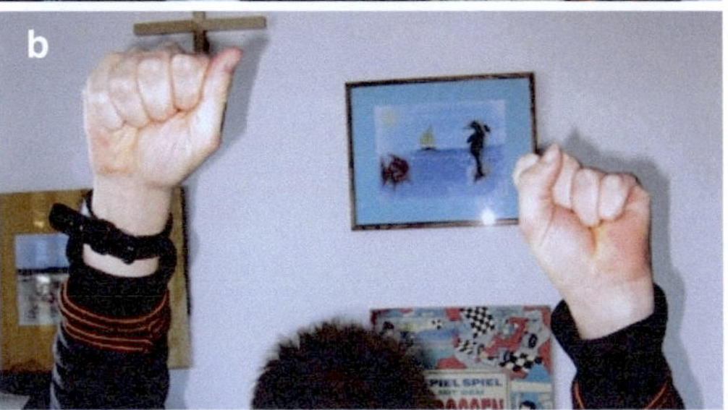

Fig. 16.11 (a, b) Late result of a combined soft tissue correction of a left-sided spastic hand and arm deformity: elbow, forearm, wrist and thumb contractures had been operated simultaneously in this young man (20 years old) with bilateral asymmetric SCP 5 years ago. The restoration of a functional hand and arm enabled him to use aids necessary for walking adequately

Thumb adduction is another part of the common flexor pronator pattern of the spastic arm and hand. It disturbs function, cosmesis and care as well.

Several types of this deformity have been described [13, 14]: adduction of the CMC joint, adduction of the MCP I joint, flexion of the IP joint and mixtures of these. In any case an exact investigation of the deformity components is necessary to define the correct surgical solution. Not infrequently, an adduction at the CMC level is associated with instability at the MCP joint in hyperextension. All components of the deformity must be treated.

Principle of the Operation

Correction of the often combined thumb malposition by recession of the shortened adductor pollicis and if unstable stabilizing the MCP joint or lengthening of a possibly shortened long thumb flexor [15]. There is always a need to consider an augmentation of the weak abductors by rerouting the tendon of the EPL (Goldner's procedure).

Surgical Technique

Release of a contracted adductor pollicis is done by a curved palmar incision at the basis of the thenar eminence and dissection of the muscle origin at the third metacarpal bone. Here the muscle with both portions is stripped off. The MCP joint of the thumb can easily be approached by an ulnar incision. The joint is opened and denuded from cartilage. Stabilization is performed by crossed K-wire fixation. Rerouting of the EPL tendon is done around the APL and EBP tendons in order to convert the EPL muscle into a thumb abductor.

Problems

Recurrence is not uncommon; overcorrection is rare.

16.6.2.7 Deformities of the Fingers (Swan Neck Deformity; Intrinsic Plus Deformity)

Indication

A hyperextension of the PIP joint with locking in extension causing problems with grasp. Intrinsic plus deformity is associated with contract flexion at the MCP joints and extension at the PIPO and DIP levels.

Operation Principle

The weak FDS muscles must be augmented, the hyperextension of the PIP joints must be limited, and intrinsic plus deformity needs a weakening procedure of the intrinsic insertions at the MCP levels.

Surgical Technique

Limiting the hyperextension of the PIP joints can be accomplished by using one slip of the FDS tendon, which should be released proximally at the ground phalanx and fixed in PIP joint flexion to the bone of the first phalanx (Swanson operation) by a pull-out suture. An alternative consists of the Zancolli procedure where a proximally and distally based strip of the extensor tendon is mobilized and transferred volarly and sutured to the flexor tendon sheath with non-absorbable sutures. A temporary paraosteal transfixation of the PIP joint in flexion for protective purposes is advisable. Any overactivity of the

intrinsic muscles in intrinsic plus position can easily be corrected by releasing the insertions of the intrinsic tendons into the extensor hood at the MCP joints according to Littler.

Problems

Loss of correction through pulling out of the sutures. Overcorrections are rare.

General Remarks

Surgical procedures aiming to treat joint stiffness or spastic paresis must always be planned using a detailed structural and functional plan. The common principles are to correct contractures and deformities and to improve range of motion, muscle strength and muscular balance.

Unstable or contracted joints should be fused. Isolated procedures are rarely used, so mostly a program for the correction of the entire upper limb is advisable. The basic underlying problems such as muscle weakness, loss of mobility and tendency towards stiffening will persist. Also the central motor deficits in spastic paresis cannot be changed by surgery.

16.7 Postoperative Management and Evaluation

Every surgeon should have close contact with the aftercare team. Postoperative care in congenital joint stiffness must take into account the healing time of the tissues and the constant tendency of movement restriction due to the underlying disorder. In every case of arthrolysis and tendon lengthenings or recessions, the extremity should be immobilized for a few days only. Then passive guided mobilization should start and appropriate dynamic orthoses should be used. From week to week, the range of motion must be increased: Sometimes intermittent manipulations under anaesthesia are necessary to regain repeat lost ranges of motion. Also in spastic paresis, postoperative treatment can be managed dynamically with additional use of dynamic splints. Cooperation of the patient with the early aftercare is mandatory. After 6 weeks for healing, protected mobilization can be replaced by regular use of the extremity and protection by functional orthotics during the day and the use of night splints. Arthrodesis must also be protected for several months postoperatively. All joints of the extremity that have not been operated must be mobilized as early as possible postoperatively to minimize the risk of immobilization weakness and new movement restrictions.

Specially tailored exercise programs including forced use and HABIT elements are possible after 8–12 weeks postoperatively. Orthotic protection has to be continued.

Every specialist team should monitor the results of postoperative care at regular intervals to detect unexpected findings early and to act timely.

Re-operations of unsuccessful results should be planned not too early. We recommend a postoperative therapy interval of at least 4–6 months after which any re-surgery might be considered.

16.7.1 Future Developments and Directions

There are some newer developments in the treatment of the upper extremity in congenital joint stiffness and spastic paresis. Unfortunately all of our conservative and surgical measures lag behind the natural worsening of muscle and joint functions. We always treat only the functional consequences to which the pathologic musculature has adapted as an essential moving force due to its high degree of plasticity. New findings about spastic muscle structure have been obtained where a shortening of maximally stretched sarcomeres has been found. Each maximum stretch of sarcomeres creates an additional weakness component.

For this purpose early assisted exercise programs with eccentric muscle-strengthening exercises may positively influence this structural muscle transformation. Stimulation of new muscle length growth by adding new sarcomeres is the goal. However, such an approach would have to be implemented at a much earlier date than presently used. This makes up-to-date information and training of the assistance professions involved urgently necessary.

Similarly a much earlier and more intense approach, possibly including motor-assisted mobilization of congenital joint contractures as a dynamic assisted early joint mobilization method, should be devised. Precisely adapted small articulated orthoses must be fitted with small yet powerful motors. The goal is to keep the secondary transformation changes of muscles, soft tissues and joints to the immobility to a minimum. Similarly early and functionally correctly indicated operations may create the prerequisites for such an early mobilization program, for example, by early relocations of dislocated joints and contracture releases.

Thus for the future, we all hope to lag less behind the secondary structural adaptive changes of tissues.

Due to the complexity of the disorders and the scarcity of patients with this disorder, it should be emphasized that all patients are supervised in specialized treatment centres. Also a closer cooperation between basic research and clinical application would be sought.

Detailed and standardized treatment programs must be devised and broadly employed. Regular follow-ups may detect problems at an early stage and improve such programs efficiently.

Also in spastic paresis problems and much earlier interventions would be advisable. Training of the parents as members of the therapy team should also be borne in mind.

References

1. Sarwark JF, McEwen GD, Scott CI. Current concepts review: amyoplasia: a common form of arthrogryposis. J Bone Joint Surg. 1990;72A:465–9.
2. Staheli LT, Hall JG, Jaffe KM, et al. Arthrogryposis—a textatlas. Cambridge: Cambridge University Press; 1998.
3. Guerin J. Difformités congenitales chez les monstres, le fetus et l'enfant. Paris: Bullet. de L'Academie de Medecine; 1882.
4. Hall JG. Arthrogryposis multiplex congenita: aetiology, genetics, classification, diagnostic approach and general aspects. J Pediatr Orthop. 1997;6B:159–66.
5. Eliasson AC, Krumlinde-Sundholm L, Rösblad B, et al. The Manual Ability Classification System (MACS) for children with cerebral palsy: scale devel-

opment and evidence of reliability and validity. Dev Med Child Neurol. 2006;48:549–54.
6. Brown JF, Robson MJ, Sharrard WJW. The pathophysiology of arthrogryposis multiplex congenita neurologica. J Bone Joint Surg. 1980;62A:291–6.
7. Bach A, Almquist E, La Grone M. Upper limb. In: Staheli LT, Hall JG, Jaffe KM, et al., editors. Arthrogryposis. Cambridge: Cambridge University Press; 1998. p. 45–50.

Further Reading

Sakzewski L, Ziviani J, Boyd RN. Efficacy of upper limb therapies for unilateral cerebral palsy: a meta analysis. Pediatrics. 2014;133:175–204.
Gordon AM, Chinnan A, Gill S, et al. Both constraint induced movement therapy and bimanual training lead to improved upper extremity function in children with hemiplegia. Dev Med Child Neurol. 2008;50:957–8.
Autti-Ramo LI, Suoranta J, Anttila H, et al. Effectiveness of upper and lower limb casting and orthoses in children with CP: an overview of review articles. Am J Phys Med Rehabil. 2006;85:89–103.
Chomiak J, Dungl P, Vcelak J. Reconstruction of elbow flexion in Arthrogryposis multiplex congenita type I: reults of transfer of pectoralis major muscle with follow-up to skeletal maturity. J Pediatr Orthop. 2014;34:799–807.
Goldner JL. The upper extremity in CP. In: Samilson RL, editor. Orthopaedic aspects of CP; clinics in developmental medicine no 52–53. London: Spastics Int. Heinemann; 1975. p. 221–57.
Van Heest A, James MA, Lewica A, et al. Posterior elbow capsulotomy with triceps lengthening for treatment of elbow extension contracture in children with arthrogyposis. J Bone Joint Surg. 2008;90A:1517–23.
Van Heest AE, Ramachandran V, Stout J, et al. Quantitative and qualitative functional evaluation of upper extremity tendon transfers in spastic hemiplegia caused by cerebral palsy. J Pediatr Orthop. 2008;28:679–83.
Davids JR, Sabesan VJ, Ortmann F, et al. Surgical management of thumb deformity in children with hemiplegic CP. J Pediatr Orthop. 2009;29:504–10.
Van Munster JC, Maathuis CGB, Haga N, et al. Does surgical management of the hand in children with spastic unilateral CP affect functional outcome? Dev Med Child Neurol. 2007;49:385–9.

17

C. Hagemann

17.1 Surgery in Nerve Injuries

17.1.1 General Information

Direct peripheral nerve injuries in childhood occur mostly because of trauma or during surgery, i.e., iatrogenic. Cutting injuries and blunt or perforating traumas as well as nerve injuries due to fractures occur. If there is no trauma, other diseases such as neuroborreliosis, Parsonage-Turner syndrome, or functional somatization disorders have to be excluded. Tumors of peripheral nerves in childhood are rare and are associated with neurofibromatosis.

The consequences of denervation are considerable. The affected area suffers atrophy, loss of sensitivity and motion, contractures, and sometimes denervation pain. If the skeleton is not fully grown, a loss of growth has to be expected (Fig. 17.1). In infancy, a 6-month persisting temporary paresis can already mean several cm of growth loss in the affected limb. The chances of success of conservative therapy are very good in neurapraxia and axonotmesis, but decrease significantly in neurotmesis and disappear in avulsion or neurotmesis far proximal of the motor end plate.

In the case of **avulsion**, there is no neuroma formation and thus no reinnervation. The main reason for the absence of neuroma formation intrathecally is the absence of Schwann cells in the central nervous system. In **neurotmesis**, even if axons are successfully sprouting through the neuroma without disorganization (which may result in cocontraction), there is a real danger of a non-occurring reinnervation despite neuroma formation if the motor end plate is very far away from the injury, since a growth rate of 1 mm per day should be assumed for sprouting axons. This may be too slow to ensure resuscitation of the paretic muscle before final atrophy if the target muscle is far distal. In this situation, nerve transfers can prevent the consequences of denervation.

17.1.2 General Considerations Regarding Indications

In the case of a cutting or perforating injury, an early operation and nerve suture up to 48 h posttrauma are is recommended. In the case of proven avulsions, there is indication for early nerve transfer, because no reinnervation is to be expected. In the case of blunt trauma, regeneration can be awaited initially. If regeneration does not appear by the tenth week and electrophysiological fibrillations and a lack of motor action potentials become apparent, the indication for surgery should be reevaluated immediately. The true extent of a lesion can often only be recognized during surgery. The sonographic evaluation

C. Hagemann (✉)
Department of Pediatric Neurosurgery, Altona
Children's Hospital, Hamburg, Germany
e-mail: christian.hagemann@kinderkrankenhaus.net

© Springer Nature Switzerland AG 2021
J. Bahm (ed.), *Movement Disorders of the Upper Extremities in Children*,
https://doi.org/10.1007/978-3-030-53622-0_17

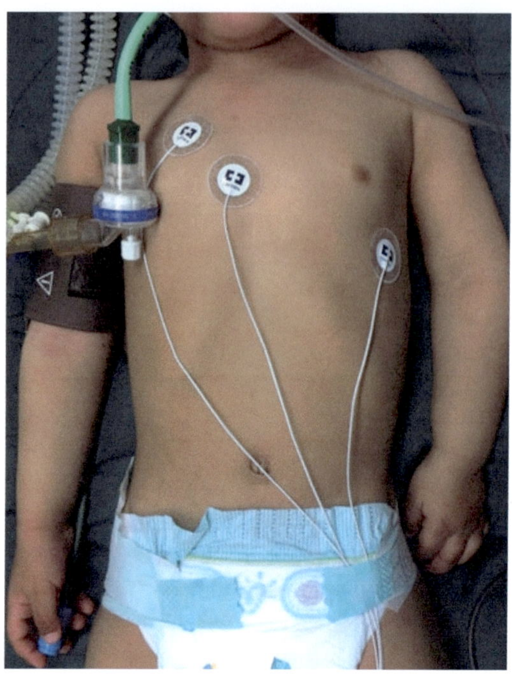

Fig. 17.1 A 14-month-old infant with total obstetric brachial plexus palsy, situation after exploration in the second month of life and transplantation of both sural nerves from C5, C6, and C7 on all trunci with avulsion of C8 and T1, partial recovery. Despite limited but pleasing reinnervation of the hand, elbow extension, and moderate elbow flexion which allows "hand-to-mouth" 1 year postoperatively, the patient developed significant loss of growth on the paretic side. For the treatment of glenohumeral dysplasia with compromised shoulder function, nerve transfer of the spinal accessory nerve to suprascapular nerve is performed at this stage. For these reasons, the decision between conservative and surgical therapy in infants and children has to be evaluated very carefully

of such lesions becomes better and better due to increasing image quality and investigator experience. The preoperative strategy has sometimes to be adapted to the intraoperative conditions during exploration. Even blunt injuries of a higher degree can show the necessity for nerve grafting. Nerve stimulation (pre- and postlesional) and intraoperative sonography (caliber jump, intraneural edema, continuity of fascicles) help in the intraoperative decision-making.

In some cases a simple decompression or neurolysis is sufficient, e.g., in compressing hematomas, osteosynthesis material, or scar tissue. Seventy-two hours after neurotmesis at the latest, Waller's degeneration has occurred distally of the

injury, and the distal stumps of motor nerves can no longer be stimulated in the situs, and the distal stumps must be assigned purely anatomically, which might be troublesome in cases of several affected nerves, trunci, or extensive soft tissue defects. Usually no direct end-to-end suture without tension is possible if the distance is more than a cm after excision of a neuroma. Anastomoses under tension are useless; the anastomosis should always be able to move through the passive motion without tension. In the case of complete discontinuity of a nerve, the nerve stumps retract within a few days, and direct nerve sutures are usually no longer possible; a nerve graft has to be interposed.

In complete neurotmesis, far proximal from the motor end plate or central in the sense of avulsion, the consequences of denervation are very likely. For example, a complete lesion of the ulnar nerve in the armpit area, despite an immediate successful suture, is likely to lead to atrophy of the ulnar nerve-dependent intrinsic hand muscles, because the distance (and thus time) of regeneration may be longer than what the atrophy requires for irreversibility. At a certain point, a denervated and atrophied muscle can no longer be resuscitated despite the reappearance of axons. According to some authors, this "point of no return" is 12 months after disconnection; others regard 18 months as the final time frame. In cases where avulsions or damage far from the motor end plate are present, nerve transfer techniques should be considered early. In the child shown in Fig. 17.2, an ulnar supercharge was additionally performed [1].

17.1.3 Direct Nerve Surgery (Neurolysis, Decompression, Transplantation/Grafting)

The **decompression** of a paretic nerve or plexus by removing dislocated osteosynthesis material, bone fragment, or hematoma is a clear indication for early surgery. After decompression, the nerve is inspected and checked sonographically and by intraoperative nerve stimulation. An external **neurolysis** is usually only necessary in the case

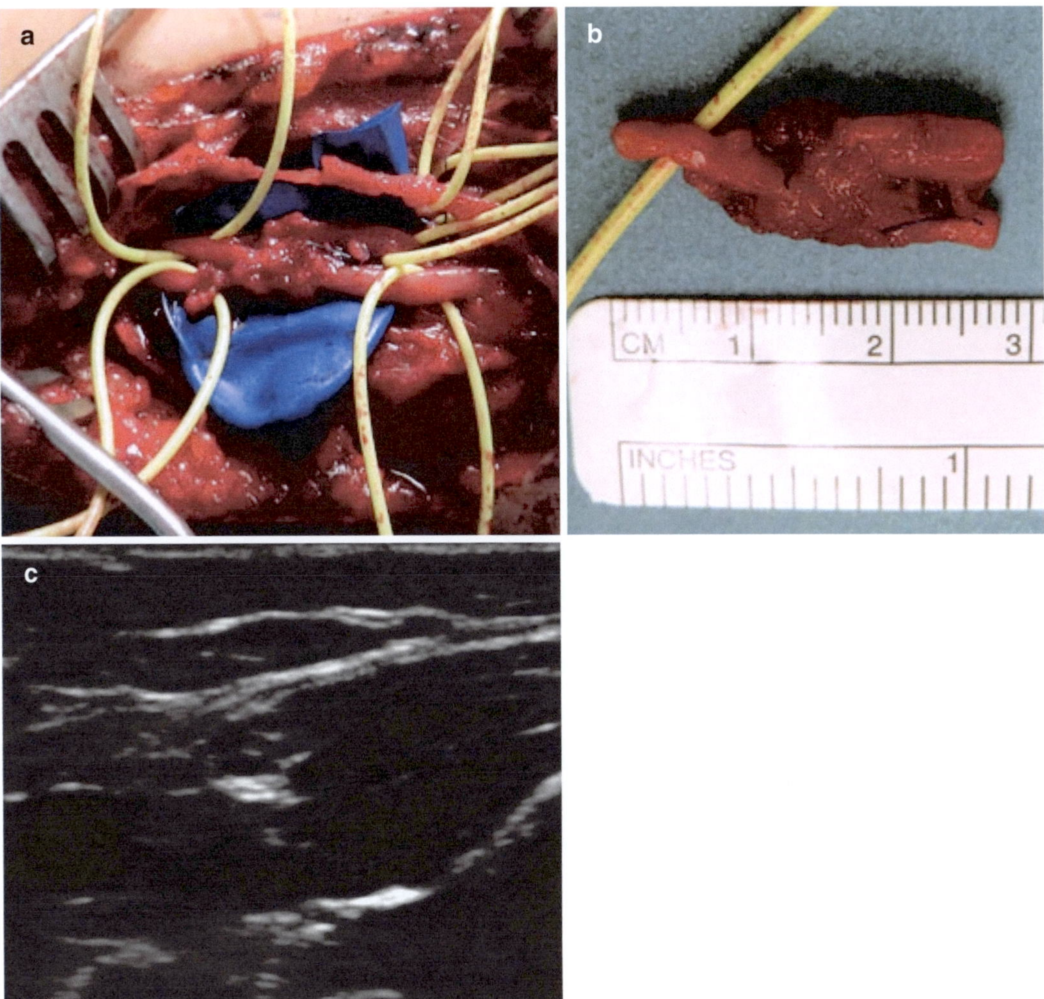

Fig. 17.2 (**a–c**) An 8-year-old boy 4 weeks after dissection of the ulnar and cutaneus antebrachii medialis (MABC) nerves 40 cm proximal of the wrist, complete loss of function. (**a**) After excision of the conglomerate neuroma, 4 cm MABC were anastomosed as a tension-free graft end-to-end in the ulnar nerve. The distal MABC was connected end-to-side to the sensitive aspect of the median nerve. (**b**) Neuroma corresponding to the presurgical ultrasound findings. (**c**) Preoperative ultrasound with the distal stumps of the MABC and ulnar nerve

of earlier injury and scarring. In principle, neurolysis can also take place within a nerve. Attention should also be paid to the connective tissue around the nerves, referred to by Hanno Millesi as paraneurium, as it is important for the gliding of the nerves during each movement.

If in surgery there is obvious necessity for **nerve grafting**, this can be carried out over the entire or partial cross section of a nerve ("split repair"). The neuroma is removed into the region of healthy fascicles, and it is advisable to control the extent of resection histologically or sonographically. If a nerve has been disconnected some time ago, fibrosis complicates the preparation, and the proximal stump is retracted and bulged due to sprouting axons. After a few weeks, nerve grafts of several cm are usually necessary to gain anastomoses without tension.

As **donor nerves**, the sural nerves are particularly suitable, but sensory branches of the cervical plexus or sensory nerves of the arm may also be harvested as grafts (Fig. 17.3). The collection

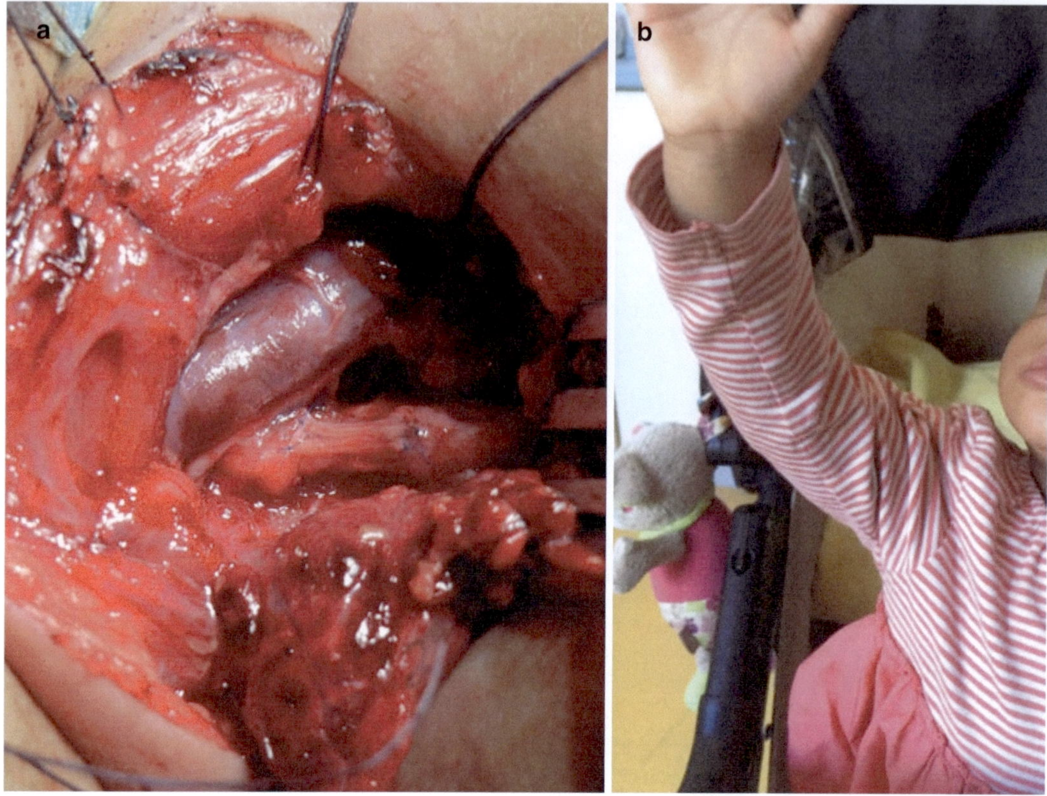

Fig. 17.3 (**a, b**) Upper obstetric brachial plexus palsy with neuroma C5, avulsion C6. (**a**) Situation after transplantation of grafts from cervical plexus (1.3 cm, target elevation). Oberlin transfer (target elbow flexion) and nerve transfer of the suprascapular nerve to spinal accessory (target shoulder external rotation) in the same session. (**b**) Functional outcome after 12 months

site should depend on the patient's wishes, surgical demands, and individual in situ possibilities (how long and how thick to graft?). In nerve grafting on the upper arm, cutaneous branches of the same arm are preferred in order to avoid additional comorbidity on the unaffected healthy limb. In plexus lesions the sural nerves are predominantly used.

17.2 Nerve Transfers

17.2.1 General Information

The first operations with nerve transfers were already carried out at the beginning of the twentieth century, and larger series were published in the course of the century by some pioneers.

Noteworthy in this context are the publications of Adolf Stoffel, Herbert John Seddon, Rolfe Birch, Algimantas Narakas, and Hanno Millesi.

The principle of nerve transfer involves the redirection of healthy axons into a paralyzed nerve leading to the paretic muscle. One disadvantage is the deficit of the donor, whereby predominantly redundant fibers are used for nerve transfers. One advantage is the short reinnervation time, as many nerve transfers may be performed very close to the target muscle and motor end plate. Successful nerve transfer of a paretic muscle in situ is probably superior to muscle-tendon transfer ex situ in terms of function. In the case of nerve injuries, the regeneration must be evaluated individually, and, if necessary, an indication for nerve transfer vs. direct nerve surgery (neurolysis, decompression, grafting) has to be decided at one point. Nerve transfers should be executed 3–6 months after injury for best results in cases of insufficient regeneration. However, successful nerve transfers later than 18 months after injury have been described, with decreasing results due to increasing irreversible atrophy. Only in the case of avulsions nerve transfer should take place as early as possible, as no regeneration has to be expected.

In paresis of elbow flexion, the **Oberlin transfer** technique transfers fascicles from the median nerve and ulnar nerve to the biceps and brachialis branches of the musculocutaneous nerve and has proven successfully in a high percentage of cases. This procedure has meanwhile been reproduced by numerous publications [2, 3]. In addition to the classic Oberlin transfer for the resuscitation of elbow flexion, nerve transfers for shoulder function are in common use. The nerve transfer of the suprascapular nerve to the spinal accessory nerve for external rotation [4] and the nerve transfer of the medial triceps branch of the radial nerve to the axillary nerve for elevation [5] have proved successful. In the area of the forearm, strategies are also being developed for nerve transfer in the treatment of paresis of the median, ulnar, and radial nerves. These strategies can also be used in other circumstances, like arthrogryposis or flaccid myelitis.

17.2.2 Nerve Transfer in Plexus and Distal Nerve Palsies

Donor nerves for extraplexic motor axons in the shoulder area are the spinal accessory nerve, intercostal nerves, and the contralateral C7 root [4, 6, 7]. For subtotal **plexus palsies**, intraplexic transfers are also available, which are performed predominantly in the area of the divisions and fascicles of the brachial plexus, for example, the nerve transfer of the medial pectoral nerve to the lateral fascicle.

For distal **nerve palsies**, nerve transfers are also used successfully. In case of palsy of the ulnar nerve, the intrinsic muscles of the hand can be reanimated by an **ulnar supercharge** transfer

of the distal anterior interosseous nerve to the deep motor branch of the ulnar nerve [1]. Pronation is retained due to pronator teres innervated by the median nerve. Palsy of the median nerve may be treated by nerve transfer of radial nerve fascicles of the branch to extensor carpi radialis brevis to the anterior interosseous nerve and fibers from the supinator branch to the pronator teres branch. In radial nerve palsy transfers from median nerve branches to the flexor carpi radialis and superficial flexor digitorum to the posterior interosseous and extensor carpi branches of the radial nerve are recommended. Susan Mackinnon [8] described such strategies also in combination with tendon transfers.

17.2.3 Example of a Rare Indication: Nerve Transfer in Arthrogryposis Multiplex Congenita

Arthrogryposis multiplex congenita (AMC) is a multifactorial and heterogeneous complex of symptoms in which prenatal joint contractures occur. With AMC, all or some extremities of an individual can be affected. Observations concerning the neuroanatomy of AMC have already been described, and nerve transfers have been performed [9]. Since the clinical constellations of AMC are so diverse, only a few of these cases can be considered for nerve transfer.

In my opinion, there is an indication for nerve transfer in AMC if a muscle is detectable and the affected joint is passively mobile and therefore not in full contracture. In addition, a functional donor nerve must be present. Figure 17.4 shows the example of a child in whom only the two upper extremities were affected by AMC. At the time of surgery, there was minimal contracture of the elbow joint on both sides with a detectable biceps in sonography. Hand function was good; therefore, there is decision to perform an Oberlin transfer bilaterally. The elbow flexion was detectable from the fifth month postoperatively, from the ninth month elbow flexion against gravity. These results were reproduced in other children with AMC [10].

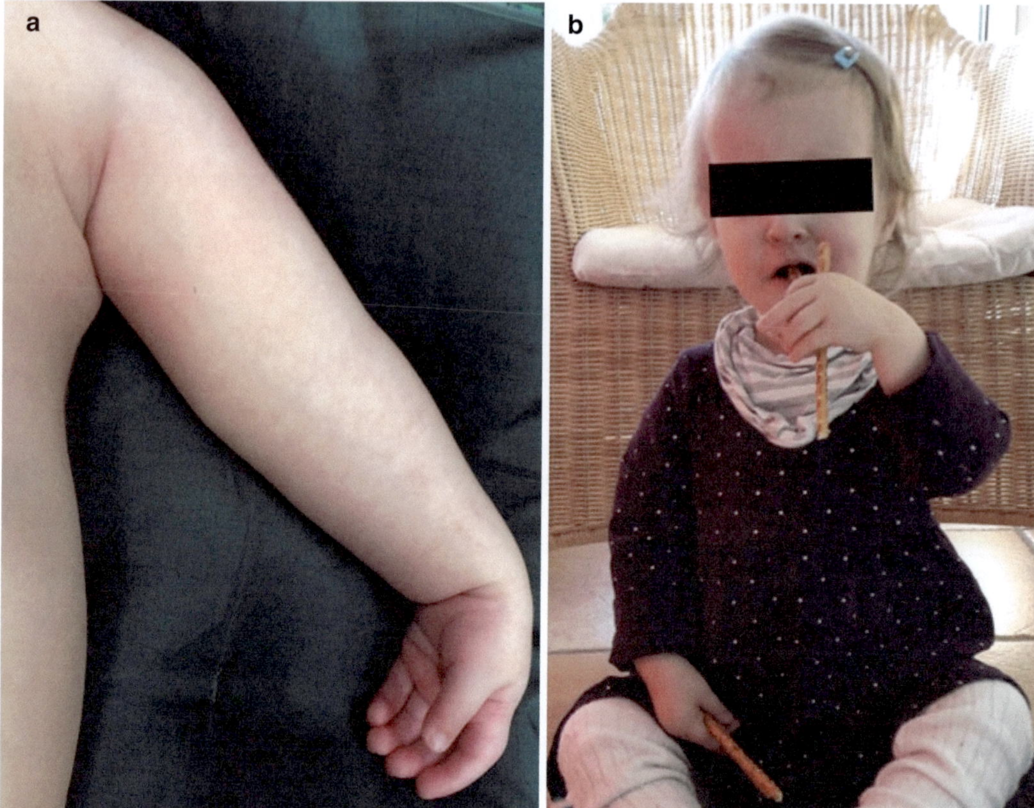

Fig. 17.4 (**a**, **b**) A 3-month-old girl with arthrogryposis multiplex congenita. (**a**) The girl shows good finger and wrist function as well as triceps and shoulder, but no active biceps (missing skin fold). (**b**) Independent hand-to-mouth movement 1 year after Oberlin's transfer

17.2.4 Sensory Nerve Transfer

In contrast to the resuscitation of paretic muscle by nerve transfer, which is impossible after final atrophy and fatty degeneration of the muscle, sensory nerve transfer can be successful even after years. Special focus is put on the area of the hand to achieve protective sensation in the thumb, index, and small finger. Sensory nerve transfers are capable to modulate denervation pain. In anesthesia of the small finger due to injury of the ulnar nerve, sensory fascicles of the median nerve ("third webspace transfer") or the lateral cutaneus antebrachii nerve are suitable for nerve transfer [8, 11, 12]. In anesthesia of the radial thumb and index area, the lateral cutaneus antebrachii (LABC) nerve might be transferred to the superficial radial nerve.

17.3 Nerve Surgery in Pediatric Compression Syndromes

Idiopathic nerve compressions in children are rare. Most of the cases in the early pediatric age are due to mucopolysaccharidosis (MPS) or multiple hereditary exostoses (MHE). In teenage years, classic compression syndromes such as neurogenic "thoracic outlet syndrome" or carpal tunnel occur rarely.

17.3.1 Idiopathic Compression Syndromes and TOS

A neurogenic **thoracic outlet syndrome** (TOS) in adolescents is often enforced by posture or selective exercises that lead to hypertrophy of the biceps and deltoid muscle, but not to strengthening of the vertebral and scapuloverte-bral muscles. Some of these teenagers are iden-tified by their habitus, and they are unable to present the ventral arm elevation over the hori-zontal plane. Such symptoms should first be treated by manual therapy with postural exer-cises to strengthen the spinal column and scapu-lovertebral muscles as well as nerve mobilization exercises. If a neck rib can be detected in such a child, it should be borne in mind that it has been present since birth; initially, a risky resection should be avoided in favor of conservative ther-apy. US surgeons perform decompression of neurogenic TOS only if the symptoms persist despite 6 months of physiotherapy. In the oper-ated patients, hypertrophic scaleni or periplexic fibrosis can be found as causes in addition to cervical ribs.

Idiopathic **upper limb nerve compression syndromes** in childhood are very rare, but show the same symptoms as in adults. An unusual case reported by Mackinnon suffered from pronator syndrome in the forearm, triggered by a hyper-flexed arm posture during sleep. This sleep posi-tion led to severe pain in the forearm, which was misjudged as cerebral dystonia probably due to the rarity of such a compression syndrome in childhood. The girl was effectively helped by decompression of the median nerve in the prona-tor tunnel. In principle, the symptoms are exactly the same as in adults with night pain and pares-thesia in the specific nerve area, but children are usually less able to describe their symptoms elo-quently. Pain is followed by atrophy of the depen-dent muscles. Taking the history regarding preferred sleeping position is always advisable in these patients, since simple positioning methods or orthoses can already enable symptom relief, similar to adults. The speed of nerve conduction is obligatory in diagnostics; surgical indications for decompression should only be made after conservative treatment or when symptoms and psychological stress are pronounced. Surgical techniques such as endoscopic vs. minimal inci-sion vs. wide exposure are discussed extensively in the literature.

17.3.2 Mucopolysaccharidosis

Mucopolysaccharidosis (MPS) is a hereditary lysosomal storage disease in which the enzy-matic degradation of mucopolysaccharides is dis-turbed. The reported incidence is around 1:29,000. Seven types are distinguished accord-ing to their characteristics and dynamics. The MPS types I-H (**Hurler-Pfaundler syndrome**) and II (**Hunter syndrome**) are particularly fre-quent in developing carpal tunnel syndrome; in the case of Hunter syndrome, over 90% of chil-dren are affected and in Hurler-Pfaundler syn-drome over 70%. The MPS types III (**Sanfilippo syndrome**) and IV (**Morquio syndrome**) develop compression syndromes rarely.

For differential diagnosis it is important to note that MPS often leads to instability or steno-sis of the craniocervical junction and the upper cervical spine. The craniocervical junction should be evaluated by MR tomography, and additional sleep laboratory examinations should be carried out to exclude central apnea. Neurophysiological examinations (nerve con-duction velocity/sensory evoked potentials) also play an important role. In case of carpal tunnel syndrome in MPS, the indication for wide open decompression is evident.

In contrast to the classic "adult carpal tunnel," in which the minimal invasive endoscopic surgi-cal technique represents an alternative according to some authors, MPS should be decompressed using a long incision because the recurrence rate is significantly increased due to the permanent further deposition of MPS in the tendon compart-ment. The procedure may also have to include a tenosynovectomy and a decompression of the Loge de Guyon, because instead of an isolated constriction in the area of retinaculum flexorum, there is a much more longitudinal form of steno-sis, in which the increased pressure on the median nerve and partly also on the ulnar nerve is not caused by the retinaculum alone, but in the com-partment of the tendons due to MPS deposits around the tendons. Due to the underlying dis-ease, the deposition of mucopolysaccharides in the tendon compartment continues, so that some

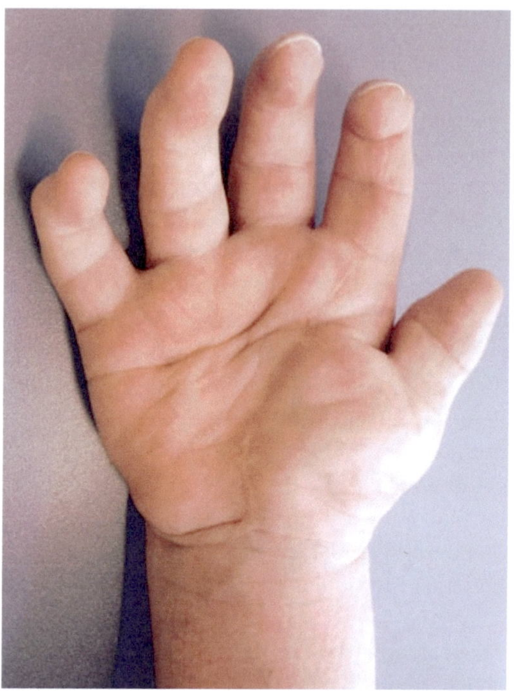

Fig. 17.5 A 17-year-old MPS type II patient, condition after carpal tunnel decompression with very short incision without tenosynovectomy 4 years ago at another institution. The patient was craniocervically decompressed and stabilized 3 years ago. Severe pain and hypesthesia. A planned revision with decompression of the median nerve and the ulnar nerve with tenosynovectomy over a longer incision could not be performed due to MPS-related intubation problems. The wider decompression was performed later under local anesthesia. The anesthesia of MPS children is associated with significant morbidity and mortality and should be carried out by specialized centers only. For this reason revision surgery must be avoided: long incision and thorough decompression are superior to minimal invasive approaches in this particular disease

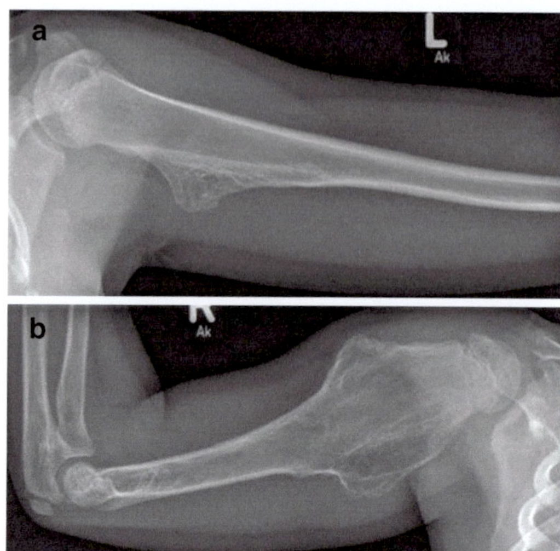

Fig. 17.6 (a, b) Examples of cartilaginous exostoses at the humerus with compression of the radial nerve. These two patients present numerous other exostoses on their legs

patients have to undergo two or even three operations, especially if an endoscopic or too short incision was performed during primary surgery (Fig. 17.5). This also applies to MPS patients with enzyme therapy or after bone marrow transplantation.

17.3.3 Multiple Hereditary Exostoses

Multiple hereditary exostoses (MHE) disease is an autosomal dominant pathology in which cartilaginous osteochondromas occur at the metaphyses during growth. The incidence is reported to be 1:50,000. The patients show between 1 and over 20 exostoses during growth. Due to the immediate proximity to the physes, deformations of joints and tubular bones can occur, and peripheral nerves, especially in the area of the knee and shoulder, are compressed (Fig. 17.6).

In the case of clinical signs of nerve compression, the corresponding nerve should be decompressed after electrophysiology and imaging and the exostosis removed as far as possible. In the same session, a Blount clamp for growth guidance may be implanted by the pediatric orthopedics if required. The use of a tourniquet is contraindicated in patients with MHE, as unknown microexostoses in the tourniquet area are able to cause pressure-related nerve damage and paresis. Hereditary exostoses also occur in the spine.

17.4 Selective Neurectomy in Focal Spasticity or Neuroma Pain

Selective or complete neurectomy is a destructive procedure that any neurosurgeon will primarily avoid. There are two indications for which partial or complete neurectomies are indeed useful: spasticity and neuroma pain.

17.4.1 Focal Spasticity

In order to reduce the tone of a spastic muscle effectively, a selective partial neurectomy of the branches to the target muscle of about 75–80% of the fiber count is necessary.

If less than 50% of the fibers are cut, the method is not sufficient, and there will be spastic rebound within short time. It is mandatory to isolate the motor branch close to the target muscle; a selective partial neurectomy should not be performed in a mixed nerve or trunci; otherwise deafferentiation pain may occur [13]. In contrast to conduction block or botulinum toxin application, a selective neurectomy is irreversible.

It takes thorough examination and experience to decide if a spastic muscle is suitable for a selective partial neurectomy. Some patients use their spasticity for certain movements and may not be able to perform this movement if the focal spasticity is reduced by neurectomy. Global spasticity is much more common than focal spasticity and is not suitable for selective neurectomy (Sect. 17.5). Before a selective neurectomy is indicated, treatment with botulinum toxin in the target muscle should be carried out in order to simulate the effect of the intervention. Alternatively, a conduction block of the motor nerve could be administered, but this is usually far more difficult than the application of botulinum toxin intramuscularly. Selective neurectomy should not be performed early, but after conservative therapy (orthoses, physiotherapy, Botox) before contractures occur.

Depending on the target muscle, the motor branches of the nerve are isolated close to the motor endplates and cut to 75–80%. Due to anatomical variations, incisions are required to be rather long because all branches of the specific target muscle must be visualized and addressed. In the case of focal spasticity in the biceps muscle, for example, the musculocutaneous nerve is dissected in the same fashion as for an Oberlin transfer to identify all 1–3 branches for neurectomy.

17.4.2 Neuroma Pain

Neurotomy of sensitive skin nerves may be indicated in cases of neuroma pain. Neuromas of mixed deep-seated nerves are not suitable for neurectomy but neurolyzed or transplanted. Neuromas can occur after traumatic or iatrogenic injuries of superficial nerves, e.g., after needlestick injury of the radialis superficialis nerve due to difficult puncture. Neuroma pain in childhood is rare, but can cause the same severe pain as in adults. They show a positive Hoffmann-Tinel sign with pain and electric shocks in the supplied area and may be detected by sonography. Neuroma pain is difficult to control with medication, and an improvement in symptoms after a conduction block indicates the possibility for neurectomy. In the case of a neurectomy, the pain is exchanged for anesthesia or hypesthesia, if sensory nerve transfers are not performed simultaneously. In childhood, however, there is a significantly higher chance of "cross-innervation" than within adults. After the neurectomy, the proximal nerve stump is turned proximally and positioned into its soft tissue gliding area and secured in this position with fibrin.

17.5 Neuromodulation in Global Spasticity or Malignant Pain with Intrathecal Drug Pump

Far more patients present a global spasticity than a focal spasticity. In the pediatric age group, bilateral spastic cerebral palsy and less frequent dystonia are the most common conditions. There are different patterns of spasticity: tetraspasticity, hemispasticity, and paraspasticity.

In addition to conservative therapy with physiotherapy and orthoses, botulinum toxin and the oral administration of baclofen may be considered. Since the oral uptake of baclofen only leads to a very low concentration in the actual target organ, the myelon, the **intrathecal baclofen pump therapy** is a real blessing for many patients. Only 1% of oral baclofen dose applied directly intrathecal leads to a 50-fold concentration of baclofen in the cerebrospinal fluid. Thus, symptoms of systemic overdose are prevented and a better detonization is achieved. In contrast there is the risk of implantation, implant failure, and the need for regular refills. The intrathecal baclofen pump therapy is particularly suitable for

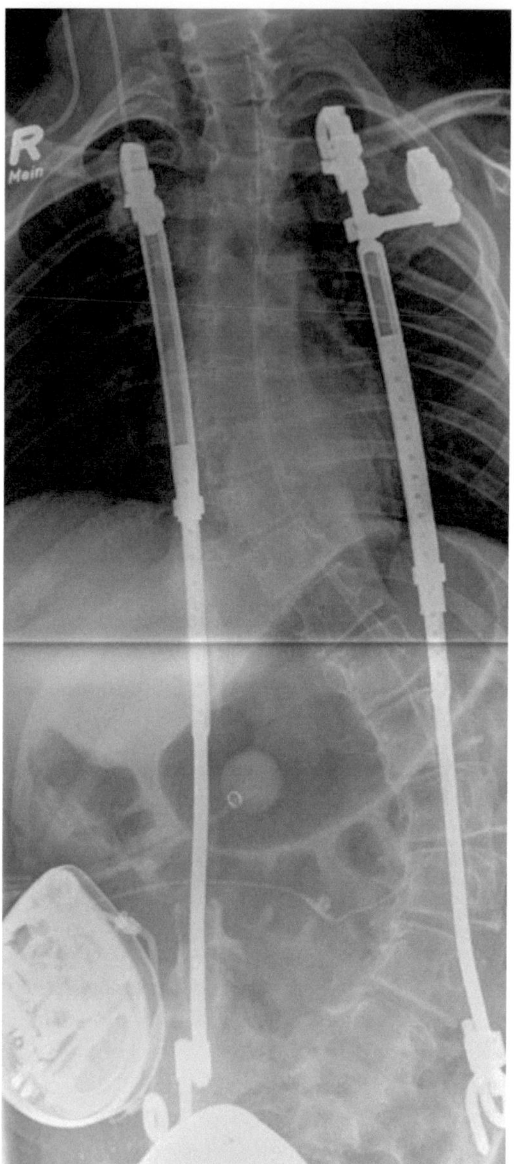

Fig. 17.7 A 12-year-old female patient with bilateral spastic cerebral palsy GMFCS Level 5, catheter position at C7/T1. Neuromuscular scoliosis treated with VEPTR, gastrostomy

patients with severe and global spasticity (Ashworth Scale 4–5, Gross Motor Function Classification Scale Level 4–5).

With intrathecal baclofen therapy, serious complications of spasticity such as pain and consequential damages (contracture, luxation, and fracture) might be avoided. Before implantation, an intrathecal testing is applied at the intensive care unit, as there are non-responders and rarely patients in whom baclofen intrathecally paralyzes the respiratory center. In principle, it is possible to position the tip of the intrathecal tube up to the cervicothoracic region to achieve detonization effect in the upper extremities (Fig. 17.7). Due to the intrathecal flow behavior of baclofen, the legs are also detonized. On the other hand, a lumbar catheter that ends below T12 cannot induce any effect on the upper extremities [14]. It is therefore necessary to consider the actual target point of the catheter tip position together with the relatives before implantation. Due to the subfascial implantation technique, implantation is achievable in very young patients [15].

In principle, pain therapy might be performed with intrathecal pumps. A few **opioids** are approved for intrathecal application. The substances act on the nociceptors of the posterior horns; a clear reduction of the dose is achieved in comparison to peroral treatment and the systemic side effects are reduced, corresponding to intrathecal baclofen. The indication is limited to malignant pain, which is fortunately extremely rare in childhood.

References

1. Davidge KM, Yee A, Moore AM, Mackinnon SE. The supercharge end-to-side anterior interosseous-to-ulnar motor nerve transfer for restoring intrinsic function: clinical experience. Plast Reconstr Surg. 2015;136(3):344e–52e.
2. Liverneaux PA, Diaz LC, Beaulieu J-Y, Durand S, Oberlin C. Preliminary results of double nerve transfer to restore elbow flexion in upper type brachial plexus palsies. Plastic Reconstr Surg. 2006;117:915–9.
3. Loy S, Bhatia A, Asfazadourian H, Oberlin C. Transferts de fascicules du nerf ulnaire sur le nerf du muscle biceps dans les avulsions C5-C6 ou C5-C6-C7 du plexus brachial. Ann Chir Main Memb Sup. 1997;16(4):275–84.
4. Bahm J, Noaman H, Becker M. The dorsal approach to the suprascapular nerve in neuromuscular reanimation for obstetric brachial plexus lesions. Plastic Reconstr Surg. 2005;115(1):240–3.
5. Leechavengvongs S, Witoonchart K, Uerpairojkit C, Thuvasethakul P. Nerve transfer to deltoid muscle using the nerve to the long head of the triceps, part II: a report of 7 cases. J Hand Surg Am. 2003;28(4):633–8.

6. Seddon HJ. Nerve grafting. J Bone Joint Surg. 1963;45B:447–61.
7. Zhang C-G, Gu Y-D. Contralateral C7 nerve transfer-our experiences over past 25 years. J Brachial Plex Peripher Nerve Inj. 2011;6:10.
8. Mackinnon S. Nerve surgery. Stuttgart New York: Thieme; 2015.
9. Bahm J. Arguments for a neuroorthopaedic strategy in upper limb arthrogryposis. J Brachial Plex Peripher Nerve Inj. 2013;8(1):9.
10. Hagemann C, Stücker R, Breyer S, Kunkel POS. Nerve transfer from the median to musculocutaneous nerve to induce active elbow flexion in selected cases of arthrogryposis multiplex congenita. Microsurg. 2019;39(8):710–14. https://doi.org/10.1002/micr.30451.
11. Oberlin C, Teboul F, Severin S, Beaulieu JY. Transfer of the lateral cutaneous nerve of the forearm to the dorsal branch of the ulnar nerve, for providing sensa-tion on the ulnar aspect of the hand. Plast Reconstr Surg. 2003;112(5):1498–500.
12. Ruchelsman DE, Price AE, Valencia H, Ramos LE, Grossman JA. Sensory restoration by lateral antebrachial cutaneous to ulnar nerve transfer in children with global brachial plexus injuries. Hand (N Y). 2010;5(4):370–3.
13. Sindou MP, Simon F, Mertens P, Decq P. Selective peripheral neurotomy (SPN) for spasticity in child-hood. Childs Nerv Syst. 2007;23:957–70.
14. Flack SH, Bernards CM. Cerebrospinal fluid and spi-nal cord distribution of hyperbaric bupivacaine and baclofen during slow intrathecal infusion in pigs. Anaesthesiology. 2010;112(1):165–73.
15. Hagemann C, Schmitt I, Lischetzki G et al. Intrathecal baclofen therapy for treatment of spasticity in infants and small children under 6 years of age. Childs Nerv Syst. 2020;36:767–73. https://doi.org/10.1007/s00381-019-04341-7.

Rare Clinical Features

18

Jörg Bahm

In few children, some leading symptoms first point in the usual, common diagnosis, but then something does not fit: some rare clinical conditions which have significance in differential diagnosis; some of these are discussed in this chapter.

We see many typical obstetric plexus pareses in our clinics, but also other motor disorders, which have given us many a riddle.

First, there are *temporary motor weaknesses* of an upper extremity with normal neonatal findings. There are no typical plexus paresis, no further diagnostic differentiation, and unclear prognosis. That is why we ask an experienced neuropediatrician for a review (Chap. 4).

One infant presented with a monoparesis of the left upper extremity—an almost typical appearance of an enlarged upper plexus palsy (Fig. 18.1). The birth history revealed a lower segment cesarian section and a malformed uterus bicornus. Could there have been intrauterine causation?

Because of insufficient motor recovery, we explored early at 3 months (Fig. 18.2) and found hypoplastic, poorly conducting upper spinal nerves, suggesting partial preganglionic lesions with remaining tissue in situ. The girl grew, the elbow was partially ankylosed, and the ulnar deviation of the wrist and slight hypotrophy of the fingers then made us think about an *atypical arthrogryposis* (Fig. 18.3).

Meanwhile I have seen three more children with similar presentation and class these as atypical arthrogryposis of the upper extremity. The lower extremities were normal, and no other organ involvement was found. They underwent early nerve or muscle transfers to activate elbow flexion and improve shoulder function successfully.

Exploration of the anterior upper arm showed whether healthy muscle tissue, which might accept reinnervation, was present, like a regular biceps and/or brachialis muscle (Fig. 18.4), which we were then able to reinnervate successfully by a nerve transfer of the Oberlin type (Fig. 18.5). If only connective tissue was found locally, we transferred a local muscle (latissimus dorsi or pectoralis major) to perform a biceps plasty. This enabled the children to develop active elbow flexion at an early age, and the sometimes slight joint ankylosis was successfully counteracted (Fig. 18.6).

However, there is still uncertainty about the exact etiology and pathophysiology, and we do not yet know exactly the indications for nerve transfer that must be imposed on these children and their parents [1].

J. Bahm (✉)

Plastic, Hand and Burn Surgery, Section for Plexus Surgery, University Hospital, Aachen, Germany
e-mail: jorg.bahm@belgacom.net,
jbahm@ukaachen.de

© Springer Nature Switzerland AG 2021

J. Bahm (ed.), *Movement Disorders of the Upper Extremities in Children*,
https://doi.org/10.1007/978-3-030-53622-0_18

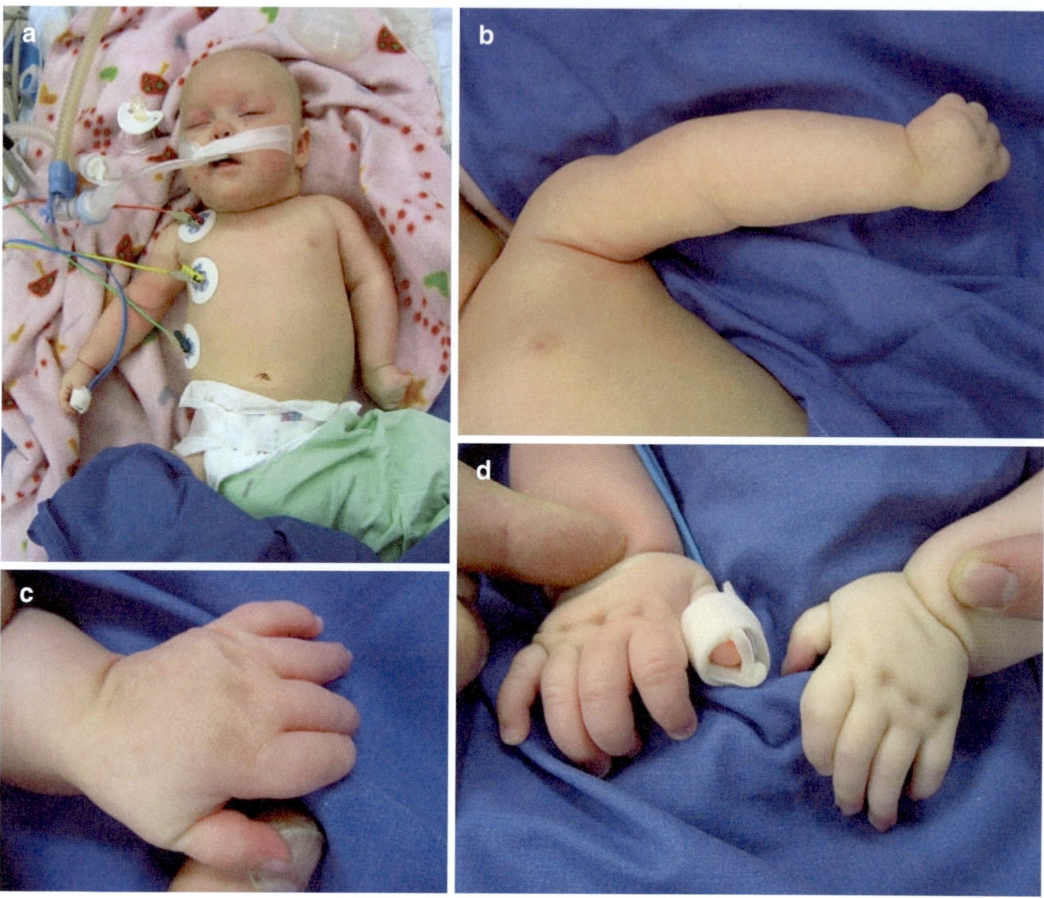

Fig. 18.1 (**a–d**) Arthrogryposis—preoperative findings: This is how the paralyzed left arm looks immediately preoperative. Note the slight axial deviation of the fingers, atypical of plexus palsy

Children who became victims of traffic accidents with *traumatic plexus damage* are difficult. These are often associated with several preganglionic avulsion-type lesions, confirmed during exploration and enhanced only by selective nerve transfers. In this situation it is a matter not only of loss of function and consenting or accompanying during and after the operation but also of helping to bear the psychological burden of the family and the child, especially immediately after the operation and during the immobilization phase.

Three other children presented with severe *shoulder amyotrophy of unclear etiology*. In one of them, a direct shoulder injury in a bouncy castle could finally be identified, responsible for a crushing of the axillary nerve in the quadrangular space of the axilla; in two others the exact accident mechanism remained unknown. In all cases, an active abduction of more than 90° against gravity was achieved by selective nerve transfer of the first motor branch to the triceps muscle onto the distal motor parts of the axillary nerve, in spite of 12 months of diagnosis delay.

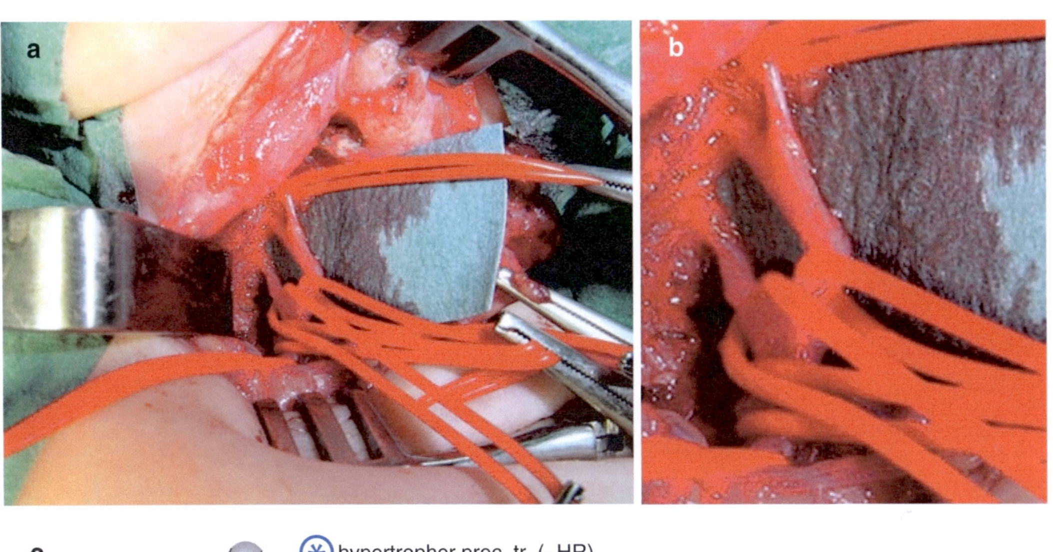

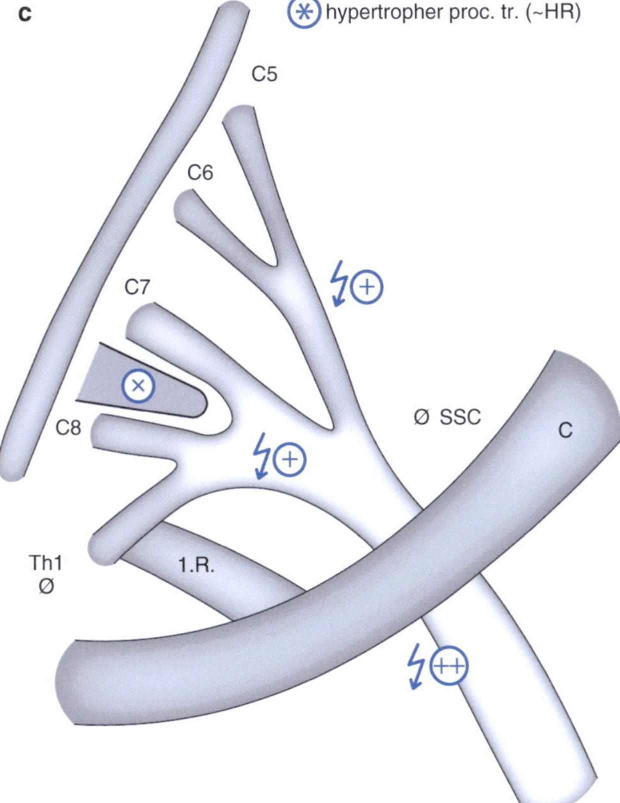

Fig. 18.2 (**a–c**) Arthrogryposis. (**a**, **b**) Intraoperative situs. (**c**) Scheme according to an operation sketch by Dr. Bahm (Appendix)

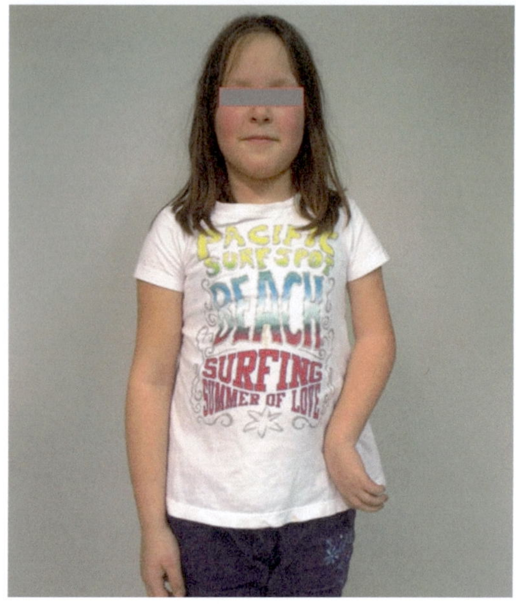

Fig. 18.3 Late development

Fig. 18.4 Exploration of the upper arm to determine whether a muscle capable of regeneration (biceps) is present

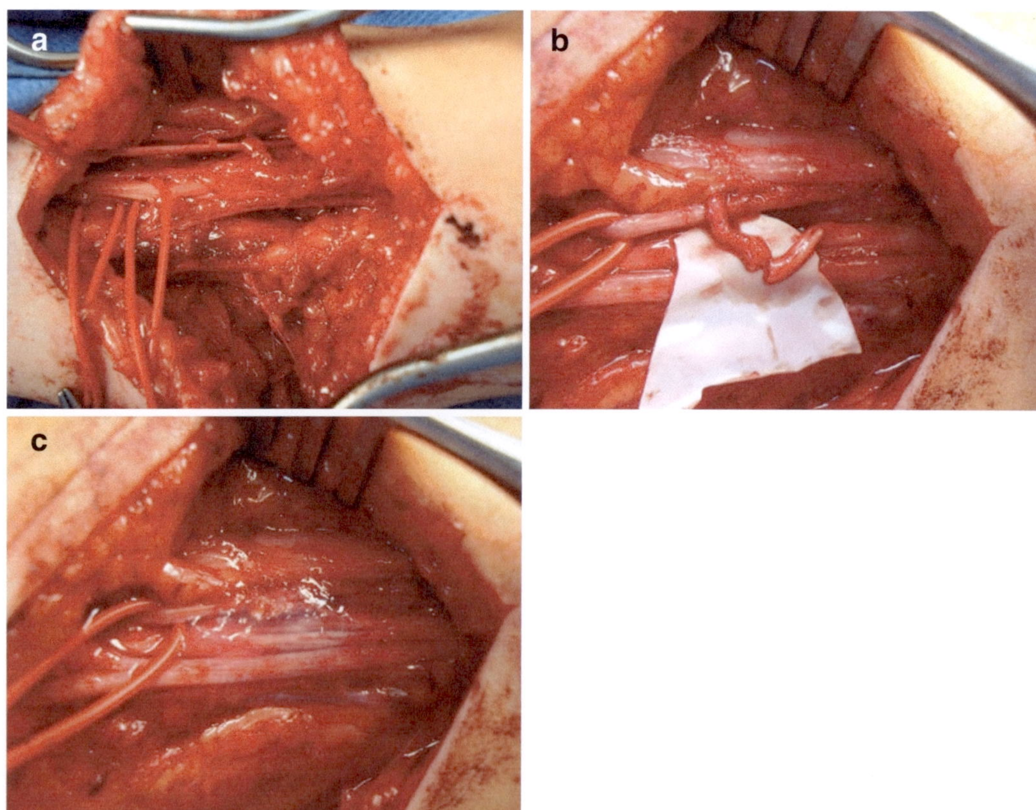

Fig. 18.5 (**a–c**) Oberlin transfer

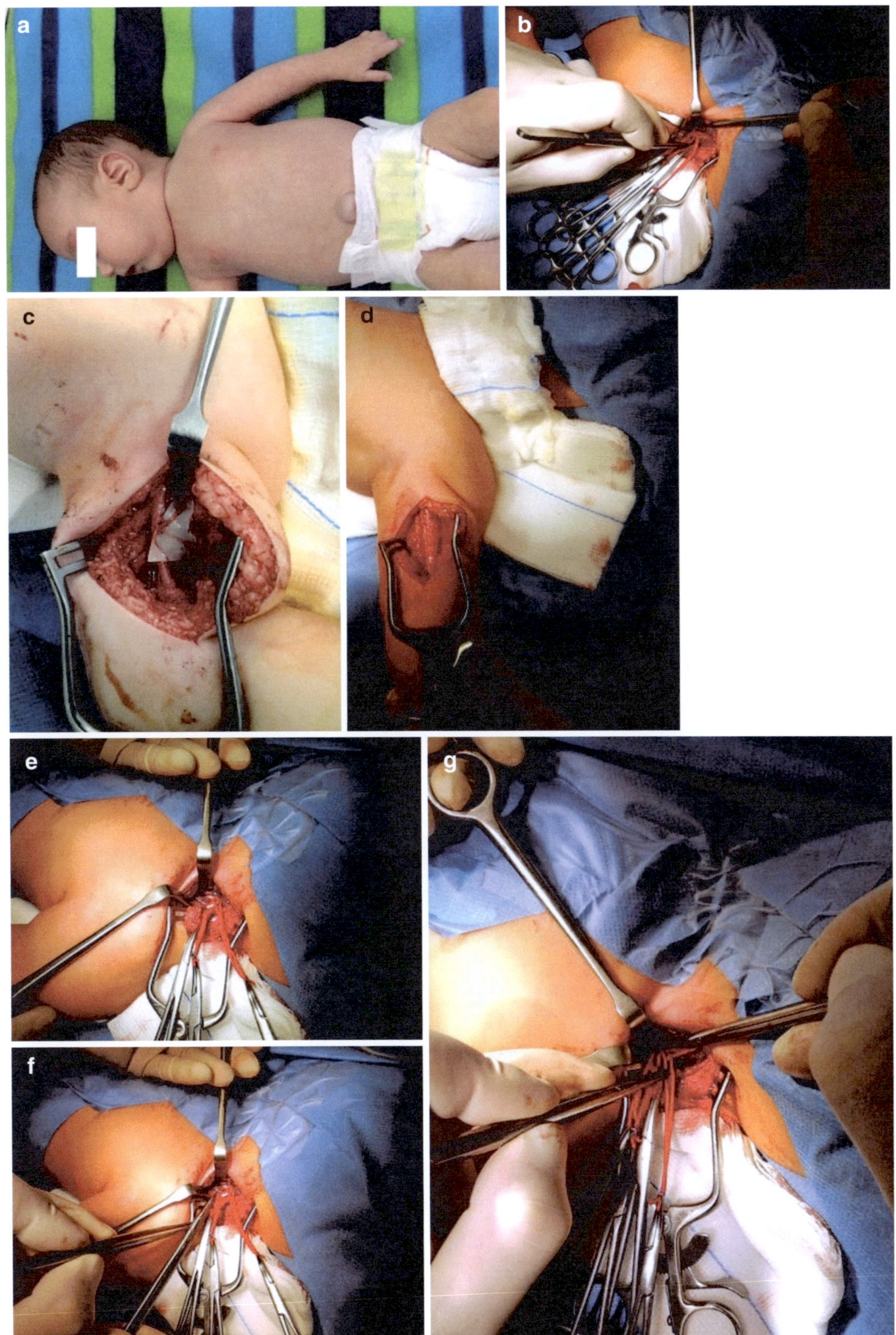

Fig. 18.6 (a–g) Exploration in arthrogryposis (second child)

A special situation also arises if a typical plexus palsy which requires operation happens in a child with *serious concomitant diseases* such as renal insufficiency, in which, in view of the overall situation, a non-operative course was followed. In this particular child, who showed satisfactory general development and acceptable arm function but a weak shoulder, we performed a local nerve transfer, using the distal branch of the XIth cranial nerve transferred onto the suprascapular nerve, a short operation lasting for 90 min and thus limiting the perioperative risks, carried out under outpatient conditions, enabling the mother herself to manage the baby's peritoneal dialysis.

Reference

1. Bahm J. Arguments for a neuroorthopaedic strategy in upper limb arthrogryposis. J Brachial Plex Peripheral Nerve Inj. 2013;8(1):9.

Anaesthesia in Infants and Young Children with Birth Traumatic Plexus Lesion: A Field Report

B. Sauerzapfe

19.1 Premedication

These patients with severe nerve damage are presented to the anaesthetist for the first time at the age of about 3 months. Patients should be healthy at this time and should not have serious concomitant diseases. Kidney or heart disease as well as metabolic problems should not be present. As these injuries occur during a difficult birth, the children often already required resuscitation and stay in intensive care units with long post-partum ventilation times and frequent examinations.

Cerebral diseases or malformations of the digestive tract can also cause problems for the anaesthetist, especially since we do not assume short interventions, but rather intervention times of 6–8 h. Fortunately, the surgical trauma is less than it would be in visceral surgery, for example. However, the duration of anaesthesia alone means that the perioperative phase must be well planned. In our clinic we assume that our patients should be at least 3 months old and weigh approx. 5–6 kg.

The *premedication consultation*—if possible with both parents—takes place on the day before the operation. First of all, it is about the overall impression of the child's stage of development. The main focus is on reassuring parents and answering their urgent questions. The examina-tion of the young patient is mainly clinical; the paediatric examination booklet should be available in order to record pathological accompanying findings.

The main focus is on the pulmonary situation. We pay particular attention to a coinjury of the phrenic nerve (upper plexus lesion with involvement of root C4). In auscultatory terms, there is often insufficient ventilation of the affected side of the lung; in anamnestic terms, there often is a longer post-partum ventilation period and/or frequent pulmonary infections.

During surgery, phrenic paresis is of secondary importance, since the effects can be minimised with an adapted ventilation pattern.

Postoperatively, the involvement of the phrenic nerve in the plexus injury considerably complicates the postoperative care of the patients, a pneumonic complication will be more frequent. Assisted mechanical ventilation is much more probable and must be addressed with the parents already during the premedication.

Laboratory findings are normally not available and necessary if the patients are properly developed and healthy except for the nerve trauma. (Laboratory values are often determined after anaesthesia has been administered; in preoperative blood collection, the difficult vascular conditions are traumatising for children and parents.)

We explain the anaesthetic procedure to the parents. In our clinic one parent may be present in the operating theatre for the anaesthetic

B. Sauerzapfe (✉)
Uniklinik RWTH Aachen, Aachen, Germany

© Springer Nature Switzerland AG 2021
J. Bahm (ed.), *Movement Disorders of the Upper Extremities in Children*,
https://doi.org/10.1007/978-3-030-53622-0_19

induction. Postoperatively, the parents can look after their child themselves in our intensive care unit, so that although there is apparatus monitoring, otherwise family-friendly conditions are created as far as possible. If the progress is regular, the child can be breastfed postoperatively; mothers are specially instructed on how to do this. A special focus in the preoperative talk is on postoperative respiratory disorders. All parents will be informed about any necessary breathing therapy afterwards.

19.2   Anaesthesia

On the day of the operation, we consider it necessary to restrict nourishment 3–4 h before the operation because of the danger of aspiration during anaesthetic induction.

The children are induced with sevoflurane in the presence of one parent; venipuncture is often problematic at this age, and therefore we only perform it on the narcotised child. We initially prefer a vein in the head area; due to the expected surgical treatment, only the healthy arm is usually available to us (often both nn. surales are necessary for transplantation). The following oral intubation is performed under deep general anaesthesia—sevoflurane and supplementation with fentanyl—without administration of a relaxant! Up to a tube size of 5 Charr. we use uncuffed tubes. The mechanical ventilation is adjusted according to the weight and is controlled and regulated by blood gas analyses after the induction. An orally inserted suction catheter Ch 6 serves to drain gastric juice for the duration of the operation, and it is taken out at the end of the operation.

The temperature probe is inserted nasally or orally to create controlled conditions.

During the operation, the surgeon places a central venous catheter into the internal jugular vein of the injured side under sight. This way we exclude a possible traumatisation of the healthy lung.

19.2.1   Positioning on the Operating Table

The head lies turned sideways to the healthy side on a head ring, which we manufacture individually with cotton wool.

Blood pressure is measured non-invasively on the healthy arm, as are pulse oximetry, ECG and stethoscope, which we stick to the healthy side of the thorax. A fresh disposable diaper is used; this allows qualitative and semi-quantitative (weight) assessment of urine production.

The *infusion therapy* follows a scheme with balanced full electrolyte solutions, which we supplement with glucose to 1–2% solution. Due to the addition of glucose, the acid-base management is almost balanced even after 6–8 h of surgery.

Intraoperatively, the anaesthetic management is individual for very different analgesic requirements due to the injury pattern. We see the greatest necessity for opioid analgesics during the removal of nerve transplants from the legs. The reconstruction of the plexus then only requires sevoflurane in a rather low concentration. This shallow anaesthesia favours extubation, which is usually possible within approx. 20–30 min after the end of the surgical suture. For analgesia, we infiltrate the graft sites with low-concentration bupivacaine; small traumatising incisions contribute to pain reduction.

At the end of the operation, *omega gypsum* (Chap. 15) is administered still under anaesthesia, to prevent the transplantation sutures from being endangered by uncontrolled movements.

This plaster is a challenge for the anaesthetist. The child's head is only accessible to a limited extent in this cast for any mask ventilation or even reintubation that may be necessary, and the neck can no longer be reclined. In addition, the immobilised arm on the thorax restricts breathing on the traumatised side. In case of a good lung function on both sides, this can usually be compensated; in case of unilateral previous damage, e.g. due to phrenic paresis, this can definitely lead to pulmonary inadequate ventilation and postoperative pneumonia.

We leave the tube after the end of the operation until spontaneous breathing is unaffected and oxygenation without additional O2 is satisfactory. The last application of fentanyl should have been done about 2 h before extubation in order to rule out respiratory depression.

19.3 Postoperative Management

Analgesics are given after *visual pain assessment* weight-adapted to the children. (To measure pain in infants, one observes the facial expression, possible defensive movements of the healthy side and screaming.) The infants are brought to intensive care unit under monitoring and are further monitored there (SaO2, RR, ECG). If necessary, analgesia is performed with novaminesulfon drops, paracetamol or ibuprofen juice.

The first food intake takes place after approx. 1–2 h with tea and, with good drinking results and if there is no vomiting, nourishment is to be continued with milk. Breastfed children can be fed directly without first giving tea; for the first meal, the anaesthetist is present to give help and to reduce the inhibitions the mothers have because of the plaster.

A weight-adapter medication sheet is visibly attached to the cot for everyone to see. It gives the written documentation of the dosages for different drugs and the handling of technical devices, which can and must be used in interventions or very rarely in case of resuscitation. This can minimise uncertainties or dose mix-ups.

On the first morning after the operation, the small patients are often surprisingly unaffected if their respiratory function was sufficient. They should do without oxygen and are taken to the peripheral ward with their parents. There is no further monitoring necessary but pulse oximetry in each shift.

For drinking control and urine and bowel movement control, we ask parents to enter this in a list. The central venous catheter is usually left for 3–4 days in order to have secure access to the venous system in the event of drinking problems or infections. It is taken out during the first change of wound dressing.

Part V

Secondary Interventions

Principles of Orthopaedic Correction

R. Stücker

20.1 Cerebral Palsy

Patients with cerebral palsy develop contractures in the upper extremities due to spastic movement disorders. Particularly affected are patients with severe disability (GMFCS levels IV and V) and patients with unilateral spastic paresis.

In the case of severely affected patients, surgical procedures are usually not directed to improve function, whereas in case of mildly affected patients or unilateral paralysis, functional improvements can be achieved by surgical procedures.

20.1.1 Secondary Shoulder Surgery

Shoulder problems in children with cerebral palsy are extremely rare. When they do occur, however, they are usually difficult to treat, and palliative aspects are the main focus. Especially patients with dystonia and athetoid movement disorders can develop shoulder dislocations, which can occasionally lead to severe pain due to increasing arthritic changes. If conservative measures including medication or botulinum toxin injections fail, surgical measures may have to be considered. The usual anterior stabilisation tech-niques can be used for painful anterior disloca-tions. In the case of increasingly painful posterior dislocations luxations, soft tissue techniques have a poor prognosis, and shoulder arthrodeses is usually the method of choice [1].

20.1.2 Elbow and Forearm

Severe spasticity may lead to flexion contractures of the elbow. The biceps muscle as a two-jointed muscle is usually responsible for the deformity. In addition, however, shortenings of the brachia-lis and brachioradialis muscles also develop. In patients with unilateral cerebral palsy, flexion contractures have cosmetic and functional sig-nificance, whereas in patients with severe dis-ease, palliative aspects are involved, e.g. when flexion contractures of 100° and more make it considerably more difficult to clean the elbow and avoid skin infections. For these severe con-tractures, a complete release of biceps, brachialis and brachioradialis muscle should be performed. Afterwards, an orthotic treatment should be pre-scribed in order to maintain the success of the operation.

Patients with hemiparesis and good function of the affected upper extremity benefit from a lengthen-ing of the biceps muscle, while patients with lim-ited function benefit from a release of biceps and brachialis muscle.

R. Stücker (✉)
Pediatric Orthopaedics, Altonaer Kinderkrankenhaus, Hamburg, Germany
e-mail: Ralf.stuecker@kinderkrankenhaus.net

© Springer Nature Switzerland AG 2021
J. Bahm (ed.), *Movement Disorders of the Upper Extremities in Children*,
https://doi.org/10.1007/978-3-030-53622-0_20

Arthrolysis of the elbow joint is usually not necessary to correct a flexion contracture. Especially when release operations are carried out towards the end of the growth phase, a sustainable result can be expected [2].

A concurrent radial head dislocation can be found in up to 27% [1]. An indication for surgery exists if there is pain or if a skin perforation of the radial head is imminent. Surgical treatments to reconstruct a radial head dislocation are usually not successful. A resection of the radial head may alleviate symptoms but should preferably be performed after the end of growth.

In addition to flexion contractures of the elbow, pronation contractures of the forearm are often encountered. Again, patients with unilateral cerebral palsy and severely affected patients with GMFCS level IV or V may be affected. The pronator teres muscle is responsible for the development of the contracture. If a release of the strongest supinator (biceps muscle) is performed as part of a surgical procedure, an increase of an already existing pronation contracture of the forearm must be expected.

Contractures are usually dynamic. Either a release of the pronator teres muscle or a re-routing of this muscle can be considered [3]. Re-routing can be used from a functional point of view to improve active supination. A transfer of the pronator teres, e.g. to the extensor carpi radialis muscle, is suitable if there is also a flexion contracture of the wrist.

20.1.3 Wrist and Hand Operations

In the so-called thumb-in-palm deformity, the correction principle consists of a release of the shortened soft tissue structures (adductor pollicis muscle) and simultaneous augmentation of the weak extensors and abductors by the brachioradialis muscle or flexor carpi radialis muscle [4]. In the case of an unstable thumb, arthrodesis of the metacarpophalangeal joint may be advisable [3].

With flexion deformities of the wrist, the flexor carpi ulnaris muscle can be transferred to the extensor carpi radialis brevis or longus mus-

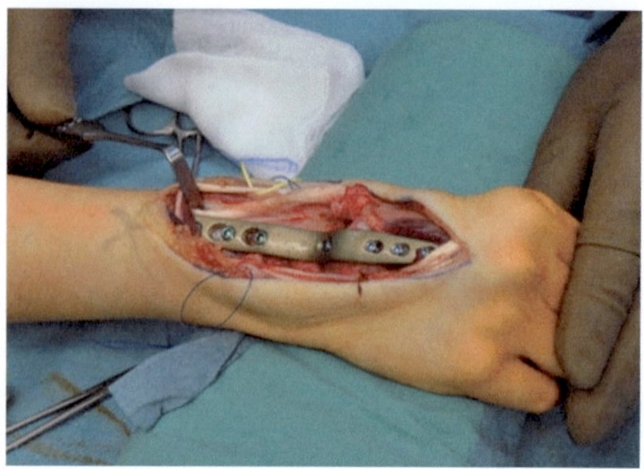

Fig. 20.1 Arthrodesis of the wrist with plate fixation

cle. If very weak finger extensors are present, the transfer can also be performed to the tendons of the extensor digitorum longus muscle [1, 3]. According to our own experience, good results can be achieved reliably. During the evaluation before surgery, it is mandatory that fingers have a sufficiently good active flexion ability.

With fixed wrist deformities, a wrist arthrodesis can also be performed to improve function. In these cases, the proximal carpal row and in severe cases both carpal rows may have to be resected. Stabilisation is then performed either with Kirschner wires or a plate (Fig. 20.1). However, a minimum of active finger flexion and extension should usually be present.

> Corrections of upper extremity deformities are not frequently necessary in cerebral palsy and are usually carried out from a palliative point of view. However, in case of unilateral cerebral palsy, functional improvements are possible after surgical procedures.

20.2 Arthrogryposis Multiplex Congenita

In children with AMC, reconstructive measures must be carefully considered, because muscle development is usually poor. However, improvements in function through osteotomies or arthrolysis can be expected in selected cases.

The following explanations refer to the typical classical arthrogryposis, also known as amyoplasia. The clinical picture with internal rotation of the shoulders, extension contractures of the elbows and flexion contractures of the wrists with adducted arms is characteristic (Fig. 20.2).

The following principles apply to orthopaedic treatment of the upper extremities: maintaining or improving joint mobility prior to measures to improve active mobility, learning bimanual functions and considering the upper extremity as a functional unit [5]. Children with arthrogryposis can develop remarkable adaptation strategies, and this must be taken into account when evaluating treatment options in order not to negatively influence function [6]. Creation of an active flexion ability of the elbow joint only makes sense if there is a certain abduction ability in the shoulder joint. Even the creation of passive mobility of the elbow is a functional gain, because a hand can be passively guided to the mouth.

20.2.1 Secondary Shoulder Surgery

The shoulder is often positioned in internal rotation and adduction due to limited mobility of the glenohumeral joint and between the scapula and thorax. Through an *external rotation osteotomy*, a significant functional improvement of the entire upper extremity can be achieved (Fig. 20.3). An osteotomy of this kind should preferably be performed either with a plate or with an external fixator, as this makes immobilisation of the extremity unnecessary. If necessary, the operation can be combined with a lengthening of the pectoralis and subscapularis muscle.

20.2.2 Surgery of the Elbow

The aim of the elbow treatment is to achieve a *flexion ability of more than 90°*. If this is not possible by conservative management during the first years of life, triceps lengthening in combination with posterior release of the elbow

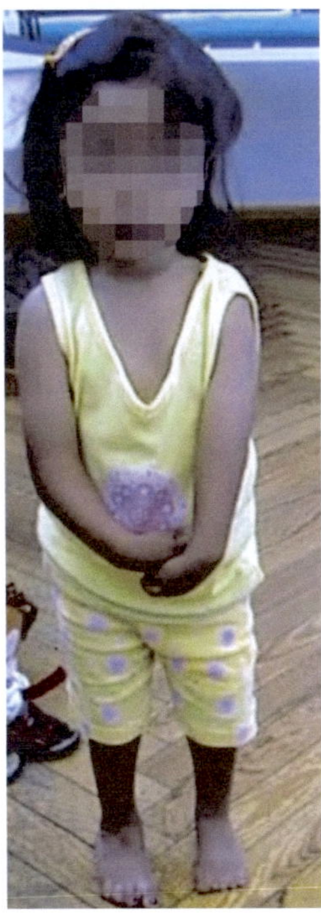

Fig. 20.2 Typical classic form of arthrogryposis

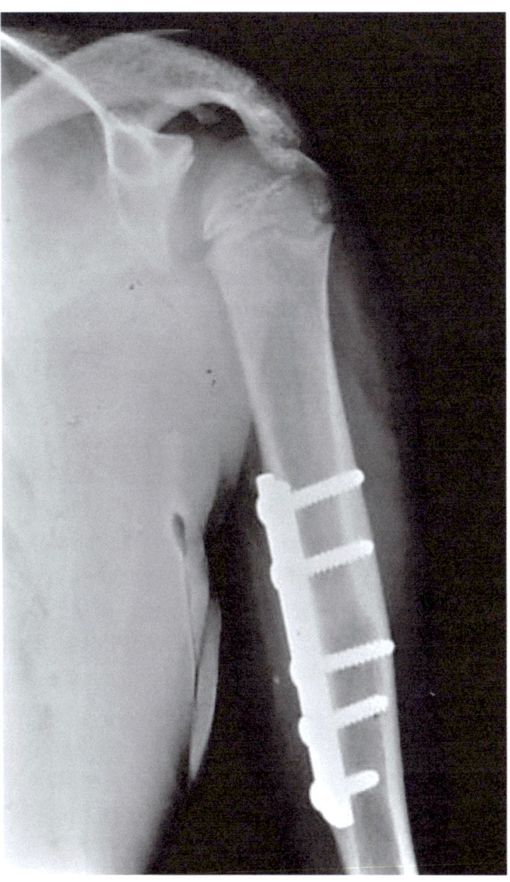

Fig. 20.3 Plate fixation after external rotation osteotomy of the humerus

is necessary. During the procedure, the ulnar nerve should be freed from the sulcus and transposed anteriorly. Extensive physical therapy is subsequently necessary because a loss of achieved flexion ability or even the development of a flexion contracture can occur. Such an operation should be performed in the first years of life. Later in life a considerable incongruency of the joint may already exist, so that a smooth hinge joint movement is difficult. In addition, this incongruency causes difficulties in maintaining the achieved joint mobility.

A number of surgical procedures have been developed to achieve active elbow flexion. Many of these processes have considerable disadvantages. Thus, a transfer of the triceps to the biceps regularly leads to a flexion contracture of the elbow joint. A transfer of the latissimus dorsi or pectoralis major muscle [7, 8] leads to considerable cosmetic problems, especially in girls. The most suitable method seems to be to the transfer of the long head of the triceps anterior to the elbow [5].

20.2.3 Wrist and Hand Operations

The wrist of AMC patients often develops a variable but *fixed ulnar deviation* and *flexion deformity*. The wrist extensors are weak and do not function. Often bony connections between the proximal and distal carpal rows are present, while the joint between radius, ulna and proximal carpal row is preserved (Fig. 20.4).

The V-shaped carpal osteotomy of the wrist with a dorsoradial base has proven very effective for correction [9]. This may have to be combined with a lengthening of the flexor muscles. A transverse incision of the forearm fascia, possibly in combination with a release of the fibrotic wrist structures, is often necessary. An alternative to this procedure is the slow soft tissue distraction with an external fixator (Fig. 20.5). According to our own experience, the surgical lengthening of the flexor muscles is usually unnecessary with this technique.

The correction of a thumb-in-palm deformity is usually successful. In addition to a release of the contracted soft tissue structures,

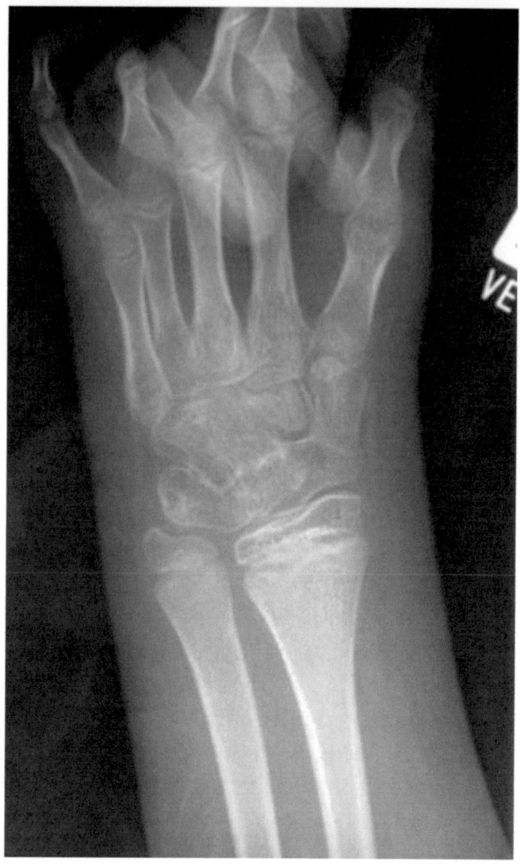

Fig. 20.4 In AMC, bony connections of the proximal and distal carpal rows are frequently present

an arthrodesis of the first MTP joint can also be considered [6].

> Conservative management has first priority in the treatment of AMC patients. Good indications for surgical procedures are an external rotation osteotomy of the humerus to correct the internal rotation of the shoulder, a posterior arthrolysis of the elbow and lengthening of the triceps to create the ability to flex and a V-osteotomy in the area of the wrist to correct a flexion deformity.

20.3 Plexus Palsy

In children with plexus palsy, reconstructions of the upper extremities may be helpful if plastic neurosurgical procedures have had an inadequate effect or if residual conditions exist that have led to significant dysfunctions.

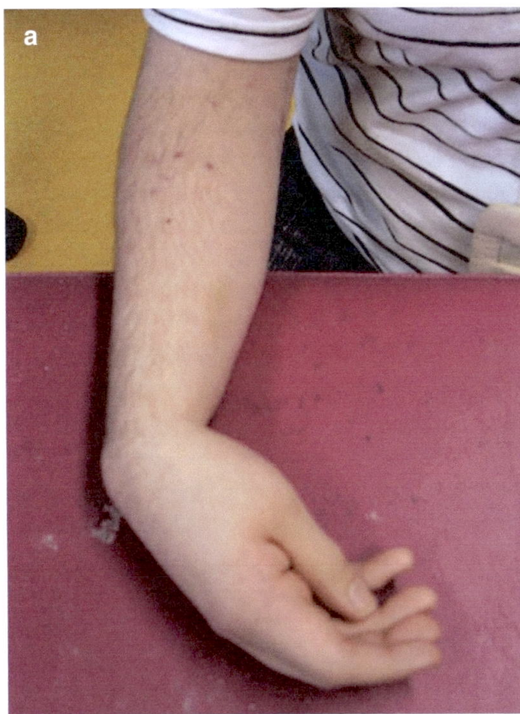
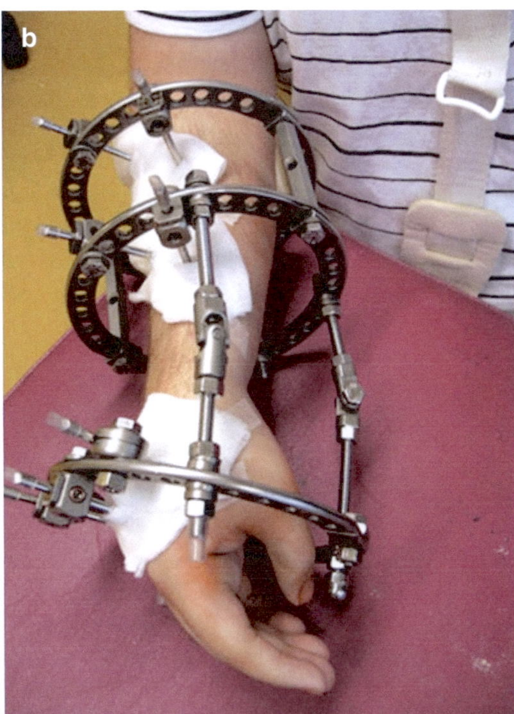

Fig. 20.5 (**a**, **b**) Patient with a typical wrist deformity before (**a**) and after (**b**) arthrodiastasis using an external fixator

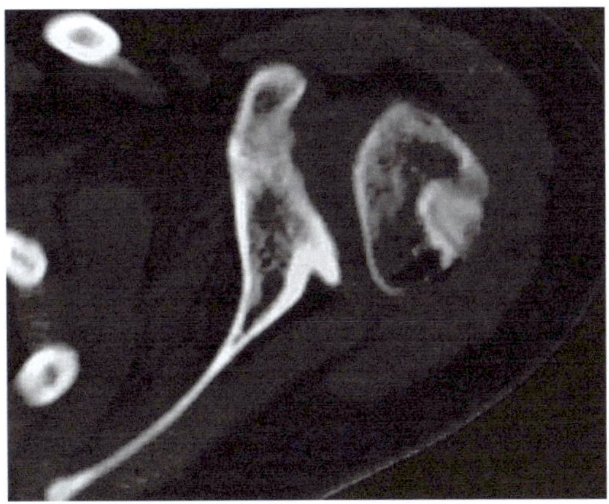

Fig. 20.6 Significant flattening of the humeral head and glenoid with resulting incongruency

20.3.1 Shoulder Surgery

When evaluating pathologic conditions of the shoulder, a distinction must be made between a congruent situation and an incongruent situation of the glenohumeral joint (Fig. 20.6). As a result of insufficient recovery of external rotators of the shoulder joint, a posterior subluxation of the shoulder joint often develops, which then leads to a deformation of the joint. The reason for this is the muscular imbalance with weakness of the external rotators with insufficient stabilisation of the posterior capsule and simultaneous contracture of the anterior structures, especially the subscapularis muscle.

In the presence of *congruency*, a transfer of the latissimus dorsi muscle to the teres minor muscle can be performed in addition to a release of the contractures. The shortened subscapularis muscle should not be lengthened at the humeral attachment but at the scapular origin. The muscular balancing together with the release of the contractures can be accomplished via an axillary approach. In a few cases, a release of the anterior

A complete recovery after plexus palsy is observed in about 50% of cases, although reports in the literature vary considerably (7–95%). However, at least 10–20% have significant functional deficits of the upper extremities. Even after early microsurgical plexus intervention, residual functional disturbances often remain, which then require various reconstruction procedures.

structures is necessary, like a Z-shaped lengthening of the pectoralis major muscle, a release of the coracoacromial ligament or a release or lengthening of the coracobrachialis muscle and the short biceps head.

In the case of insufficient joint congruency, muscle transfers around the shoulder joint should not be performed. In such cases, an external rotation osteotomy of the proximal humerus is more appropriate. In addition to improving the external rotation, this also improves the abduction ability of the affected shoulder to some extent.

20.3.2 Elbow and Forearm Surgery

Flexion contractures of the elbow often develop in combination with a persistent internal rotation malposition of the shoulder joint. When considering correcting a flexion contracture of the elbow joint, the muscle function of flexors and extensors should be assessed. If there is not sufficient active elbow extension, a relapse of a flexion contracture is likely. If active extension of the elbow is possible, a careful lengthening of the flexors and an anterior capsular release or a complete capsular detachment can be used to achieve correction.

For functional reasons, it is preferable to correct a forearm malposition to slight pronation. A severe pronation or supination malposition should be corrected. In mild cases a pronation deformity can be corrected by re-routing the pronator teres, but in severe cases osteotomies of the radius and ulna must be performed.

The same applies to supination deformities. A re-routing of the biceps tendon according to Zancolli could be considered in mild cases without active pronation, while in severe cases bony corrections must be performed (Fig. 20.7).

20.3.3 Hand Surgery

Reconstructive procedures to improve hand function are limited because the entire hand musculature and also the sensory system are usually affected and therefore tendon transfers are not

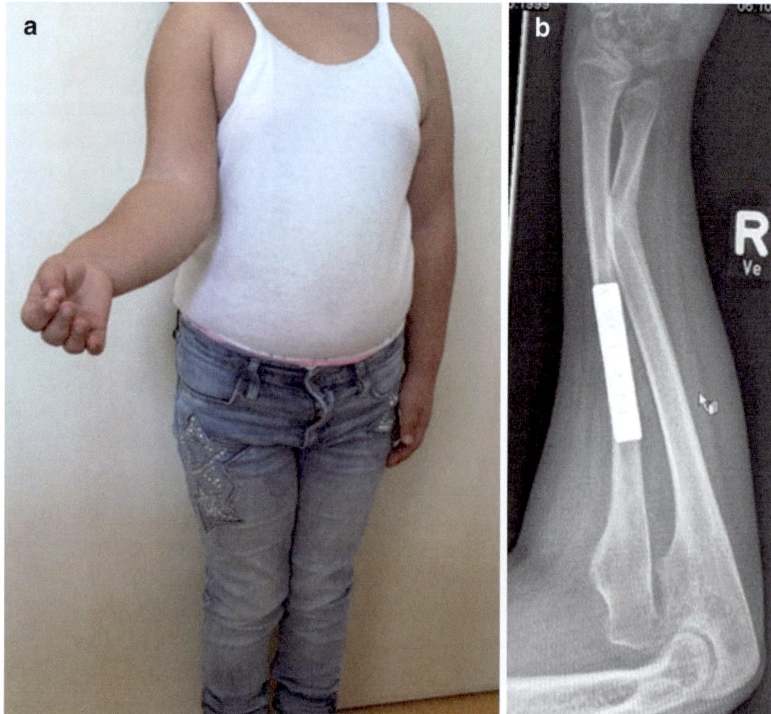

Fig. 20.7 (**a**, **b**) Severe supination contracture (**a**) and correction by rotational osteotomy (**b**)

promising. In individual cases, stabilisation of the wrist by arthrodesis can be useful in order to achieve at least a slight improvement in function.

> Operative measures to maintain the congruency of the shoulder joint may be necessary at an early stage. In case of incongruence, an external rotation osteotomy, possibly in combination with a correction of a flexion contracture of the elbow, can be useful. Severe pronation or supination malpositions of the forearm can be successfully corrected by osteotomies in the bones.

20.4 Summary

In cerebral palsy, arthrogryposis and plexus palsy, secondary reconstructive surgery of the upper extremities may be considered from a palliative point of view or to improve function. The entire upper extremity must be seen as a unit. Thus, indications for surgery around the shoulder cannot be seen separated from the situation of the elbow, the position of the forearm or wrist and possible contractures of the fingers. In patients with cerebral palsy, severe flexion contractures of the elbows, wrist contractures or a significant thumb-in-palm deformity may be an indication for surgery. In patients with unilateral cerebral palsy, surgical measures can also be used to improve function, especially in pronation contractures of the forearm, or to improve wrist function.

Children with arthrogryposis can often compensate their disability caused by contractures or muscular weakness surprisingly well. This must be taken into account when evaluating the function of the upper extremities. However, the correction of an internal rotation contracture of the shoulder or an extension contracture of the elbow or a correction of a wrist malposition can lead to functional improvements.

In patients with plexus palsy, functional disorders may remain despite early microsurgical intervention. The maintenance of passive mobility of the joints has first priority, followed by creation of active motion in the area of shoulders, elbows and wrist by surgical procedures, e.g. a transfer of the latissimus dorsi to the teres minor to improve external rotation. Possibilities to improve active elbow flexion are still limited and not always sufficiently successful.

References

1. Miller F. Cerebral palsy. Berlin Heidelberg New York: Springer; 2005.
2. Mital MA. Lengthening of the elbow flexors in cerebral palsy. J Bone Joint Surg Am. 1979;61:515–22.
3. Döderlein L. Infantile Zerebralparese. Darmstadt: Steinkopff; 2007.
4. Sakellarides HT, Mital MA, Matza RA, Dimakopoulos P. Classification and surgical treatment of the thumb-in-palm deformity in cerebral palsy and spastic paralysis. J Hand Surg Am. 1995;20:428–31.
5. Herring JA. Disorders of the upper extremity. In: Tachdjian's pediatric orthopaedics. 4th ed. Amsterdam: Saunders Elsevier; 2007.
6. Staheli LT. Arthrogryposis. Cambridge: Cambridge University Press; 1998.
7. Carroll RE, Kleinmann WB. Pectoralis major transplantation to restore elbow flexion to the paralytic limb. J Hand Surg Am. 1979;4:501–7.
8. Zancolli E, Mitre H. Latissimus dorsi transfer to restore elbow flexion. J Bone Joint Surg Am. 1973;55:1265–75.
9. Ezaki M, Carter PR. Carpal wedge osteotomy for the arthrogrypotic wrist. Tech Hand Up Extrem Surg. 2004;8:224–8.

Jörg Bahm

21.1 Introduction

Once the actual nerve damage has healed and the process of nerve regeneration is completed, a more or less balanced muscle equilibrium develops over time which, together with other factors such as skeletal development, determines the maturation of the affected limb in the adolescent.

The observed functional impairments of muscle weakness, imbalance and bone and joint deformities are best sorted topographically and should of course never be considered in isolation, but in terms of their long-lasting effects on the entire limb.

The problems and operations described in the following are usually aimed at *improving function*. Only a really *useful increase* in function justifies an indication for operation; however, especially during puberty with increased attention to the body image, there arise also questions about the correction of the appearance, mostly in the sense of "making the affected arm inconspicuous", the appearance of which should best match the other, unaffected extremity. This can help the adolescent to improve social integration:

"I do not want to attract attention by the changed position of my arm".

In the following, we consider the most common limitations from proximal to distal (mostly after infantile plexus lesion; [1, 2]), whereby proximal problems have a more global influence on the movement pattern: the shoulder orientates the hand in space in the long term, and a loss of strength in the proximal musculature especially in the adolescent, when limb weight increases, may induce not only a reduction in the range of movement but also load-dependent pain and early arthritic changes. Demy [3], in a retrospective survey, showed that the shoulder region is the most common problem area in young adults.

21.2 Shoulder

21.2.1 Medial Rotation Contracture of the Shoulder and Glenohumeral Dysplasia

The most common abnormalities observed in all age groups are the medial rotation contracture (MRC) of the shoulder and glenohumeral dysplasia (GHD).

Especially in the case of C 5-6 and C 5-6-7 lesions in children, a progressive rotational imbalance of the shoulder often occurs both in operated and spontaneously regenerating injuries, probably due to insufficiently balanced

J. Bahm (✉)
Plastic, Hand and Burn Surgery, Section for Plexus
Surgery, University Hospital, Aachen, Germany
e-mail: jorg.bahm@belgacom.net,
jbahm@ukaachen.de

© Springer Nature Switzerland AG 2021
J. Bahm (ed.), *Movement Disorders of the Upper Extremities in Children*,
https://doi.org/10.1007/978-3-030-53622-0_21

medial rotational force provided by the earlier and better regenerating subscapular muscle. Only in severe and complete lesions, in the paralysed shoulder, is this imbalance absent and the glenohumeral joint passive range of motion (ROM) unaffected.

As with two unequal teams in a tug of war contest, first a medial rotation posture develops, because of imbalance between a strong subscapularis and weak infraspinatus muscle, with initially free passive ROM of the glenohumeral joint. This progressively leads to medial rotation contracture (MRC, Fig. 21.1).

The glenohumeral joint, which is mainly controlled by a balanced muscle system, undergoes morphological constraints: the humeral head rotates medially and subluxates posteriorly, and the glenoid adapts itself in such a way that a rather posterior located socket, frequently called pseudoglenoid although it is lined by hyaline cartilage, develops and the true anterior glenoid withers away. The humeral head becomes fixed itself in this medially rotated, posteriorly subluxated position with a permanent, not antagonized traction of the subscapular muscle. This change in local biomechanics influences both the shape of the joint partners in the growing joint (flattening of the humeral head, delayed ossification of the epiphysis, multiple deformation possibilities of the glenoid) and their arrangement (changing also the version of the humeral head and glenoid). Moreover, there is, too, the variable extent of injury at birth, to bone, joint and muscle, quite evident when there is a connatal glenohumeral posterior dislocation [4].

The most conspicuous aspect is the **dysmorphia of the glenoid** (Fig. 21.2, classification according to [5–7]), where a flattened or even convex glenoid or a distinct double shell formation with a biconcave structure or a double facet can occur and becomes visible in the CT/MRI, depending on the extent of the posterior pseudoglenoid, combined with an increasing retroversion of the

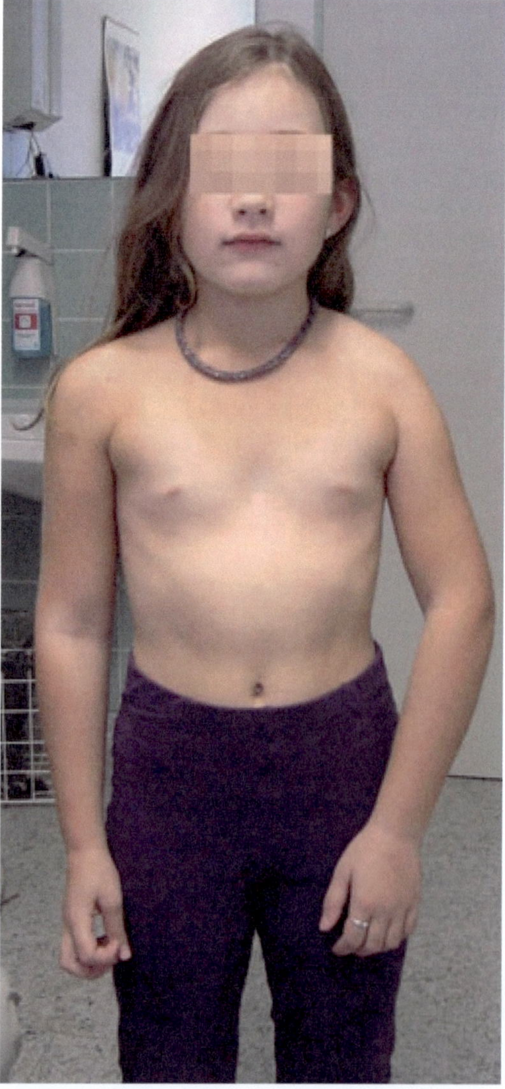

Fig. 21.1 Medial rotation contracture: clinical observation of the internally rotated basic posture of the arm

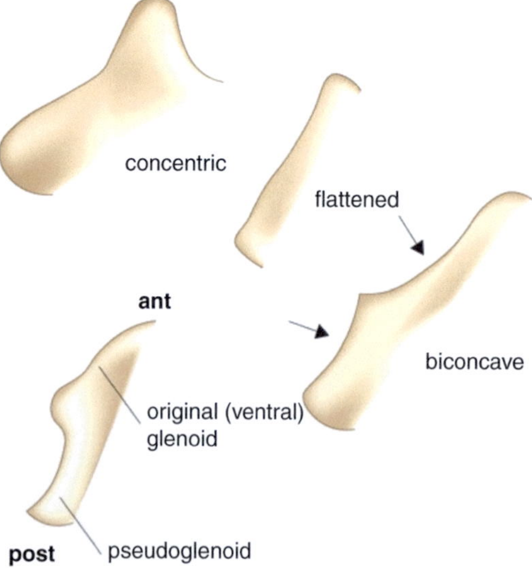

Fig. 21.2 Classification according to Waters/Birch

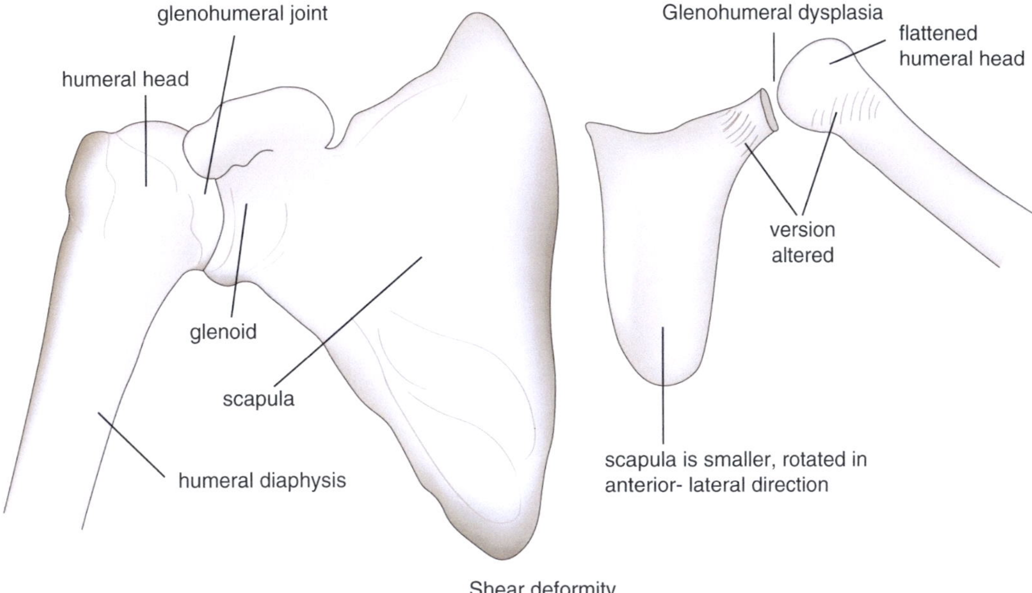

Fig. 21.3 SHEAR deformity

humeral head. This leads to a complex dysmorphic joint in late adolescence and young adults.

In addition, this altered morphology also affects the transferred leverage forces on the shoulder blade (dorsal or inferior contractures) and must also be seen in connection with rare but complex hypoplasias and malpositions of the entire shoulder blade ([8]: SHEAR (scapular hypoplasia and external and anterior rotation) deformity; Fig. 21.3).

Restriction in the passive and active range of lateral rotation indicates this change, especially passive lateral rotation (pLR) in an adducted arm (ADD) position (Fig. 21.4): Imaging will add objective morphologic data (MRI or ultrasound in the younger child as cartilage can be better visualized; CT and 3D CT in the young adult) (Fig. 21.5).

The surgical strategy is summarized in Table 21.1. In the newborn, rare peripartal traumatic dorsal humeral head subluxations [4] must undergo a closed reposition under anaesthesia and an external rotation plaster for 4 weeks as early as possible. This strategy will allow to better follow the recovery of the active movements under subsequent congruent joint conditions and also to counteract the medial rotation malposition during the recovery period of the lateral rotators

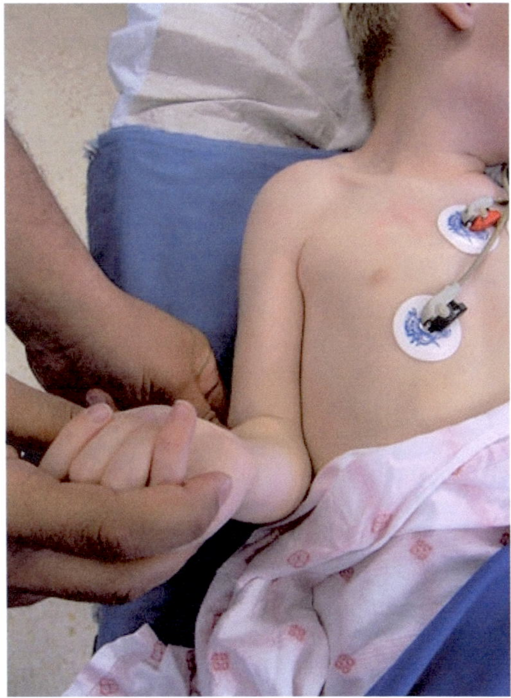

Fig. 21.4 Restriction of passive lateral rotation (pLR) with adducted arm

by regular stretching exercises of the joint with the adducted arm, performed by therapists and regularly educated parents (Fig. 21.6).

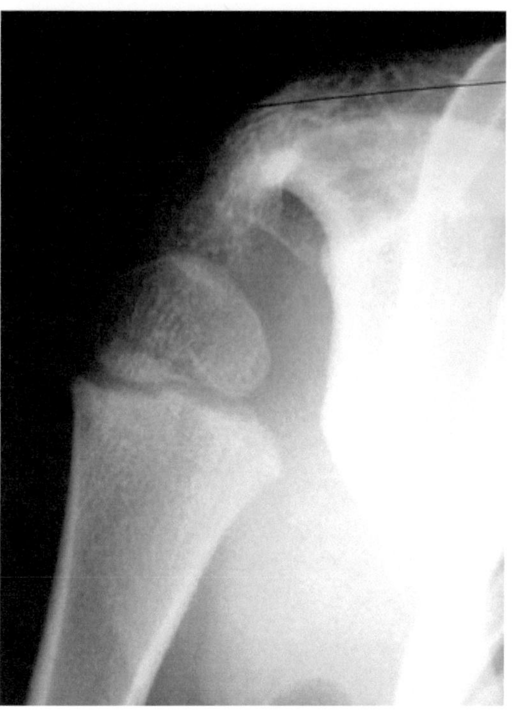

Fig. 21.5 Imaging prior to a shoulder release (Fig. 5.4)

With **children over 2 years** with fixed MRC (pLR [ADD] under 30°), the passive range of movement must be improved by an operative anterior shoulder release (Fig. 21.7) or by a detachment of the subscapular muscle from the front of the shoulder blade by a lateral approach ("subscapular slide") so that recovering lateral rotators subsequently act on a mobile congruent joint.

If **1 year after joint release** there is still no improved active lateral rotation, the latter can be augmented by a muscle transfer of the latissimus dorsi and teres major muscle ([9]; Fig. 21.8) or a pectoralis major tendon rerouting. A nerve transfer to improve the reinnervation of the suprascapular nerve, transfer of the distal branch of the accessory XI nerve to the suprascapular nerve may be considered first.

When with **increasing age** the secondary changes caused by the dislocation become irre-

Table 21.1 Strategy of treatment for medial rotation contracture (mrc)

Timing	Therapeutic actions
As early as possible	(Re-)establish glenohumeral congruence, i.e. in case of subluxation of the humeral head, immediate closed reposition under anaesthesia and 1-month immobilization in adduction-external rotation
	Extend the passive lateral rotation capacity through stretching exercises (if under 30° with the arm adducted) or maintain its level
Before 2 years of life	If anterior shoulder contracture with limited passive lateral rotation does not resolve through conservative measures: anterior shoulder release
	If uncompensated activity of the M. subscapularis dominates: botulinum toxin
	If the active lateral rotation remains weak: neurotization of the N. suprascapularis by means of N. accessorius
After 2 years of life	Shoulder release if necessary, but there exists already frequently a glenohumeral dysplasia
	Strive for muscle equilibrium, if necessary muscle transfer (Hoffer) to strengthen the lateral rotation
	Testing later nerve transfers
About 6 years of life	Humeral osteotomy in lateral rotation
	Muscle transfer only when potential motors are strong (good proportion between muscle mass and arm weight)

versible, the movement sector can be shifted more from an excessively medially rotated area to the lateral rotation sector (Fig. 21.9) by a humeral osteotomy moving the distal segment into the desired arc of rotation. This can be achieved by open transverse diaphyseal osteotomy with plate osteosynthesis, or percutaneous osteotomy and external fixation. The glenohumeral joint situation remains unchanged. The intervention does not lead to an extension of the active or passive range of movement, but instead to a transfer of the movement arc into a more useful, more natural range, which also results in a simplification of other movement sequences, in particular the hand-to-mouth movement (Fig. 21.10).

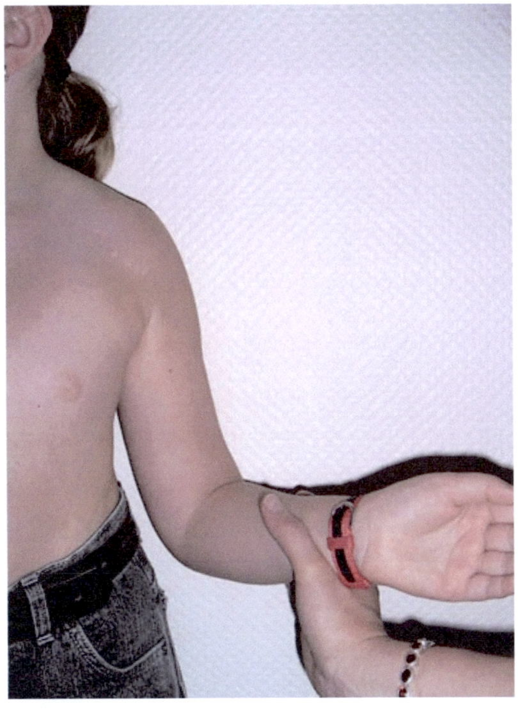

Fig. 21.6 Exercise to enhance passive lateral rotation while stretching the anterior joint capsule and the subscapular muscle

Targets are:

- Early detection of the medial rotation tendency and thus prevention of joint deformation
- Early surgical correction by a release to limit dysplasia in case of joint incongruence
- Best possible improvement of the passive and active range of motion, preferably by expanding the range of motion (Fig. 21.11), otherwise at least by transferring the motion sector to a more useful one

In our practice over 20 years, this dynamic joint dysplasia is the most frequent and most serious secondary problem after birth palsy. Too often, it is not recognised and diagnosis is delayed. This leads to far-reaching consequences regarding the impairment of rotational movements, the severity of joint dysplasia and later lasting functional limitations and pain problems. In the young adult, shoulder sequelae with fixed joint dislocation and arthritic pain are the most challenging to treat.

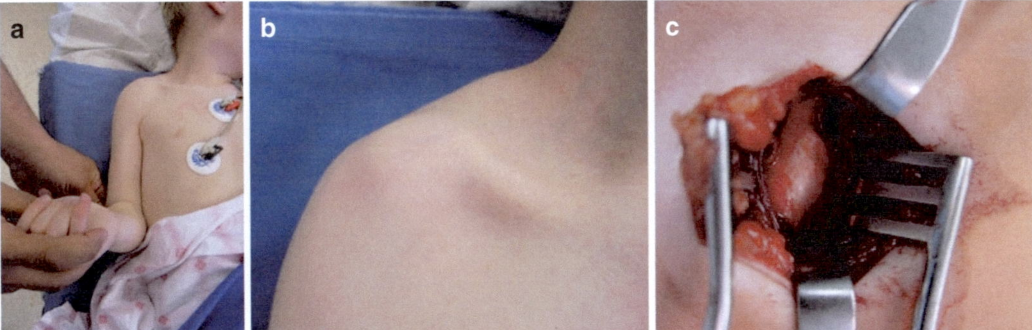

Fig. 21.7 (**a–j**) Anterior release. (**a**) Preoperative functional test about the passive lateral rotation capacity of an already anaesthetised child. (**b**) Prominent subcutaneous coracoid. (**c**) Deltopectoral access to the coracoid. (**d**) Resected coracoid. (**e**) Immediately postoperatively, the lateral rotation ability of the shoulder is improved. (**f**) Repositioned humeral head. (**g**) Suture of the subscapularis tendon and the common tendon of pectoralis minor and coracobrachialis. (**h**) Postoperative plaster of Paris splint. (**i, j**) Postoperative function

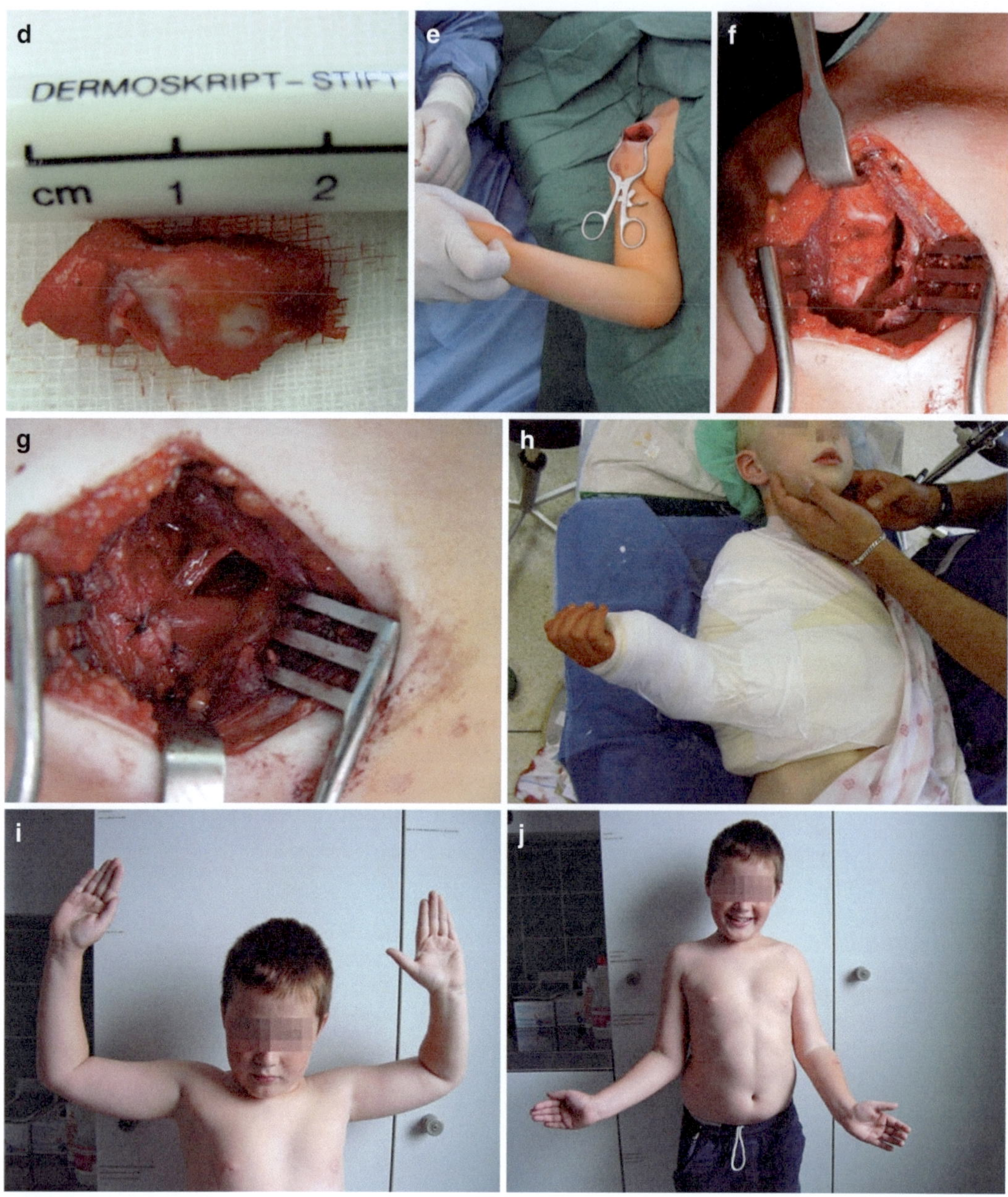

Fig. 21.7 (continued)

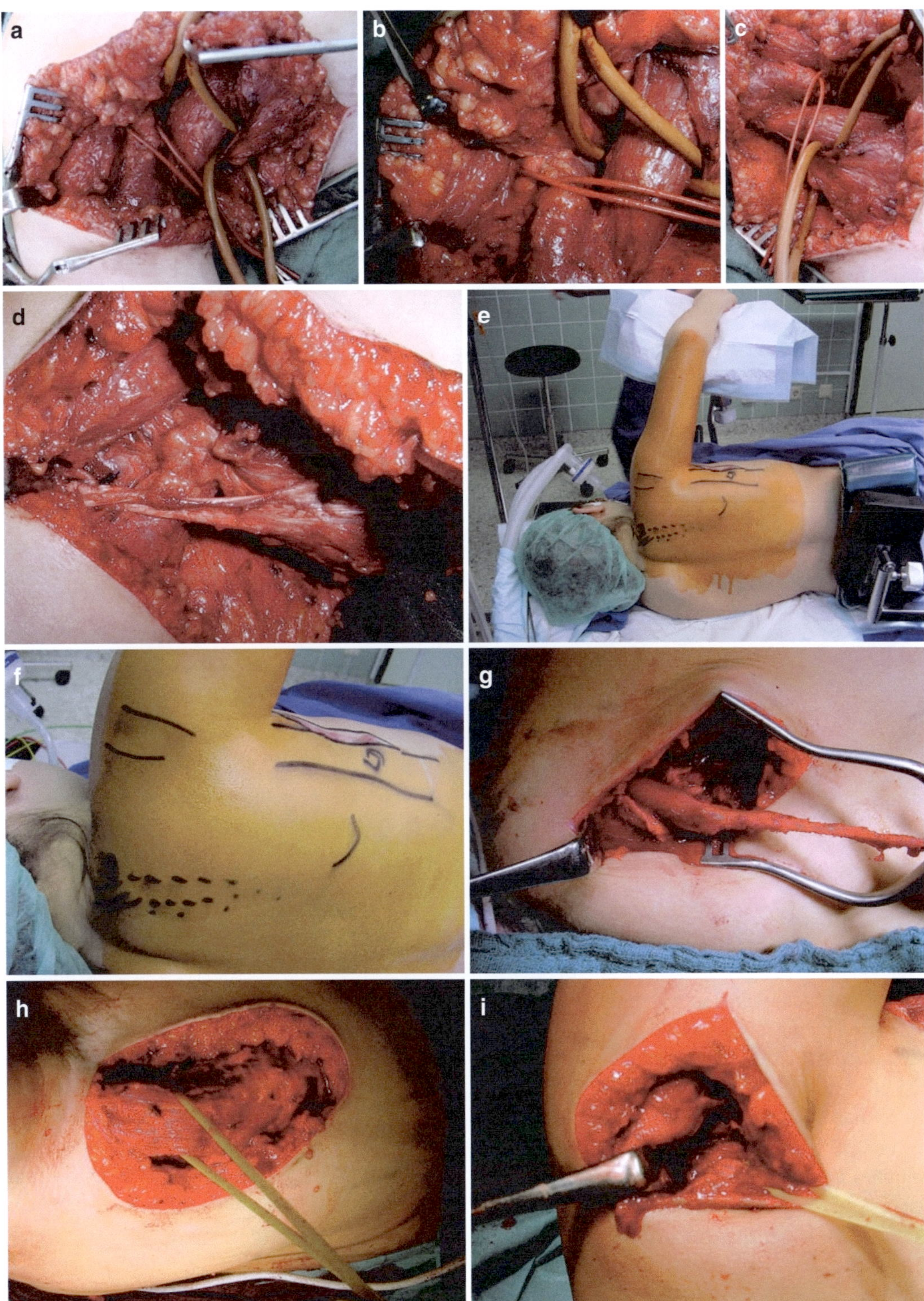

Fig. 21.8 (**a–i**) Muscle transfer (Hoffer) (**a–c**) Selective preparation of the approach of M. latissimus dorsi and M. teres major. (**d**) Tendon fixation at the humeral head. (**e, f**) Positioning and cutting plan with selective transfer of both muscles. (**g–i**) Specific transposition of both muscles in order to control the external rotation separately when the upper arm is adducted or abducted

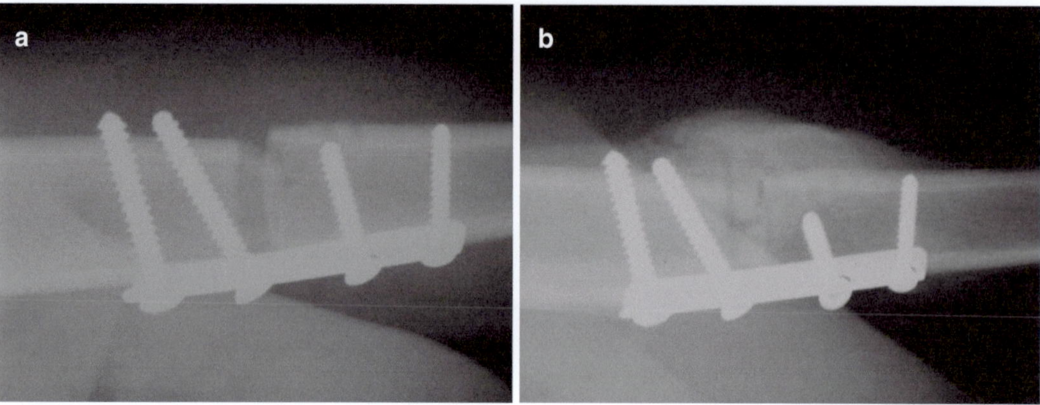

Fig. 21.9 (**a**, **b**) Humeral osteotomy

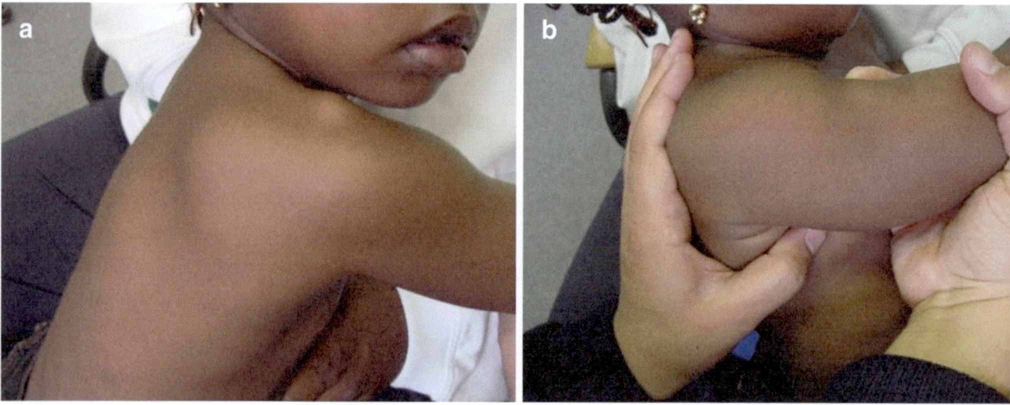

Fig. 21.10 (**a**, **b**) Postoperative shoulder contracture

21.2.2 Weakness in Abduction

Isolated muscle hypotrophies and loss of strength in the individual movement directions can be improved by muscle transfers. A limited antepulsion (flexion) of the shoulder due to weakness of the pectoralis major muscle is rarely augmented. A permanent weakness of abduction (due to the combined losses of deltoid and supraspinatus muscle) can only be moderately corrected by a **cranial M. trapezius transfer** (Fig. 21.12) or by a pedicled **M. teres major transfer** (Fig. 21.13). The gained functional improvement is poor. This is why everything should be done in the primary phase for a good reinnervation of the axillary **and** suprascapularis nerve, either by direct reconstruction of the upper trunk (especially with a possible direct suture) or by elective nerve transfers to the axillary and suprascapular nerves.

In young adults with otherwise completed reconstruction program who present with very poor active shoulder function, active abduction below 30°, hardly any active lateral rotation, the active movements of the scapula should be tested and, when passive and active scapular mobility is good, these motion forces may be transferred to the entire arm by glenohumeral arthrodesis: Especially in young adults, the follow-up results [10] show a significant increase in active shoulder function, combined with a stable joint situation of the otherwise caudally luxating glenohumeral joint. Serratus anterior and trapezius muscles as scapular stabilizers must be normal for this operation.

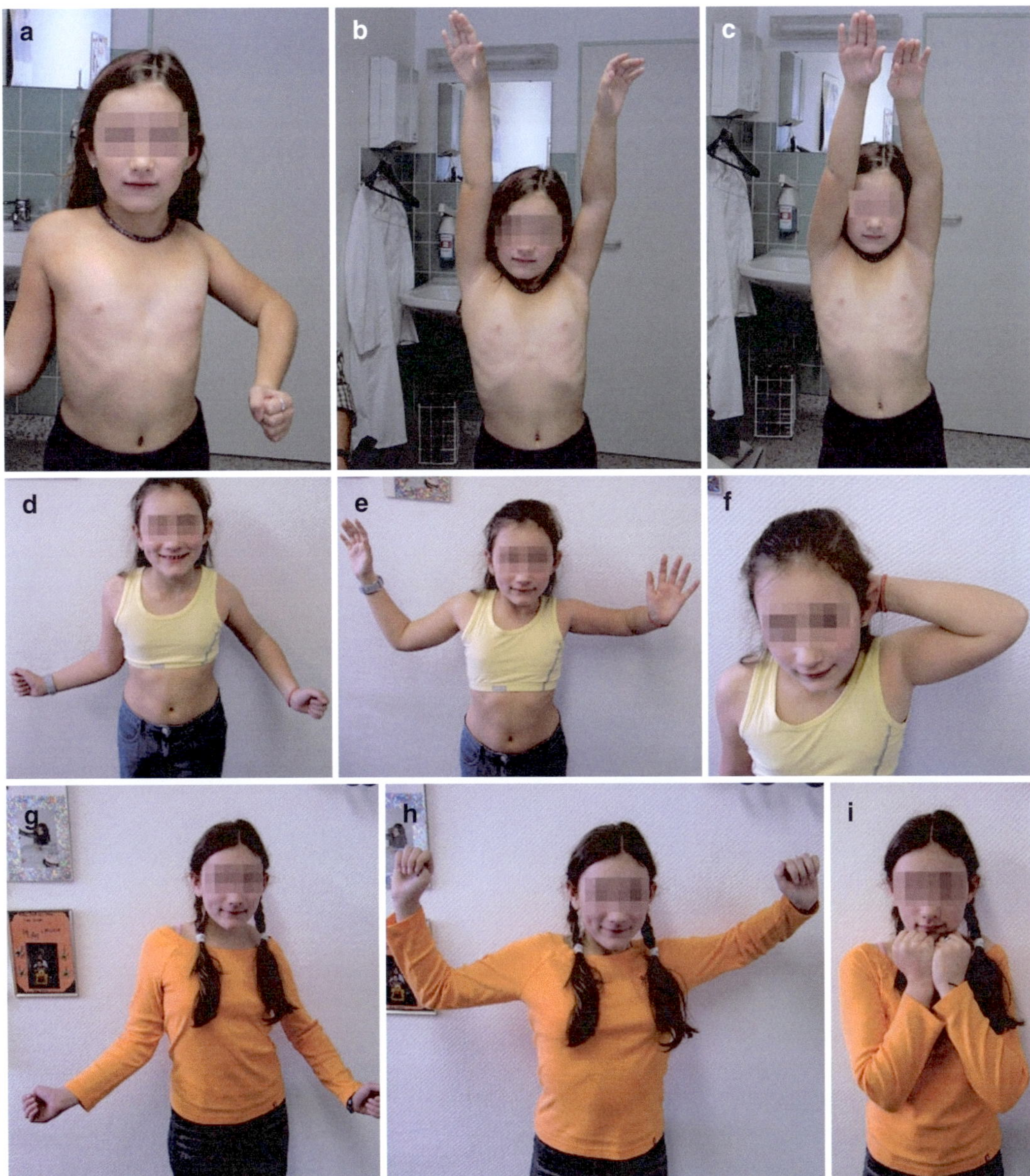

Fig. 21.11 (**a–i**) Corrected movement pattern

21.2.3 Shoulder Contractures

We differentiate between anterior, posterior and inferior contractures, meaning hardened soft tissue bridges that impair passive, and therefore active, joint mobility.

The **anterior contracture** corresponds to a deltopectoral narrowness which is associated with the medial rotation malposition described above (Fig. 21.14).

The **posterior contracture** refers to a stiffening of the dorsal capsule area of the glenohumeral joint without pathological fibrosis in the posterior deltoid muscle. We think that these act as levers on the incongruent glenohumeral joint with a posterior subluxated humeral head.

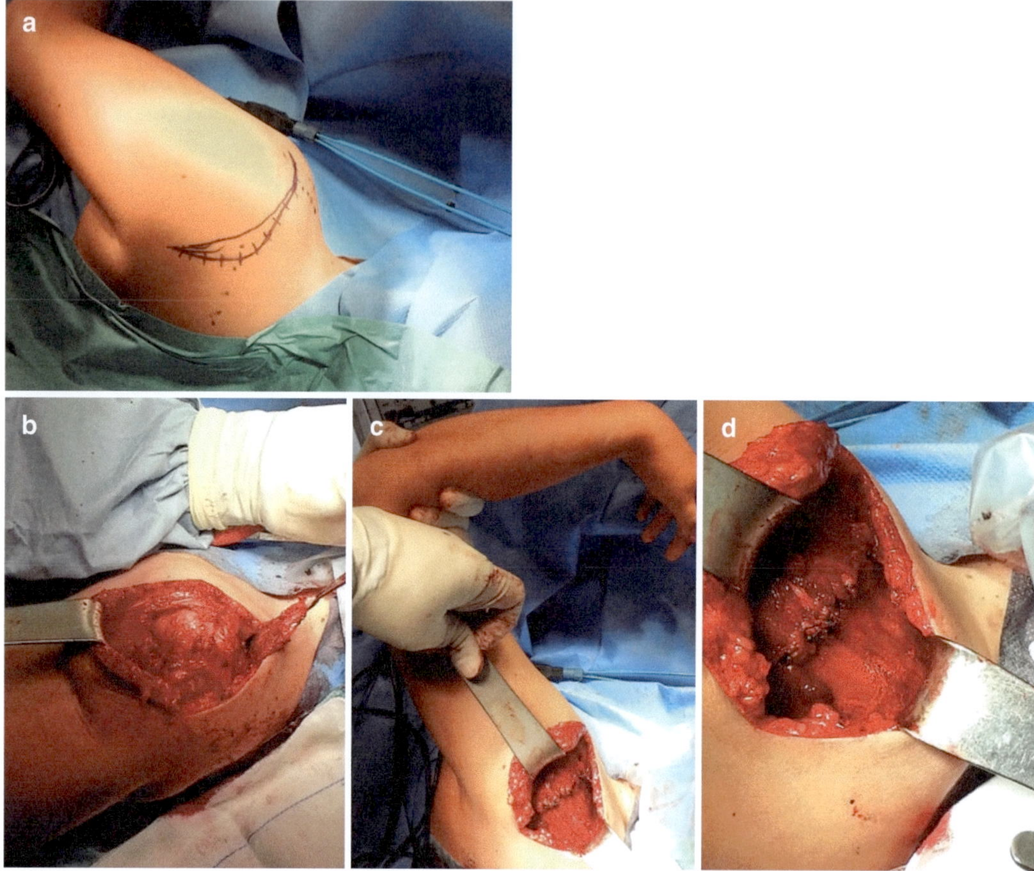

Fig. 21.12 (**a–d**) Cranial trapezius transfer

The contracture pulls the scapula outwards and backwards together with an anteversion and medialization of the humeral head, like a scapula alata. But this is not a consequence of serratus anterior muscle palsy that could be corrected neurosurgically or by muscle transfer. In this condition, we usually tolerate the protruding shoulder blade, inform the parents and recommend stretching exercises of the posterior capsule-ligament apparatus at the most for small children (Fig. 21.15).

The **inferior contracture** corresponds to a clearly palpable hardening at the lower angle between shoulder blade and upper arm and a local, strand-like thickening of the muscle fascia of the latissimus dorsi muscle, which we some-times defined and excised during an operation for transfer of this muscle (Fig. 21.16).

21.3 Elbow

The elbow is not only moved by the flexors and extensors but also integrates the proximal radio-ulnar joint (and in particular the radial head) and the torques of pronosupination and their pathological changes (Fig. 21.17). In addition, the effects of pathological muscle coactivations caused by mixed reinnervation within a lesion of the upper and middle trunk, thus affecting both the elbow flexors and extensors, are well seen at the elbow level.

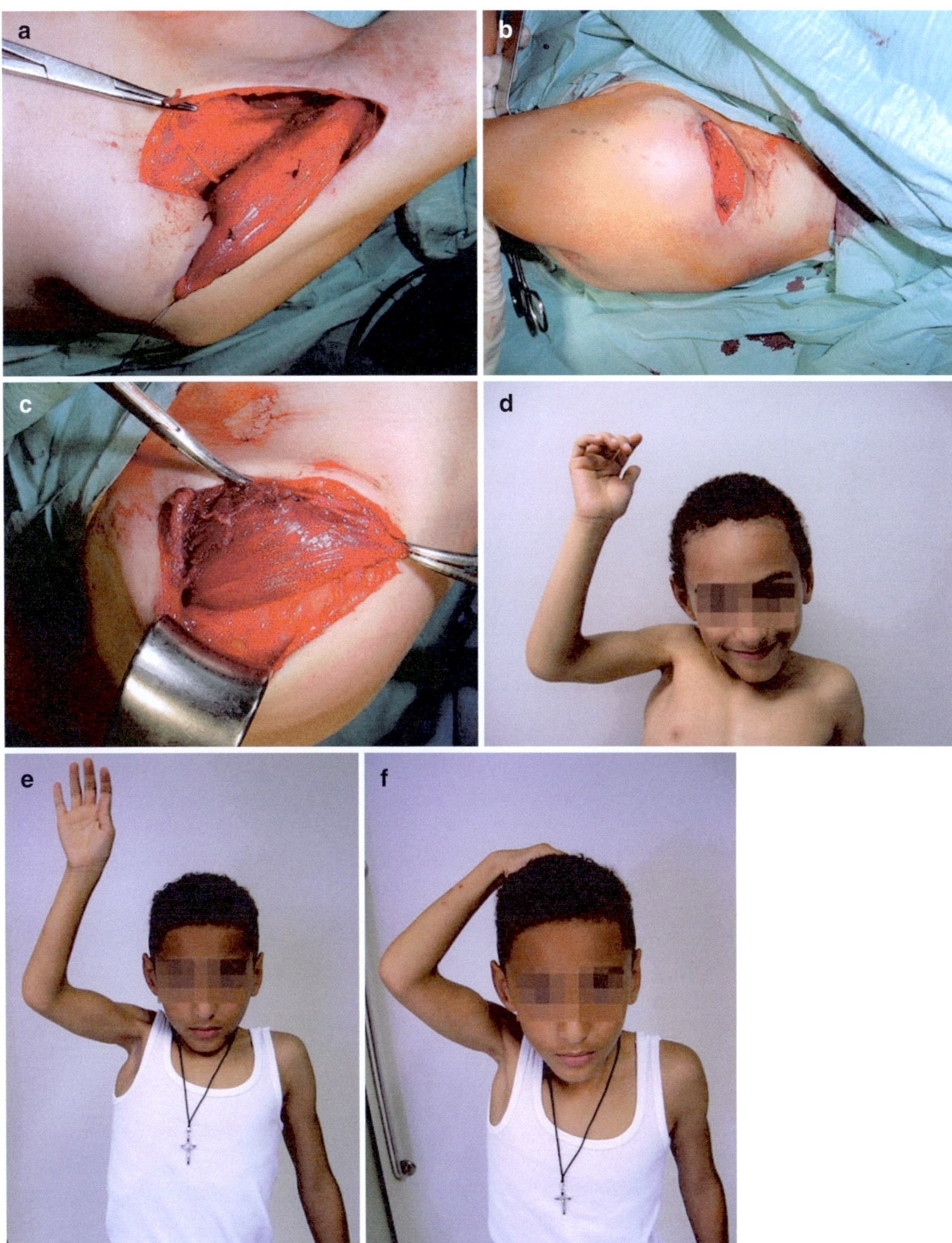

Fig. 21.13 (**a–f**) M. teres major transfer

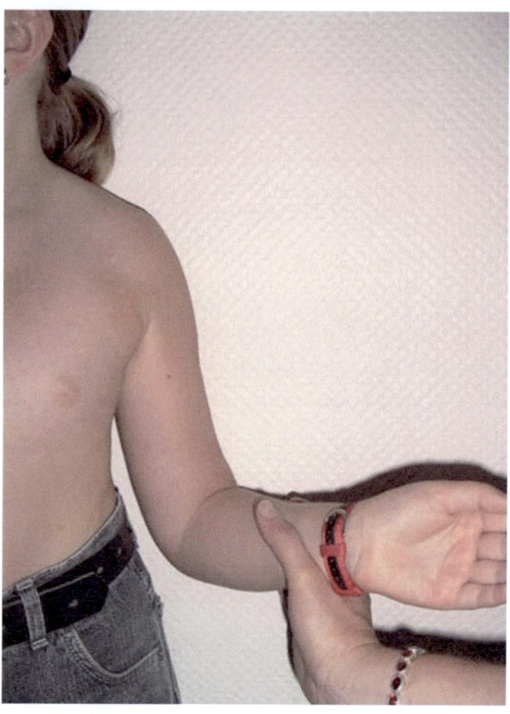

Fig. 21.14 Anterior contracture, stretching exercises

21.3.1 Cocontractions

These pathological coactivations of the antagonistic flexors and extensors lead to a characteristic dynamic movement pattern in which, after an initial good start of flexing, the motion "gets stuck" as the extent of movement increases. It is slowed down by a simultaneously activated, increasingly active elbow extension.

Non-invasive surface EMG measurements of the two antagonists have clearly identified this and shown how the application of botulinum toxin in the M. triceps terminates the coactive movement pattern and significantly improves active elbow flexion.

It should be mentioned here that a cocontraction may also be physiological (and allows us, e.g. to position the flexed arm in a certain position in space) and that here we only consider and treat pathological coactivations after proximal nerve damage, which led to a mixed wiring of the motor nerve fibres to the antago-

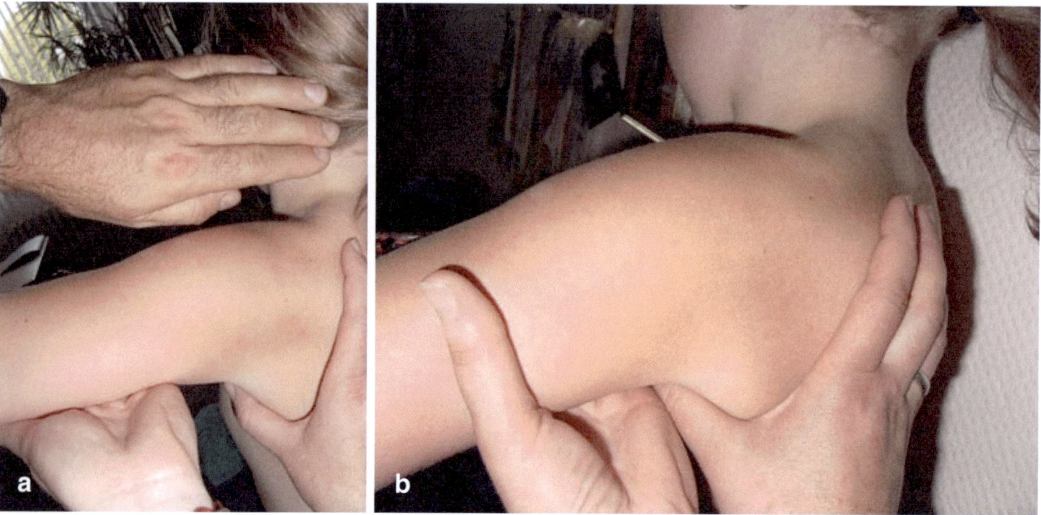

Fig. 21.15 (**a, b**) Posterior contracture, stretching exercises

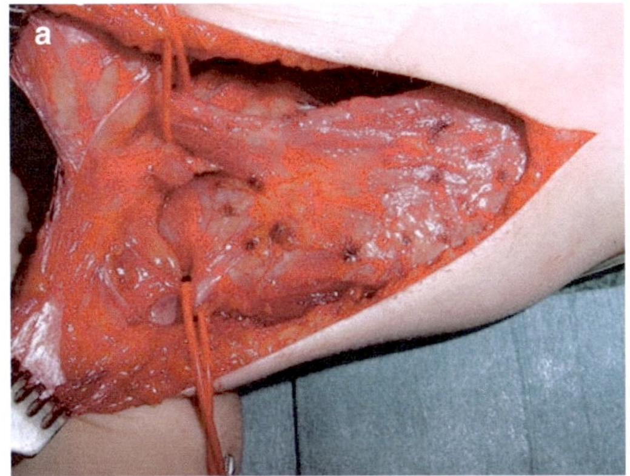

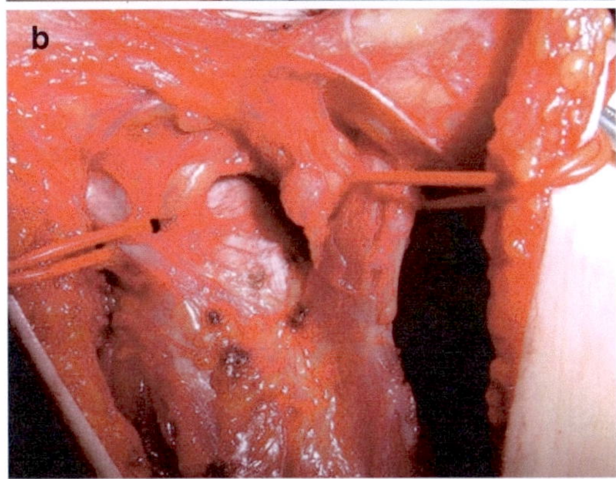

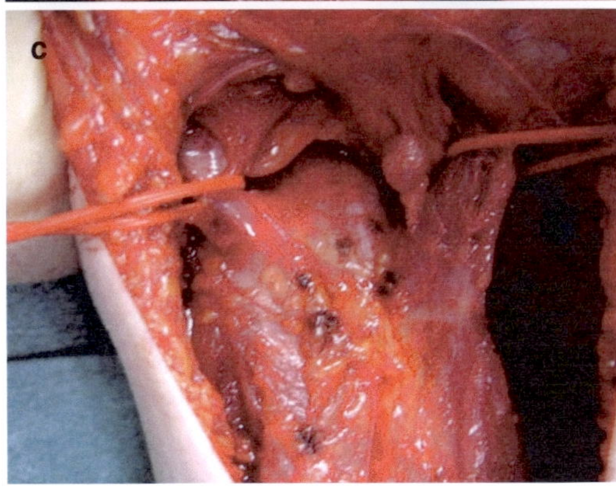

Fig. 21.16 (**a–c**) Inferior contracture, surgical site

nists. We also hypothesize that the sensory pathways, especially the deep afferents, get mixed in such a neuroma formation. It is pleasing to note that this problem of pathological coactivation is rare after nerve reconstructions. It often reacts positively to botulinum toxin treatment.

21.3.2 Elbow Flexion Weakness

Paralysis of the elbow flexor muscles requires a pedicled transfer of the latissimus dorsi muscle or by a free gracilis muscle transfer.

In children up to 2 (or perhaps even 3) years of age, local exploration of the anterior arm can be used to check the nerve supply to the biceps and brachialis muscle. Both motor branches originate from the musculocutaneous nerve. As a local nerve transfer, either both or one of the motor branches can be upgraded by an Oberlin transfer.

It is important to consider the distinct role of the two flexor muscles separately: The brachialis muscle is rather a "starter" of flexion with the arm stretched out (in this position the biceps tendon cannot develop any moment of force), but this function is supplemented by any forearm muscle with humeral origin, like pronator, FCU, ECRL or ECRB. The biceps muscle becomes active only after an angulation of 30° and then performs the entire extent of forearm flexion; it is also a strong supinator. Accordingly, a primary or secondary nerve transfer electively focuses on the respective aspect of movement initiation or powerful maintenance.

Fig. 21.17 Pathophysiology of the elbow joint

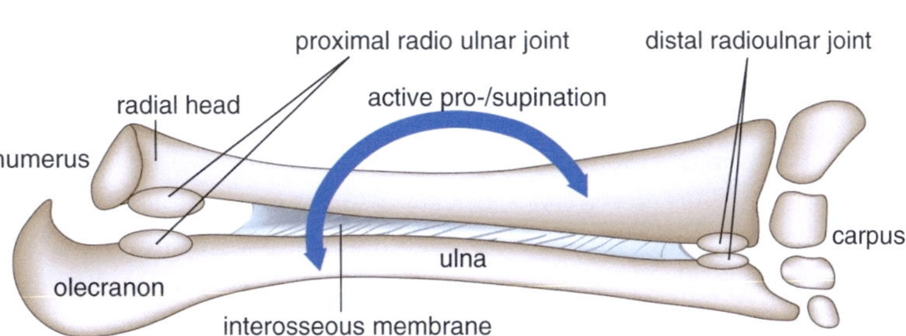

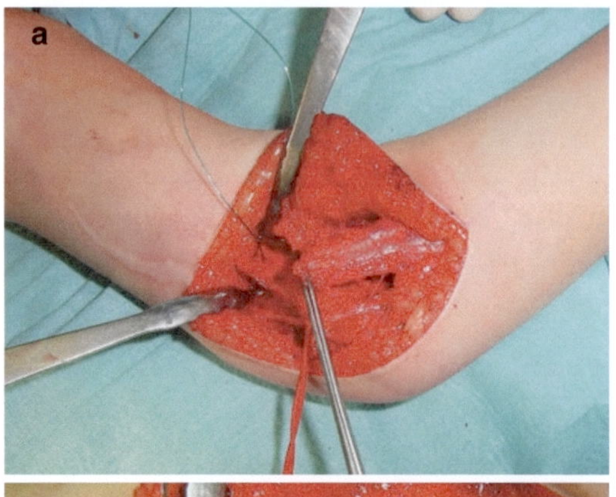

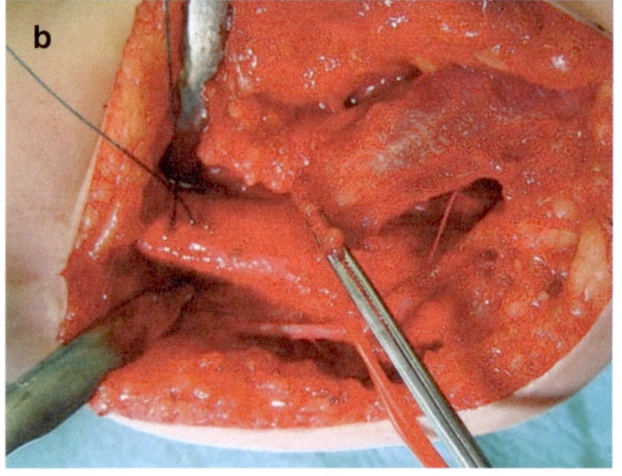

Fig. 21.18 (**a, b**) Steindler transfer

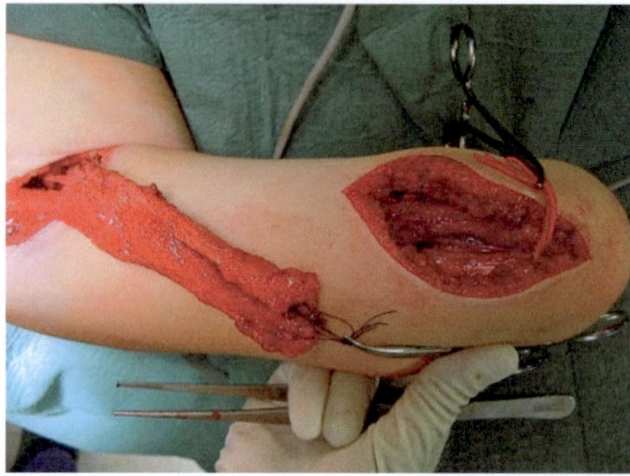

Fig. 21.19 Triceps plasty by M. latissimus dorsi transfer

In rare cases nowadays, especially when no other muscle donor is available and the forearm flexors are strongly developed, a good improvement of the flexor start can be achieved by proximalization of the ulnar muscle attachments on the distal humerus according to Steindler, however with the danger of a progressively developing flexion contracture (Fig. 21.18). Elbow dislocation and growth plate disturbance have also been reported with this rather debated operation.

21.3.3 Extension Weakness

The lack of reinnervation of the triceps leads to a reduced stretching force, which can also be increased by a pedicled latissimus dorsi transfer (or theoretically also by the transfer of the posterior part of the deltoid muscle, extended with fascia) (Fig. 21.19). This weakness should be identified and addressed as it probably promotes stretch inhibition and increasing flexion contracture, caused by the chronic muscle imbalance.

21.3.4 Permanent Stretch Deficit and Flexion Contracture of the Elbow

Usually during the first school years, the imbalance at the elbow becomes so noticeable that a slight bending posture of the elbow occurs and is noticeable to the parents. Often the fixed flexion is only 20–30°, for the time being without functional consequence. Here, a dynamic stretch orthosis at night (so as not to hinder daily activities) counteracts further deterioration. Serial plaster of Paris splints, carefully applied and followed, may be a valuable alternative.

Pronounced contractures of more than 60° must be surgically corrected and usually require a lengthening of the brachialis muscle via an access in the elbow crease, sometimes including even the brachioradialis muscle (rarely the biceps tendon), with simultaneous anterior capsulotomy (with preservation of the collateral ligaments so as not to endanger the stability of the elbow). However, this procedure is associated with a high recurrence rate, and there is also the danger of weakening the power of active elbow flexion by massively loosening the brachialis muscle. Accordingly, this procedure is indicated only hesitantly, after splint treatment and with good patient compliance. In any case, small stretch deficits in older, almost adult children can be tolerated, as this deficit seems to stabilize beyond puberty.

21.3.5 Radial Head (Sub)luxation

In a few children, anterior subluxation of the radius head (Fig. 21.20), which we believe is associated with the traction of the distal biceps tendon, becomes apparent clinically or in a routine x-ray of the elbow (Fig. 21.20).

Clinically, the first visible phenomenon is the piano key phenomenon when the radius head jumps in and out of the joint. As long as it is repositionable, there is no urgent need for action, since normally there is no functional limitation and even the limited prosupination in these children does not seem to suffer from this translation.

Things become more problematic when over the years the growing proximal part of the radius, which is no longer subject to the constraint of the proximal radioulnar and elbow joint, moves beyond the joint in a radial-dorsal direction, into dislocation. At some point the completely dislocated radial head impresses as a subcutaneous, bony bulge on the distal upper arm and blocking pronosupination.

Previous attempts to stabilize the radial head after open reduction only by reconstructing the annular ligament or by displacement of the distal biceps tendon to the ulna are unfortunately inadequate—often a relapse occurs.

A permanent and stable solution is inconceivable without an understanding of the three-dimensional bone growth and the dynamic forces acting on the proximal radial head, not only during flexion and extension of the elbow but also during pronosupination, when there is rotational movement and accompanying translation (see § 21) and the stabilisation of the radial shaft between the proximal and distal radioulnar joints (Fig. 21.21) [11].

Since in larger children the proximal radial shaft often grows beyond the capitellum, and therefore joint reconstruction then may only be achieved by means of an osteotomy, we have switched in these surgical cases to combine an open joint exposure and reposition with a three-dimensional proximal radial shaft osteotomy, in a way that the ultimately free radial head is first replaced into its spherical bearing and then the radial shaft is shortened and slanted so that a plate osteosynthesis leaves the head congruent both in the neutral position and in the pronated forearm (which in the joint promotes anterior subluxation) (Fig. 21.22): This means that the dislocating forces must be neutralized intraopera-

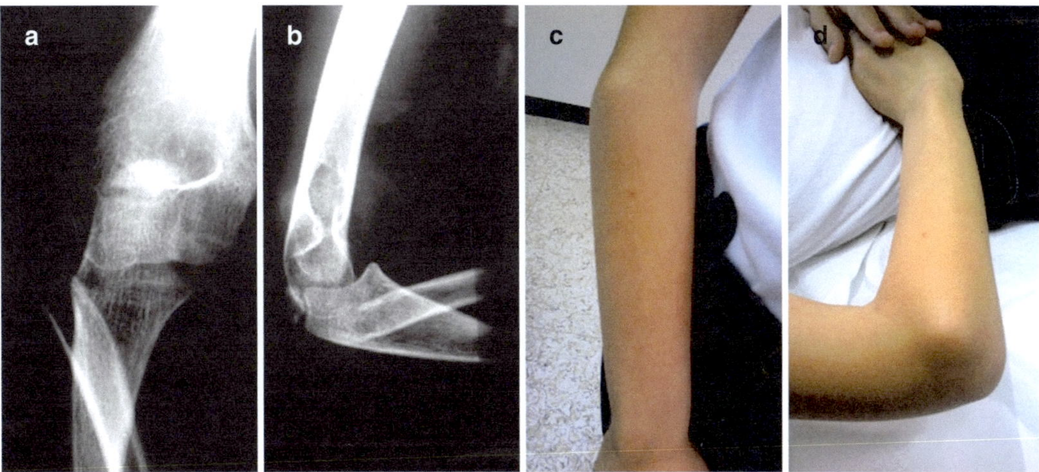

Fig. 21.20 (**a**–**d**) Ventrally subluxated radius head. (**a**, **b**) X-ray. (**c**, **d**) Clinic

Fig. 21.21 Pathophysiology of the radial head (sub)luxation

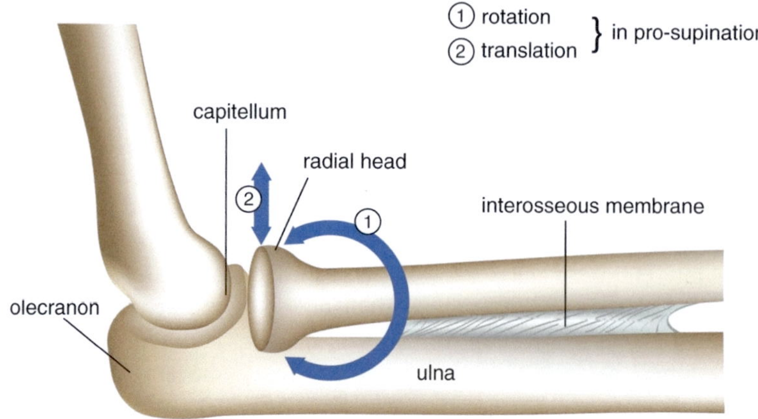

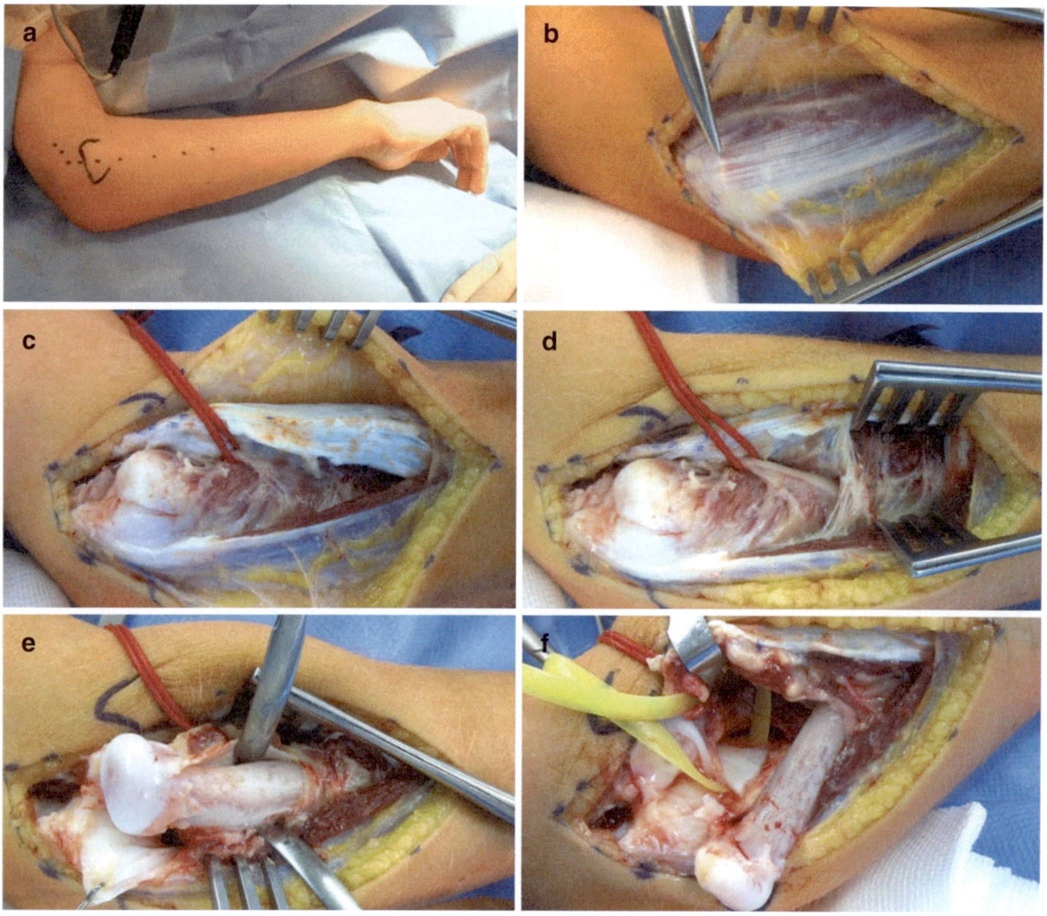

Fig. 21.22 (a–k) Open correction

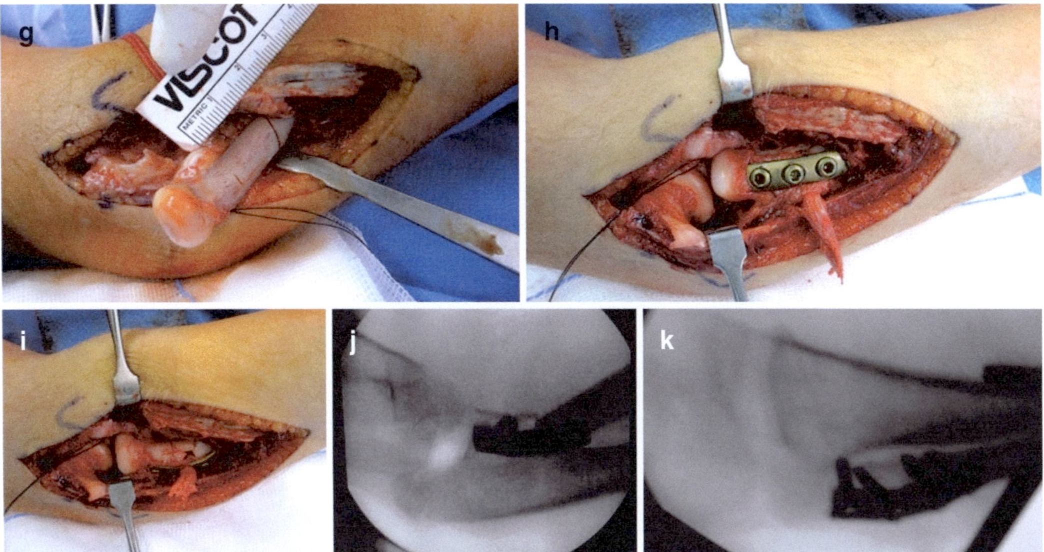

Fig. 21.22 (continued)

tively in all rotational positions of the radial shaft and that we also support the active supination postoperatively (e.g. by a tendon transfer of the brachioradialis muscle) so that the tendency to anterior subluxation is eliminated dynamically by an improved balance of the active forces. The annular ligament is nevertheless reconstructed in the best possible way; usually sufficient connective tissue is found after cranial dissection; otherwise a new ligament can be formed by a strip of muscle fascia harvested from the distal triceps muscle. The distal biceps tendon is transferred onto the ulna. Our long-term results to date show that joint congruence can be maintained (Fig. 21.23), but that passive and active pronosupination are not automatically consistently improved. It seems that the desire to promote congruence is rather fulfilled by a stronger active pro- and supination.

The stabilizing effect of the interosseous membrane, which, together with the muscle tandem of pronators and supinators, provides the dynamic background, should not be underestimated.

An improved surgical technique, based on a more detailed understanding of pathophysiology, will certainly bring progress in the coming years. We believe that the condition requires active, operative treatment. In late presentations with a clearly dislocated radial head and blocked prosupination, usually in a fixed pronation position, there is considerable functional impairment.

21.4 Forearm Rotation (Prosupination)

A good knowledge of the physiology and pathophysiology of forearm rotation is essential to understand the various limitations and their correction.

The involved anatomical structures are the two radioulnar joints (proximal and distal), which play proximally into the elbow joint and distally into the wrist joint and the interosseous membrane between the two forearm bones, the middle third of which reacts particularly to immobilization with contracture. Then there are the antago-

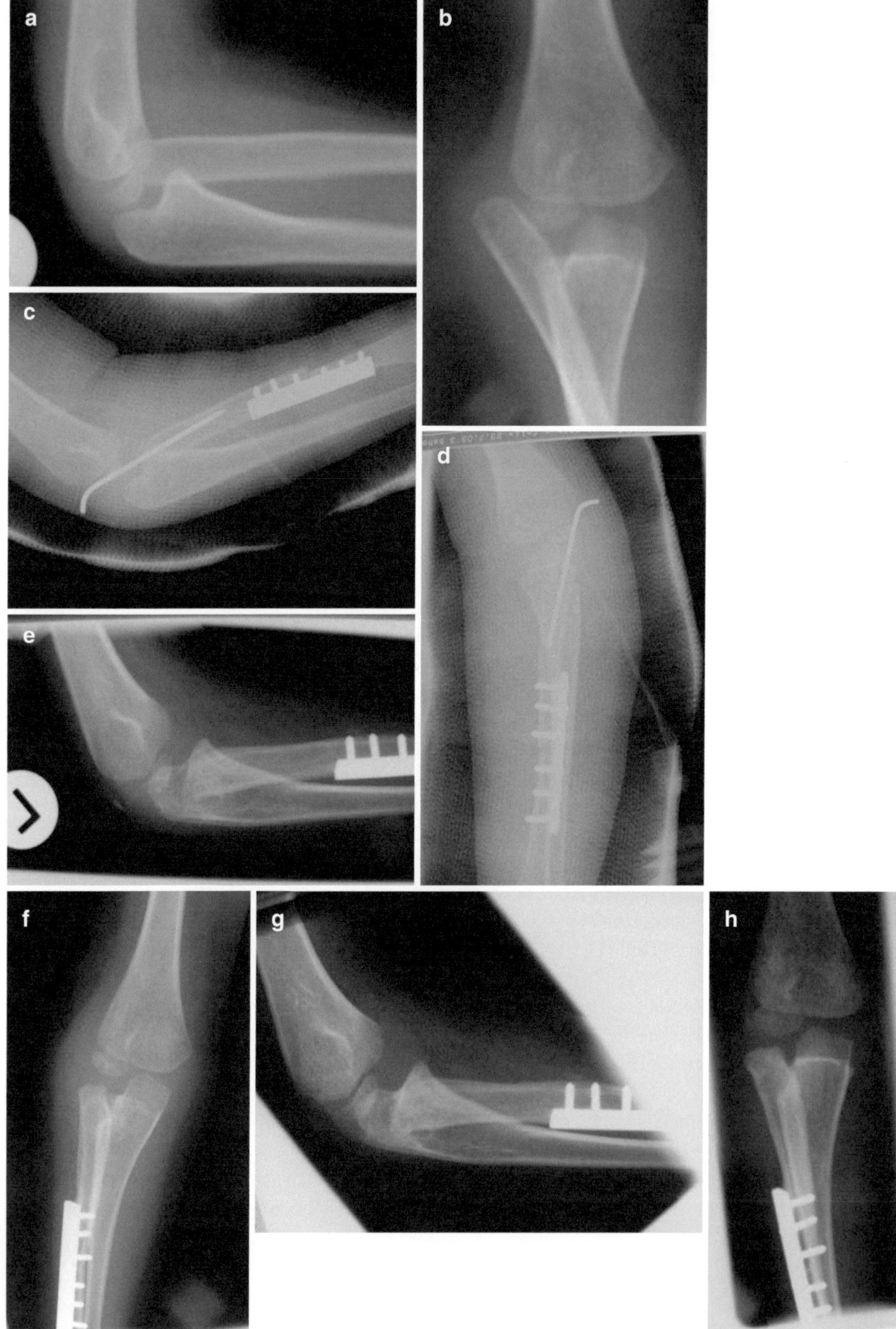

Fig. 21.23 (**a–h**) Long-term result in x-ray image

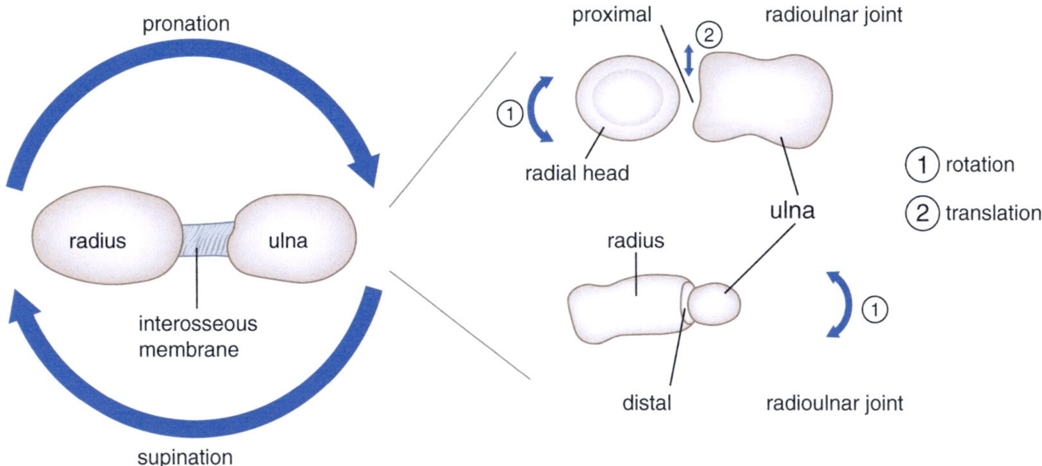

Fig. 21.24 Biomechanics and pathophysiology of prosupination

nistic muscle groups of the pronators, pronator teres and quadratus muscles, both innervated by the median nerve, and supinators, supinator and biceps muscles (Fig. 21.24).

In adolescent children with neurogenic disorders, we find not only paralysis affecting the dynamic balance of prosupination but also shrinkage of the interosseous muscle and bone or joint changes, including luxation of the radial head (see above).

When analysing and treating the malpositions listed below, we must take all these aspects into account, in order to avoid inadequate correction and recurrence as far as possible.

21.4.1 Biomechanics of Prosupination and Radioulnar Joints (Fig. 21.24)

The rotational balance of the prosupination is maintained by the regulated force applied by the individual muscles. In the normal child's upper limb, it is possible to move almost 90° in the direction of supination (palm upwards) or pronation (palm downwards). This maintains an elastic interosseous membrane and ensures balanced growth of both long bones and the small radioulnar joints, which allow the rotation of the radius around the ulna. In addition to the rotational

movement of the radial head, the accompanying anteroposterior translation must also be taken into account. The uncompensated forward amplification of this translation together with uncompensated pronation may lead to anterior subluxation of the radial head if the ligament structures and other dynamic elements cannot hold the head in its spherical bearing.

21.4.2 Supination Contracture

This malposition and the resulting forearm contracture is the more frequent pathology of the forearm after birth palsy; after a spastic movement disorder, pronation contracture occurs more frequently.

The interosseous membrane shrinks in this position of the forearm bones, and the palm of the hand shows "expectantly" upwards, which has caused this malposition the concise but unattractive term of the "beggar's hand" (Fig. 21.25).

If a passive, freely movable prosupination has been obtained, an active pronation can be achieved by a dynamic procedure using a tendon transfer; if the forearm position is fixed, the membrane must first be loosened over a long distance before a tendon is put on. Here the result is usually difficult to predict, so that in these cases a static correction with rotary osteotomy of the radial shaft in pronation is often preferred.

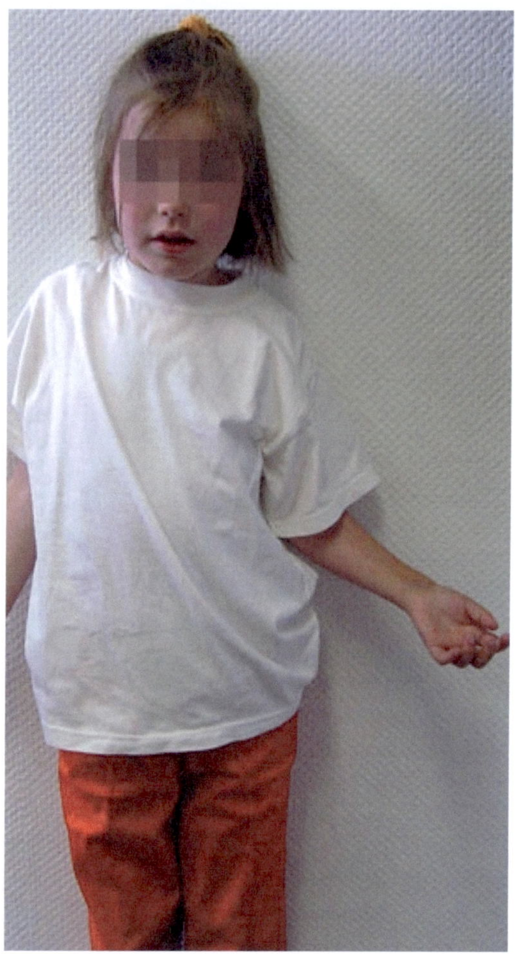

Fig. 21.25 Beggar's hand

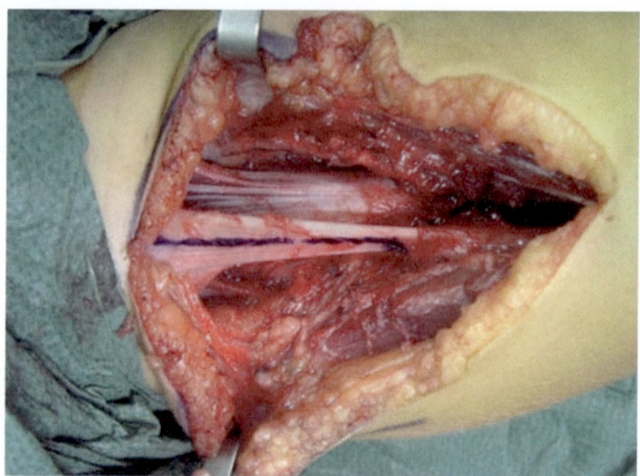

Fig. 21.26 Zancolli rerouting of the biceps tendon

Considering tendon transfers, pronating rerouting of the distal biceps tendon is possible using the Zancolli technique ([12]; Fig. 21.26), so that the activated biceps muscle pronates the radius (and no longer supinates as before). Another possibility is the pronating rerouting of the tendon of the brachioradialis muscle ([13]; Fig. 21.27).

Radius osteotomy is usually performed at the easily accessible transition from the middle to the distal third of the shaft, whereby 60° to more than 90° rotation may be necessary to move from a complete supination to a light pronation: 90° from the complete supination position to the neutral position, plus 20–30°pronation. If a relapse occurs nevertheless, the supinator muscle may have to be lengthened or an osteotomy of both long bones may have to be planned. This osteotomy even might be repeated, in case of recurrence of posture.

21.4.3 Passive Movement Restriction and Interosseous Membrane

If there is a severe passive restriction of movement, the interosseous membrane must be split intraoperatively in any case. Postoperatively, the partially regained extent of movement must be maintained either by passive rotation exercises or, and better, by the remaining muscle power. This presupposes residual capacity in both the pronators and supinators, which is usually not the case. It is also rare in these "muddled" situations that muscle donors are available for augmentation of one or the other rotational movement, let alone for both.

Here it must be taken into account that prosupination motion acts very close to the bone, overall the radius, and only a few donors for musculotendinous transfers are available (biceps and brachioradialis muscles). Otherwise, only a weakening of the already weak antagonist can be considered (lengthening tenotomy of the pronator teres muscle or supinator muscle, as practised in spastic movement disorders). Therefore, the static correction due to a radial osteotomy with a more predictable position result is often preferred in these circumstances.

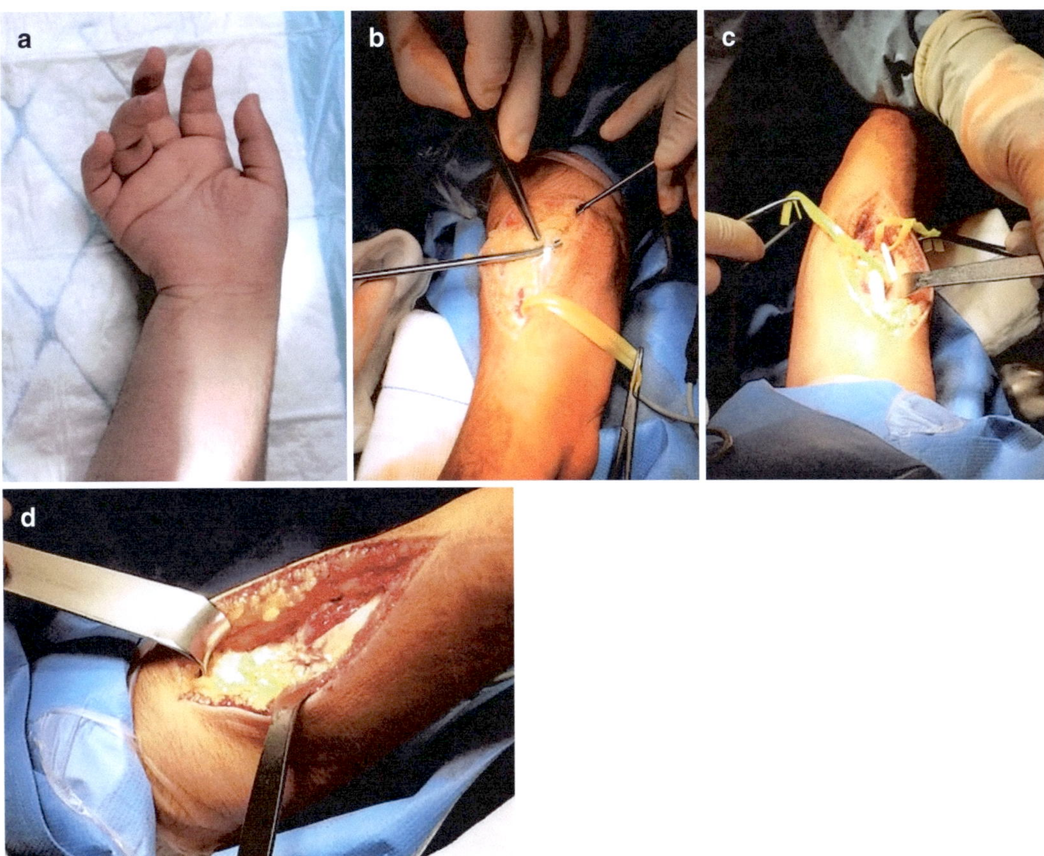

Fig. 21.27 (a–d) Brachioradialis rerouting according to Özkan

21.4.4 Combination with the Subluxation of the Radial Head

From the above it follows that problems of subluxation of the radial head, which are pathophysiologically related to pronosupination, should never be analysed or corrected without considering forearm rotation. Only the ignorance of the translational forces on the radial head during pronosupination probably leads to the policy addressing only the anterior pull of the biceps tendon. The important supinating effect of biceps tends to reduce the radial head. According to our knowledge, rather the hyperpronation pushes the radial head out of its spherical bearing. There is an analogy with the shoulder, where the posterior subluxation of the humeral head is associated with increased and unopposed medial rotating force.

21.4.5 Distal Ulnar Malformation

If the wrist deviates ulnarly, one first thinks of an imbalance of the wrist extensors (radial and ulnar) or of a functional superiority of the flexor carpi ulnaris (FCU) muscle. Astonishment arises when the x-ray of the wrist (Fig. 21.28) shows a clearly hypoplastic, non-ossified ulnar head without a developed distal radioulnar joint. Even if this explains the malposition, we lack both the cause and a consistent therapeutic approach [11].

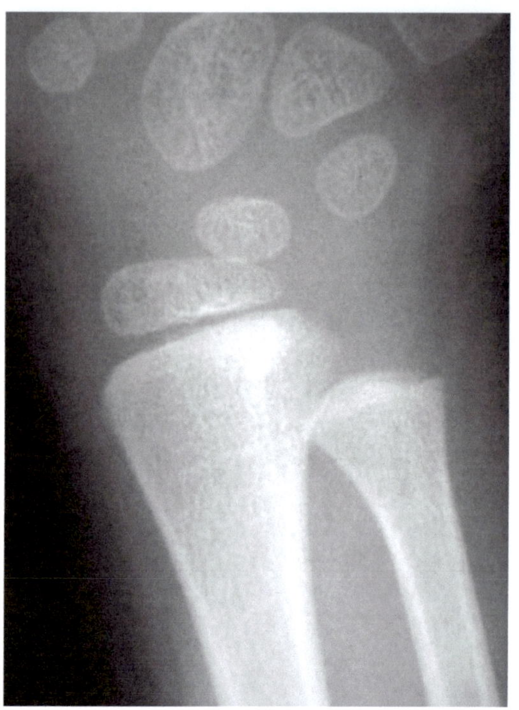

Fig. 21.28 Distal ulnar hypoplasia

Several hypotheses can be considered:

- Hypoplasia in the context of severe damage to the distal ulnar nerve (which, however, is not clinically plausible in these children).
- Hypoplasia due to an unclear circulatory disorder. We have not used angiography in these cases.
- Bony maldevelopment due to a primary tendon imbalance that causes the carpus to incline ulnarly.

Due to the absence of a radioulnar joint, prosupination is also restricted both passively and actively in the long term.

For treatment, one can consider distraction measures with an external mini fixator. Arthrodesis in analogy to the Sauve-Kapandji method is probably out of question for the growing child. There is also no reliable tendon rearrangement that could restore the dynamic imbalance to improve the overall wrist and hand function, although an occasionally observed prolapsing ECU tendon, acting then as an ulnar devi-

ator, has been successfully transferred to the APL tendon with considerable gain of function (Birch 2019, personal communication). Özkan developed a similar technique [14].

21.5 Wrist

21.5.1 Dropped Hand Position: Lack of Wrist Extension

In small children, this is compensated by a nocturnal, volar positioning splint, which should leave the fingers free. At the age of 4 or 5 years, a tendon transfer of the pronator teres muscle or flexor carpi ulnaris muscle to the extensor carpi radialis brevis muscle can be performed, which, with sufficient donor muscle strength, achieves a good active wrist extension of 20–30° over the neutral position (Fig. 21.29). If the extension of the wrist is adequate but metacarpophalangeal finger extension is weak, the pronator teres mus-

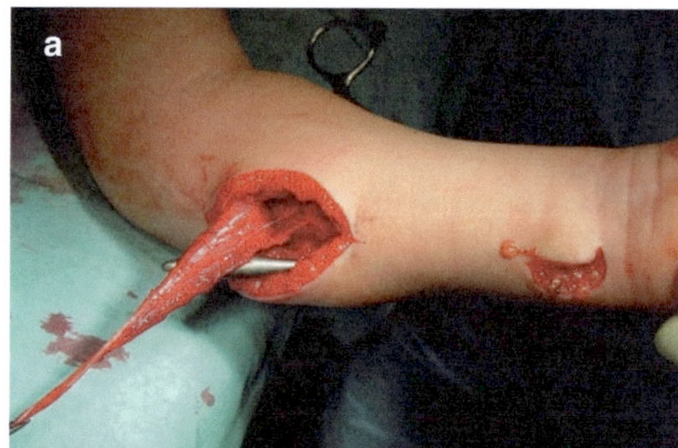
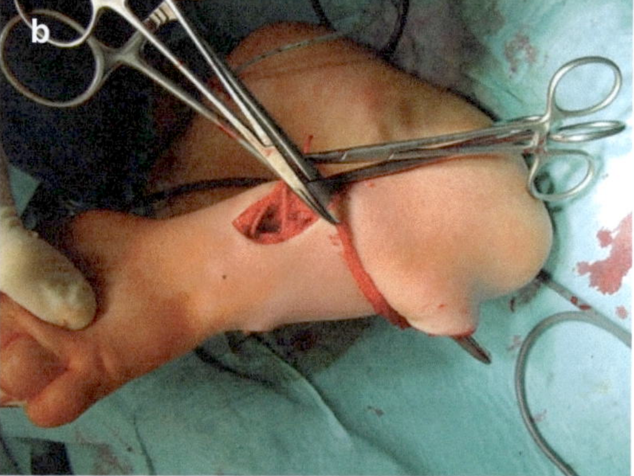

Fig. 21.29 (**a, b**) Tendon transfer of the flexor carpi ulnaris muscle to the extensor carpi radialis brevis muscle

cle or flexor carpi ulnaris muscle is transferred directly to the tendon of the extensor communis muscle.

21.5.2 Ulnar Deviation of the Wrist

See at Sect. 21.4.

21.5.3 Tenodesis Effect

This refers to the use of active wrist extension and flexion to achieve passive closing and opening of the fingers, simply because the flexion path increases with active wrist extension and thus the tension on the flexor tendons (thus the fingers flex) and vice versa with active wrist flexion, but also while "dropping" the wrist into gravity, the fingers open automatically by stretching the metacarpal joints and the grip can be released (Fig. 21.29). Therefore, wrist arthrodesis should only be indicated as a last option in these patients.

21.5.4 Wrist Arthrodesis in a Growing Child

This last option is used when the tendon transfers are insufficient or for other reasons, as in a severe Volkmann contracture in a wrist flexion position, when the straightening of the wrist cannot be achieved otherwise. The aim is now to achieve stiffening through bony adhesion without damaging the growth zone in the metaphysis. Accordingly, the inserted plate or the external fixator [15] must spare this zone (Fig. 21.30) and the synthesis material must be removed early.

21.6 Hand

Surgical hand corrections are usually performed on older children and usually correspond to classical reconstruction procedures known from adult hand surgery. Here we will deal specifically with some special features.

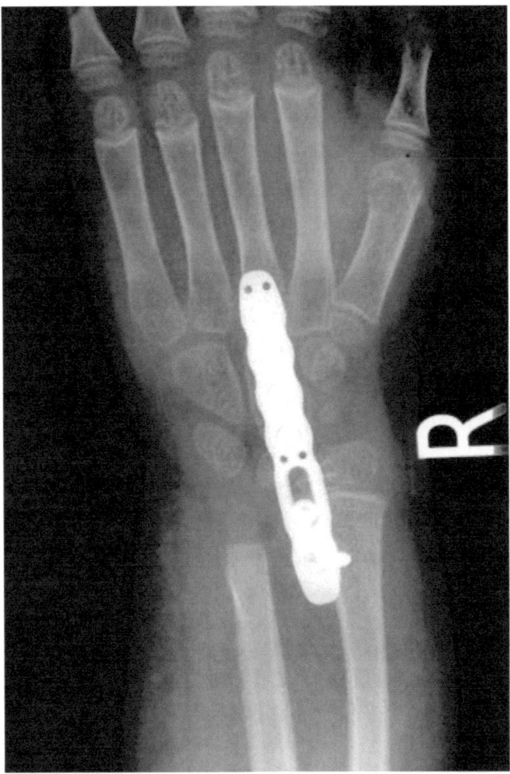

Fig. 21.30 X-ray image of a wrist arthrodesis in a child with osteosynthesis material which is sparing the metaphysis

21.6.1 Sensory Disturbances

These are difficult to determine for small children, but they occur more frequently than we generally assume. Dry skin, undetected injuries (burns), or chewing or tearing off the nails indicate a disturbed sensitive perception. Also the neglect of the entire extremity, the non-inclusion, often has to do with the disturbed afferent return to the brain.

Pain seems rare. Some parents state that their child complains about painful arm sensations during fever attacks, with and without external tactile stimuli.

Even multiple root tears do not seem to lead to neuropathic pain in babies and toddlers, not even in the course of the disease. Hypothetically, we can associate this with an immature sensitive switching system, involving the thalamus.

21.6.1.1 Resensibilisation

There are several **nerve transfers** that can be used to supply important areas (especially on the hand and fingers: ulnar hand edge, sensitive supply area of the median nerve with the three radial finger three-point grip) by redirecting a functioning sensitive nerve branch.

Donor nerves are the cutaneous divisions of the intercostal nerves especially the second, which gives the intercostobrachial nerve into the axilla and which normally sensitively innervates the inner side of the arm, and also the cutaneous division of the musculocutaneous nerve, which is found radially in the volar elbow crease, close to the biceps tendon.

Recipient nerves are either the lateral head of the median nerve or the distal, cutaneous part of the ulnar nerve at the distal wrist, anterior to the deep motor branch. It is known from plexus surgery in adults that these sensory nerve transfers help to relieve neuropathic pain in root tears, especially C8 and Th1.

21.6.1.2 Sensibility Training

As part of the postoperative therapy for all children with peripheral nerve damage, sensory rehabilitation is often neglected, either due to a lack of patient compliance or lack of techniques. For further reading, we refer to the excellent work of Lundborg [16] and Spicher [17], which point to the importance of cortical plasticity and multimodal influence on the reorganization in the sensory cortex during therapy.

21.6.2 Bending Weakness

Children with severe complete proximal nerve damage (total plexus palsy, arthrogryposis) often have a weak or differently differentiated flexion force of the long fingers even after primary nerve reconstruction. A tendon transfer of extensor carpi radialis longus (ECRL) muscle can only globally improve the flexion power of all fingers, enhancing a global fist closure movement.

21.6.3 Overstretching of the Metacarpophalangeal Joints

In these hands, the lack of recovery of the intrinsic musculature also leads to an uncompensated overstretching of the metacarpophalangeal joints, which subsequently ends in a claw-like finger flexion that is by no means functional. It is important to ensure good passive motion ability of the metacarpophalangeal joints at a very early stage, as this is the only way to reconstruct global gripping in the medium term: at first flexion of the metacarpophalangeal joints to 90° and then flexion of the metacarpophalangeal and distal joints to make a fist. Equally important here is a wrist that is stable in the neutral position, as otherwise the finger flexors pull the wrist into a flexed position and thus deprive the finger joints of significant flexion force.

21.6.4 Restoration of a Global Fist Closure by a Free Functional Muscle Transfer

In rare cases, after complete plexus palsy with insufficient motor innervation of the hand, or after severe Volkmann contracture, global finger flexion can be restored by a muscle transfer to the forearm if the wrist is stabilized, a certain active finger extension exists to open the fist and thus allows the release of objects, and the hand can also be integrated due to a basic sensibility.

Only the latissimus dorsi muscle (if it is sufficiently innervated and eutrophic) can be considered as the local donor muscle; otherwise a free M. gracilis transfer from the thigh must be planned (Chap. 22).

Motor donor nerves are either the spinal accessory XIth nerve or a distal redundant motor donor as in a Volkmann contracture, where the proximal peripheral nerves are healthy. The spinal accessory nerve must then first be extended into the proximal forearm with a cable graft using an entire sural nerve (and its reinnervation may take 8–12 months and checked by biopsy).

Afterwards, the free functional muscle transfer is carried out as a second surgery in two teams. While the first team harvests the muscle out of the thigh, the second team prepares the receptor site in the forearm identifying connec-tion points for the vessels, nerves and flexor tendons.

The muscle is then separated from its local circulation (beginning of the ischemia period), transferred and immediately connected to the arterial and venous vessels by microsurgery (end of the ischemia period), and then the nerve and tendons are coapted (Fig. 21.31).

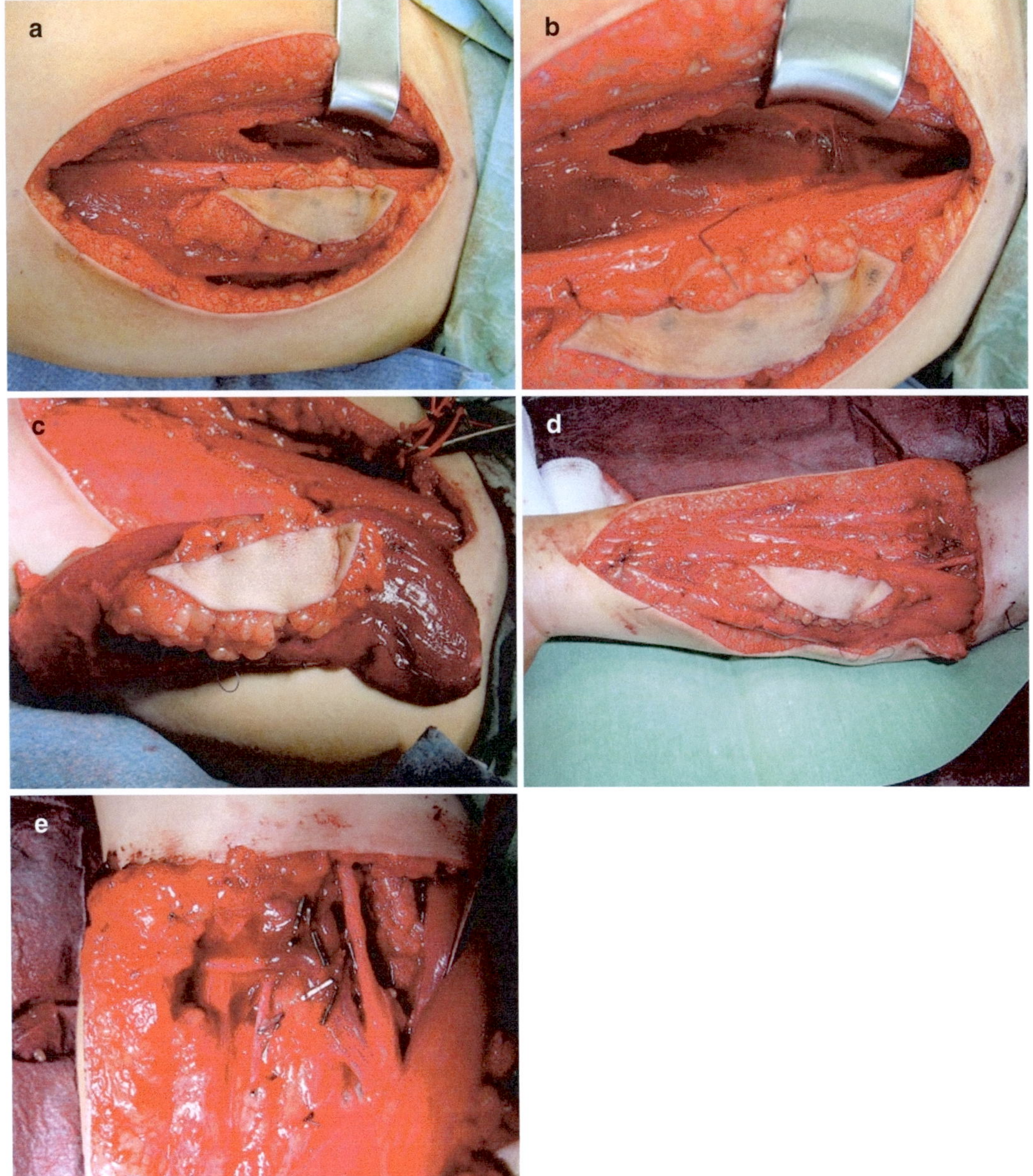

Fig. 21.31 (**a–e**) Free M. gracilis transfer. (**a**) Flap harvest from the proximal thigh. (**b**) View towards the proximal vascular nerve bundle. (**c**) The "free" flap. (**d, e**) In the recipient's site

We have reviewed our cases [18]; in the long-term observation, we have found out that even with apparently minimal use of these mostly severely damaged hands, a hypertrophy of the transferred gracilis muscle occurs in the course of time, which confirms motor integration.

We have found that the progressive response of the muscle and its increasing function do not pose a particular problem for the children and the therapist.

Of course, such an elaborate surgical microsurgical procedure must be discussed in detail with the parents and the young patient; and in particular the microsurgical risk with possible loss of muscle due to circulatory insufficiency must be addressed.

References

1. Bahm J. Die Folgen der geburtsassoziierten Plexusparese im Kindes- und Jugendalter: Motorisches Ungleichgewicht, Fehlhaltung und Wachstumsstörung. Obere Extremität. 2014;9:78–83.
2. Bahm J. Die kindliche Armplexusparese—Eine aktuelle Übersicht sekundärer Operationsverfahren. Handchirurgie Mikrochirurgie Plastische Chirurgie. 2004;36(1):37–46.
3. Demy C. Séquelles de lépaule chez le jeune adulte opéré après lésion obstétricale du plexus brachial. Travail de Master en kinésithérapie. Lüttich: HEPL; 2013.
4. Schmelzer-Schmied N, Ochs BG, Carstens C. Die Schulterluxation beim Neugeborenen. Orthopade. 2005;34:454–61.
5. Kambhampati SLS, Birch R, Cobiella C, Chen L. Posterior subluxation and dislocation of the shoulder in obstetric brachial plexus palsy. J Bone Joint Surg. 2006;88B:213–9.
6. Waters PM, Bae DS. Effect of tendon transfers and extra-articular soft-tissue balancing on glenohumeral development in brachial plexus birth palsy. J Bone Joint Surg. 2005;87A:320–5.
7. Waters PM, Smith GR, Jaramillo D. Glenohumeral deformity secondary to brachial plexus birth palsy. J Bone Joint Surg. 1998;80A:668–77.
8. Nath RK, Paizi M. Scapular deformity in obstetric brachial plexus palsy: a new finding. Surg Radiol Anat. 2007;29:133–40.
9. Hoffer MM, Wickenden R, Roper B. Brachial plexus birth palsies—results of tendon transfers to the rotator cuff. J Bone Joint Surg. 1978;60A:691–5.
10. Chammas M, Goubier JN, Coulet B, Reckendorf GM, Picot MC, Allieu Y. Glenohumeral arthrodesis in upper and total brachial plexus palsy. A comparison of functional results. J Bone Joint Surg Br. 2004;86(5):692–5.
11. Bahm J, Elkazzi W, Schuind F. Forearm problems in obstetric brachial plexus palsy. In: De Smet L, Schuind F, editors. Difficult problems and Complications at the Forearm (FESSH 2012 Instructional Course Book). Montpellier: Sauramps Medical; 2012.
12. Bahm J, Gilbert A. Surgical correction of supination deformity in children with obstetric brachial plexus palsy. J Hand Surgery. 2002;27B(1):20–3.
13. Ozkan T, Aydin A, Ozer K, Ozturk K, Durmaz H, Ozkan S. A surgical technique for pediatric forearm pronation: brachioradialis rerouting with interosseous membrane release. J Hand Surgery. 2004;29A:22–7.
14. Özkan T, Aydin HU, Berköz Ö, Özkan S, Kozanoğlu E. 'Switch' technique to restore pronation and radial deviation in 17 patients with brachial plexus birth palsy. J Hand Surg Eur. 2019;44(9):905–12.
15. ElKazzi W, Bahm J, Schuind F. Wrist arthrodesis in children—a new technique: case presentation. Hand Surg. 2014;19(2):275–9.
16. Lundborg G. Nerve injury and repair. 2nd ed. New York: Churchill Livingstone; 2005.
17. Spicher C. Manuel de rééducation sensitive du corps humain. Genève: Editions Médecine et Hygiène; 2003.
18. Bahm J, Ocampo-Pavez C. Free functional gracilis muscle transfer in children with severe sequelae from obstetric brachial plexus palsy. JBPPNI. 2008;3:23.

Non-neural Microsurgery in Children

22

Jörg Bahm

As in adults, the short ischemia tolerance of the transferred muscle must be taken into account, which requires a patent vascular anastomosis within 6 h.

Published surgery series are small, and the authors do not usually go into the "tips and tricks" that lead to better success or a low rate of flap loss [1].

In our opinion, the following special perioperative circumstances must be considered—they concern the **anesthesiological perioperative regimen** [2]:

- Good room and patient temperature to prevent vascular narrowing or spasm
- Sufficient peri- and postoperative analgesia
- Maintaining good circulating blood volume and stable, non-fluctuating blood pressure conditions, avoiding vasoconstrictive drugs for temporary blood pressure increase
- Good understanding between the surgeons and the anesthesia team

Since children always have healthy blood vessels, even if they are rather small in the flap area, a special antithrombotic prophylaxis after vascular suture is not actually necessary; aspirin 100 mg seems sufficient. Consensus recommendations on perioperative management usually do not specifically address small children, but provide valuable general information on dealing with vasospasm, volemia, and the questionable benefit of blood plasma expanders [2].

An inpatient follow-up period of at least 7 days is generally used.

In case of problems with the blood supply to the skin island (especially in very obese children with a thick subcutaneous fat layer and few perforator vessels), an early, emergency revision is recommended to check the anastomoses and to assess the muscle blood circulation: We had several cases in which the muscle was well supplied with blood during the revision and functionally survived even though the skin island had to be discarded, which thus made further postoperative clinical monitoring impossible. Blood circulation monitors based on Doppler would certainly be very helpful here.

Examples from our patient series of free gracilis muscle transfer were already described in Chap. 21. The selective nerve transfers with small donor and recipient nerves, such as Oberlin transfer in a 4-month-old infant, the few end-to-side nerve anastomoses, and the pedicled muscle transfers in small children belong to this technical category, since the neurovascular bundle must

J. Bahm (✉)

Plastic, Hand and Burn Surgery, Section for Plexus Surgery, University Hospital, Aachen, Germany
e-mail: jorg.bahm@belgacom.net,
jbahm@ukaachen.de

© Springer Nature Switzerland AG 2021
J. Bahm (ed.), *Movement Disorders of the Upper Extremities in Children*,
https://doi.org/10.1007/978-3-030-53622-0_22

also be prepared microsurgically. Unusual transfers, for example, for biceps replacement in arthrogryposis, must be performed within the first year of life (Chap. 18).

Each microsurgical team will follow its own guidelines based on patient type and experience; however, for a variety of technical procedures, the number of patients remains rather low.

I am therefore very pleased that in the next chapter Richarda Böttcher from Berlin will present her procedures.

References

1. Bahm J, Ocampo-Pavez C. Free functional gracilis muscle transfer in children with severe sequelae from obstetric brachial plexus palsy. JBPPNI. 2008;3:23.
2. Kremer T, Bauer M, Zahn P, Wallner C, Fuchs P, Horch RE, Schaefer DJ, Bader RD, Lehnhardt M, Reichert B, Pierer G, Hirche C, Kneser U. Perioperatives Management in der Mikrochirurgie-Konsensus Statement der Deutschsprachigen Arbeitsgemeinschaft für Mikrochirurgie der peripheren Nerven und Gefäße. Handchir Mikrochir Plast Chir. 2016;48:205–11.

Secondary Microsurgery

R. Böttcher

23.1 Introduction

Elective microsurgical procedures include reconstructive operations on vessels and nerves as well as free tissue transplants. In children, this form of therapy is mainly used for specific clinical pictures and injury sequelae. Frequent locations for application of free tissue transplants are congenital combined soft tissue defects of the face and neck region. Beside, so-called free flaps are used in contractures, in traumatic and iatrogenic soft tissue defects and for functional reconstruction. Irrespective of this, vessels and nerves can be reconstructed using microsurgical techniques. A more recent development relatively rare for children are so-called neurotizations, in which muscles are reinnervated by coapting functioning terminal nerves or single fascicles to the supplying nerve.

23.2 Indications

23.2.1 Overview

The potential of reconstructive microsurgical interventions in children are little known due to their rarity and the associated low representation in scientific literature. For most indications, a therapy assessment is carried out without consideration of microsurgical reconstructive options. Functional deficits, malformations and contractures are accepted as irreversible consequences of the underlying disease. It would be advantageous to include the plastic-reconstructive microsurgical options in the treatment considerations at an early stage and on interdisciplinary basis.

Aspects for the indication result from age and general state of health of the child, the type of current functional impairment, potential contractures and growth restrictions due to soft tissue loss and the donor site morbidity but also from the expected compliance of the family. Microvascular elective procedures do not guarantee success. Evidence-based statements about the functional and aesthetic outcome are generally not possible. For this reason, the weighing of indications in close consultation with parents and the treating paediatricians and neuropaediatricians is of essential importance. Parents need to know that they have a responsible role to play in long-term follow-up, similar to the care of a burn injured child.

In reconstructive microvascular surgery, the following aspects are essential for **indication** and **treatment selection**:

- Age of the child at the time of the intended procedure
- Concomitant diseases, in particular cardiovascular diseases and coagulation disorders

R. Böttcher (✉)
Unit for reconstructive Surgery of Brachial Plexus Injuries, Tetraplegia and Spastic Disorders,
Unfallkrankenhaus Berlin,
Panketal, Germany
e-mail: richarda.boettcher@wmanage.de

© Springer Nature Switzerland AG 2021
J. Bahm (ed.), *Movement Disorders of the Upper Extremities in Children*,
https://doi.org/10.1007/978-3-030-53622-0_23

- Size and location of soft tissue defects
- Contractures
- Innervation deficits
- Spasticity, flaccid paralysis, dyskinesia
- Familiar aspects, parental compliance
- Potential progression of the underlying disease

While microsurgical reconstructive procedures isolated on vessels or nerves do not cause any significant donor site morbidity and no major intraoperative volume loss, the choice of the flap and the intraoperative conditions also play an important role for the indication of free tissue transplants. It should be noted that the thickness, dimension and combined tissue quality of the flap must meet the requirements in the recipient area. The length of the required flap pedicle, usually containing artery, one to two veins and potentially a nerve, must also be taken into account when selecting the flap. In modern perforator flaps such as the anterolateral thigh flap (ALT) the pedicle often have only a very delicate and limited length even in adults, so that their use in children seems unsafe.

Frequent in children are **contractures** due to compartment syndromes in which cross-joint contractures cause a movement disorder. A typical example is an elbow contracture after open humerus fracture near the elbow with compartment syndrome. Here the active extension in the elbow joint is not possible, although a largely uninjured triceps muscle is present. In these cases, contracture release combined with appropriate soft tissue coverage results in improved motor function.

Other diseases require the transplantation of functioning "active" muscles with neurovascular anastomosis. A large musculocutaneous free graft with the option of a nerval coaptation is the **musculus latissimus dorsi graft**. The complete removal of this muscle does not lead to a functional deficit. Another option for a free functional musculocutaneous flap is the **musculus gracilis**. Due to its long and slim shape, it can be used for functional reconstructions in cases without the need for extensive coverage [1].

Details of the various flaps are given in Table 23.1.

23.2.2 Diseases

Depending on the underlying clinical picture, various aspects must be weighted in the indication (see above). Based on the pathogenesis, the following indication groups can be identified.

23.2.2.1 Early Innervation Deficits

These diseases include primarily the obstetric traumatic **plexus lesions**. Depending on the extent of the nerve deficit and the postnatal dynamics of the reinnervation, primary nerve reconstructions within the first year of life are useful. In addition to neurolysis and nerve transplants, neurotizations close to the muscle are also possible, in which the end branch of a functioning nerve or a fascicle is coapted close to the muscle to an injured distal nerve. The remaining movement disorders and functional deficits become apparent in the further course of the disease, which can no longer be influenced by nerve reconstructions due to the prolonged latency since the nerve damage occurred. This results in indications for free functional muscle transplants that assume an isolated function. The prerequisite for these muscle transplants is therefore the presence of an uninjured donor nerve to which the motor nerve branch belonging to the transplant can be coapted, which is not necessary for the original function. The typical graft in these cases consists of one or two neurovascular gracilis muscle flaps [2].

Also children with **arthrogryposis** whose limitations are due to neurogenic causes may belong to this group of indications. First reports of neurotisations of the musculocutaneous nerve in arthrogryposis by a fascicle from the ulnar nerve and/or median nerve sound encouraging and show children with increasing active elbow flexion.

23.2.2.2 Congenital Muscular Diseases

Also in this group, there are children with arthrogryposis, in which the muscular loss is in the

Table 23.1 Common free tissue transplants for reconstructive surgery of the extremities in children

Name	Combined tissue quality	Zuschnitt	Donor site	Pedicle	Can be used as an "active" free muscle graft (nerve!)?
M. latissimus dorsi	Muscle, skin island possible	Large expansion, oval to oblong	Dorsolateral thoracic aspect, usually primary closure possible	Arteria thoracodorsalis, N. thoracodorsalis, option for long preparation up to the axilla (origin from species axillary)	+
M. gracilis	Muscle, lifting with skin island possible	Thigh length, slender	Inside of femur, primary closure	Short pedicle arising from arteria femoralis profundus, Nerve branch from n. obturatorius	+
Fibula	Bone graft with muscle cuff, limited option for skin island	Depending on age at least 5 cm length	Lateral lower leg	Arteria fibularis (peronea)	–
Anterolateral thigh flap (ALT)	Skin, if necessary fascia	Large extension, oval to spindle-shaped	Primary closure limited	Limited perforator branches from the ramus descendens arteria circumflexa femoris lateralis, variable	–
Toe graft	Complete	Anatomical	Foot	Long, sensory nerve coaptation	+ (Replacement of thumbs and/ or fingers)
Scapular/ parascapular flap	Skin, subcutaneous tissue, combination with bone graft possible	With children rather thick, elliptical, therefore unusual		Arteria subscapularis	–

foreground. Since in arthrogryposis uninvolved functioning donor nerves for free muscle transplants can only rarely be identified, local surgical proceedings such as tendon and pedicled muscle transfers are significantly more frequent. Other neuromuscular diseases also generally belong to this group, although the rapid progression of most of these diseases limits surgical reconstructions. Most surgical procedures will only have temporary effects, so that the effort and morbidity of the procedures should be confined. Tenodeses which, for example, minimize the effects of intrinsic misinnervation are often useful.

23.2.2.3 Congenital Combined Nerve and Soft Tissue Defects

The **neonatal compartment syndrome** is a combined severe clinical picture that occurs before birth but is rarely recognized as such [3]. Pressure in the compartments of the muscle groups leads to a progressive circulatory disorder. The exact triggering factors are still unknown today and are highly likely to be multifactorial. Prenatal ultrasound showed the corresponding changes in the tissue already several hours before birth. The neonatal compartment syndrome presents itself postnatally in the form of ensanguined blisters and pallor on the affected extremity. The malposition of the arm due to the tissue damage, is misinterpreted as a sign of perinatal plexus injury.

Like any untreated compartment syndrome, the clinical picture leads to reduced perfusion, permanent nerve damage, scarring of the muscles and skin involved and, in individual cases, loss of the extremity due to vascular occlusion. After weeks and months, severe contractures appear with soft tissue shortening, malposition and sensory loss, which can hardly be improved conservatively. For this combined sequelae, it is therefore necessary to enable a sufficiently large and well-perfused soft tissue coverage. Here is the indication for a M. latissimus dorsi transplant or, in the case of isolated soft tissue replacement, possibly an ALT flap.

23.2.2.4 Acquired Nerve Injuries

Direct nerve injuries caused by shards, knives, etc. are usually detected immediately and treated appropriately, even in small children. Nevertheless, even with these causes of accidents, the consequences of injuries that have been classified as minor can result in sensory or motor impairment remain. For example, deficiency of the ulnar nerve is often clinically not clear enough to be suspected in a small child. However, the open wound at least gives an indication of a possible injury. The situation is different with nerve injuries, which primarily occur in the context of closed fractures or iatrogenous as a result of fracture treatment. The palsy then complained of by the children is often not diagnosed despite clear clinic or misinterpreted as rehabilitation deficits. Due to the resulting delay of appropriate diagnostics, nerve reconstructions are often carried out, with serious delay and the necesstiy for nerve transplants.

23.2.2.5 Acquired Combined Nerve, Vascular and Soft Tissue Lesions

These combined injuries occur as part of polytrauma or as a result of compartment syndromes, including vascular injuries. Their consequences are permanent and can almost completely inhibit the function of an arm or leg. The strategy of operative improvement may have to include a step-by-step therapy sequence. While early neurolysis or nerve reconstruction makes sense in cases with nerve entrapment or partial nerve injuries, several authors recommend prolonged combined surgical restoration over several months until development of the scarring contracture may be finshed. This involves the complete resection of fibrously altered and shortened former muscle tissue, the lengthening of tendons and, if necessary, the splitting of the interosseous membrane. All structures of the affected region are carefully removed from the scars and necroses are removed. Nerves should also be neurolysed consequently and if nevessary interfascicular with the microscope in order to achieve the best possible reinnervation. The soft tissue defects resulting from the removal of contractures require physiological soft tissue coverage with sliding layers, so that local plastic reconstuctive options are limited for large defects, and free soft tissue transplants may also be necessary for these children.

23.2.2.6 Spastic Cerebral Palsy

Spastic cerebral palsy is generally not a domain of microsurgical reconstruction. Tenodeses, muscle transfers and myotomies are more frequently used here as surgical treatment. Superselective neurotomies of individual motor branches are rarely performed on the upper extremities in order to reduce the severity of spastic paralysis. However, they are increasingly used on the legs for the treatment of pes equinovarus. All surgical procedures are a component in multimodal therapy and can only be planned in close interdisciplinary cooperation. Also the more frequent muscle transfers cannot supersede further interdisciplinary care and therapy. Typical operations are the transposition of the flexor carpi ulnaris muscle to the tendon of the extensor carpi radialis brevis muscle, the redirection of the pronator teres muscle through the interosseous membrane to reconstruct supination and the myotomy of the adductor muscles of the thumb in combination with a plastic widening of the interdigital space.

23.3 General Information

Microsurgical interventions in children require a trained and experienced team in an appropriately qualified facility. While in case of an emergency for a microsurgical operation, e.g. a replantation, in the interest of a timely treatment, the consideration of the nearest suitable institution falls in favour, the elective highly specialized interventions should always be carried out in centres with corresponding experience. Instruments and technical equipment must enable the surgeon to prepare even the smallest structures and tiny anastomoses with the necessary safety.

For the **surgical microscope** is to demand a up to twentyfold magnification. Pediatric anaesthesiologists and the possibility of follow-up treatment suitable for children complete the therapy. From the authors point of view for all interventions with vascular involvement, the preoperative application of a **plexus catheter** will be extremely helpful. This widens the vascular periphery and reduces the risk of spastic perfusion problems. Authors also describe free flap transplants in plexus or spinal analgesia in combination with sedation [4]. A plexus catheter also offers the possibility of painless aftercare. This must be guaranteed for children, especially as they often have to expect repeated hospital treatment as a result of their basic illness.

Up to now there is no clear evidence for the effects of postoperative treatment with **acetylsalicylic acid** in the case of vascular reconstructions of the extremities and free transplants in childhood. Due to the risk of Reye syndrome, a cautious therapy assessment is recommended.

In reconstructions that are accompanied by soft tissue coverage and substantial changes in the surface contour, a **photo documentation** of the preoperative findings and the postoperative course is wise. Video sequences of playful spontaneous behaviour also make sense in order to document changes in the usability of the affected extremity. On the one hand, these serve to document the findings and are also very helpful in clarifying the changes achieved to parents and small patients. With the appropriate consent, we also use these photos and videos to explain the

therapy options to other patients preoperatively but also to refute exaggerated expectations.

23.4 Type of Operation

Depending on the indication, various aspects have to be considered when planning and performing microsurgical procedures. It is always important to keep both the body temperature of the child and the room temperature of the operating theatre at a level that promotes dilation of the peripheral vessels and prevents spasms. A muscle relaxation at the beginning of anaesthesia should be short-acting in order not to diminish the informative value of possibly necessary neurophysiological measurements by nerve or muscle stimulation.

23.4.1 Vascular Reconstructions

Secondary vascular reconstructions become necessary when traumatic or iatrogenic vascular injuries including dissections are diagnosed with delay but cause a reduced perfusion. In these cases, reconstruction with vein transplants is the therapy of choice. In children, it is usually possible to remove the corresponding venous transplant from the same limb. Large-volume subcutaneous veins whose course from distal to proximal on the later graft is documented by a marking suture before complete resection are well suited. After removal, the graft is used for arterial reconstructions in reverse flow direction so that any venous valves do not prevent arterial flow.

The anastomosis is performed microsurgically with the surgical microscope and in children usually with single-button sutures and non-absorbable monofilament sutures with a thread thickness of less than 0.04 mm (according to USP 8-0 to 11-0). Intravenous heparin application is often performed before the reconstructed vessel sections are opened. However, an evidence-based recommendation for this procedure cannot be given if the publication situation is inadequate.

23.4.2 Free Tissue Transplants

When planning free tissue transplants, the choice of the right transplant is crucial. This is based on the extend and thickness of the soft tissue defect. After resection of scar fields in contractures or post-traumatic defects, large areas may be involved, where the removal of the correspondingly large graft from the donor region may lead to the necessity of compensatory split or full skin coverage with the consequence of a further donor region. This consequence cannot always be avoided by choosing a suitable flap. Even a very large musculus latissimus dorsi graft will not be larger than 14 cm × 6 cm in the 12-month-old child. Due to the physiological thickness and the multi-layered structure of the graft, circular defects cannot be completely covered. Figure 23.1 demonstrates the difficulties involved.

In contrast to adults, it is much more important in children to lift a corresponding skin island with the free flap as large as possible.

If one covers a free muscle flap with full skin or split skin in children, the associated disadvantages of scar shrinkage and hypertrophy partially cancel out the desired effect of the free flap.

It is therefore necessary for the surgeon to be experienced in a range of different flaps and available techniques in order to select the right suitable muscle. A relevant overview of free flap transplants is shown in Table 23.1. Figures 23.2 and 23.3 show the preparation of an anterolateral tigh flap as an example of a perforator flap and the elevation of a neurovascular pedicled musculus latissimus dorsi flap, which can also be used as a functional graft.

Functional free muscle transplants with connection of the flap nerve to available donor nerves of the upper extremity are generally rare in children. In the case of complete obstetric plexus lesions, they can be considered if the early reconstructive measures have improved shoulder and elbow function and donor nerves are still available to connect the free muscle graft. The use of the contralateral C7 root using a nerve interposition is also described for children. In complete plexus lesions, this can consist of the vascularized elevated ulnar nerve of the injured side. It is

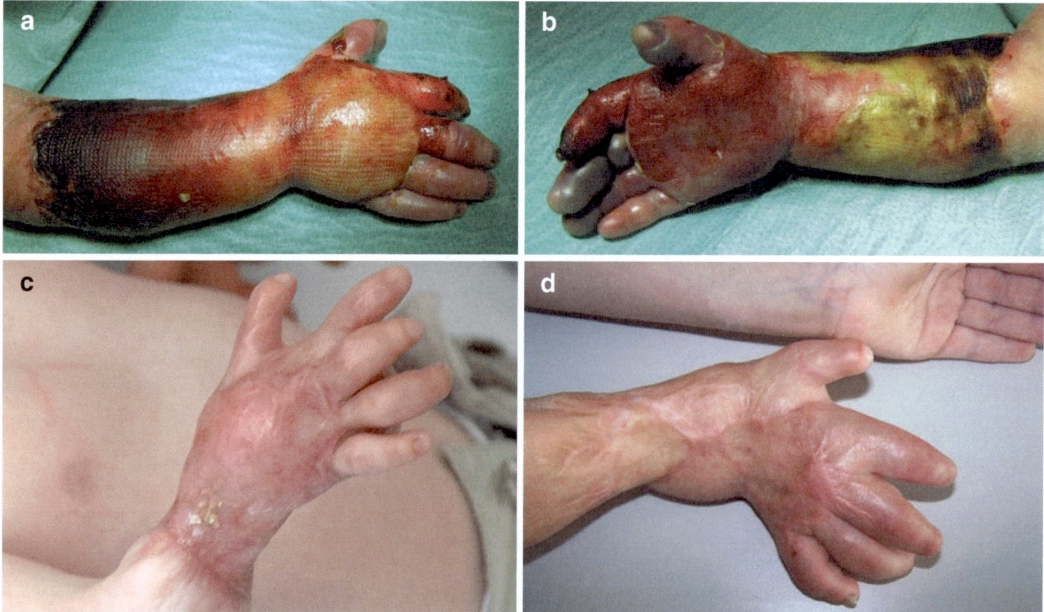

Fig. 23.1 (**a–d**) Newborn compartment syndrome. (**a, b**) Right hand of a premature infant 4 days postnatal with neonatal compartment syndrome. (**c**) The same hand at the corrected age of 4 months. (**d**) The healed M. latissimus dorsi flap, lifted to its maximum size, was needed on the flexor side to cover the reconstructed median nerve and the preserved musculature as well as the flap vessels and does not reach the extension side sufficiently

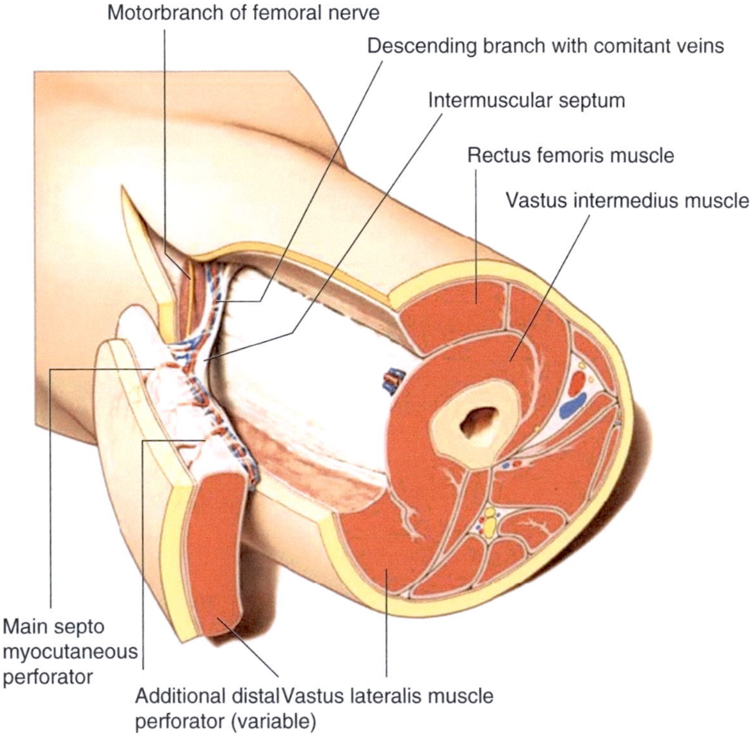

Fig. 23.2 Preparation of a free anterolateral flap of the thigh. (From [5])

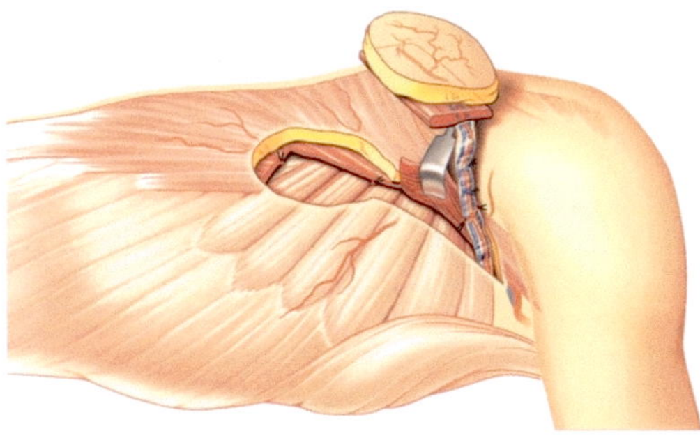

Fig. 23.3 Preparation one free neurovascular pedicled musculus latissimus dorsi flap. (From [5])

coapted to the contralateral C7 root and, after an appropriate reinsertion period, checked for the presence of sufficient axons on the residual distal stump. Then, as with any other healthy donor nerve, a free musculus gracilis graft can be attached to reconstruct a hand function. Figures 23.3 and 23.4 show the elevation of such a neurovascular musculus gracilis flap and the same after complete healing of the upper arm.

However, there is insufficient long-term data available for this technique in children to make a final assessment of the method.

A special case of free tissue transplants exists with malignant **limb tumours**. Here fibular transplants are particularly helpful to bridge defects of long tubular bones [6]. In the case of soft tissue sarcomas, it may also be useful to carry out a functional reconstruction by means of a free functional muscle graft with coaptation to the originally responsible and still preserved motor nerves. In the case of postoperative regional radiotherapy, however, the success of such an operation will be questioned due to radiation-induced fibrosis.

23.4.3 Nerval Reconstructions

Secondary reconstructive nerve surgery is significantly more common in children than in adults. In principle, the same reconstruction principles

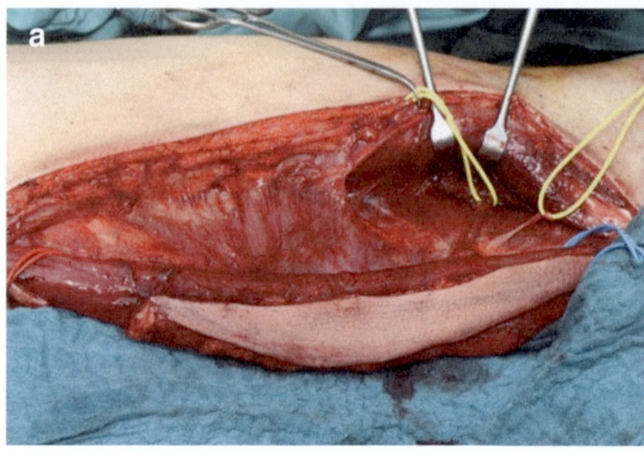
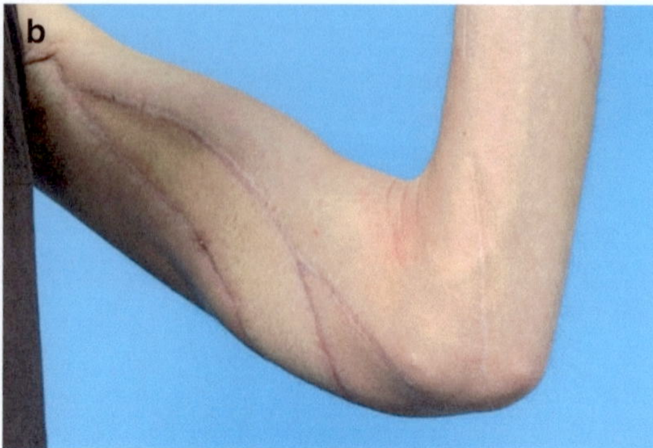

Fig. 23.4 (**a**, **b**) Lifting of a free neurovascular pedicled gracilis muscle on the medial aspect of the right thigh. (**a**) Yellow loops mark the vascular bundle of the muscle and the leading nerve branch from the obturatorius nerve. (**b**) The healed graft with large skin island on the left upper arm

Table 23.2 Secondary nerve reconstruction in children

Proceedings to the motor reinnervation	Principle	Advantages	Drawbacks
Defect bridging by graft	A injured nerve is locally reconstructed by nerve transplants	The original nerve keeps its responsibility for the respective muscle	Required transplants with potential donor morbidity
Nerve transposition, neurotization	A functioning nerve is dissected as distally as possible and coaptated to the distal stump of an injured nerve;	In the case of proximal injuries, this results in a significant shortening of the reinnervation time by proximity to the target organ	Possible weakening of the original function of the utilized nerves
Direct neurotization of a muscle	The distal branch of a functioning nerve is implanted directly into the muscle in the presumed vicinity of the motor end plates	A solution also for cases in which the distal nerve stumps are no longer presentable	

are valid (Table 23.2). For reinnervation, severed axons or fascicles require a reconstructed epineural tube and, at best, a soft, well-perfused wound environment without significant hematomas and without pressure. During the reconstruction, the residual nerve stumps must not come under tension, as this reduces the diameter of the nerve and prevents undisturbed axonal growth. Proximal nerve stumps can usually be recognized quite easily by the pronounced stump neuroma. A Waller's degeneration takes place at the distal nerve stumps, which does not entail any significant increase in circumference. In addition, some of the nerves, especially the ulnar nerve under the flexor carpi ulnaris muscle, retract considerably.

Detailed anatomical knowledge is then required in order to locate abd prepare the nerve stump.

Both nerve stumps are usually generously neurolysed and then sharply shortened until the individual soft groups of fascicles emerge unhindered from the epineural sheath as in a healthy nerve. The defect distance between the stumps is measured and bridged with nerve transplants. The nervus suralis is also most likely to be used in children. In the case of nerval reconstructions as part of plexus surgery, additional nerves from the affected arm are available. It is possible to obtain the ramus superficialis nervi radialis or the nervus cutaneus antebrachii medialis at upper arm level over a long distance.

Nerve coaptations with and without graft are generally performed under the surgical microscope with the smallest possible number of single-button sutures and fine thread.

So far no mention has been made of the possibilities offered by the **end-to-side coaptations** in reconstructive nerve surgery. Typical examples are fulminant avulsion injuries of the thumb, in which the two sensitive nerves virtually tear out of the median nerve. In such cases, the distal nerve stumps are shortened, transplanted and then inserted laterally through an epineural slit into the median nerve. In children, this method seems to work much better and to bring about a sensitive reinnervation.

23.5 Posttreatment

The direct partner of the surgeon is always the treated child [7]. His needs are in the foreground and determine the postoperative course.

23.5.1 Postoperative Treatment

The whole environment should be adapted to it. Sufficiently large family rooms are ideal. The expressly permitted stay of the child in the parental bed, a calm and possibly darkened atmosphere and painlessness guarantee the ideal conditions for undisturbed healing. For children, we almost always do without heavy plaster bandages, which often slip or lead to dismantling. Instead, well-padded soft dressings are chosen, which immobilize gently due to their volume and withstand even stubborn dismantling attacks with self-adhesive gauze dressings.

Of considerable importance is the consistent involvement of parents, whose restlessness and anxiety are always transmitted to the child. The more comprehensive and personal the education of the parents is, the more likely they are to be able to cope with the sometimes difficult first days and possible complications.

The necessary backup of **painlessness** has already been mentioned above. Pain-therapeutic visits should be carried out automatically every day after larger operations with several operation sites and should be available at any time if required. Local analgesia via a plexus catheter can be given continuously.

Manipulation of well-fitting dressings should be kept to a minimum, although free flap transplants require the creation of a "dressing window" for perfusion control. A well-known and established procedure for monitoring free transplants is explained to the parents and then consistently applied. The colour of the skin island, tissue turgor, felt temperature and reperfusion are documented under light pressure. This takes place for example in the first 48 h hourly, afterwards further 2 days two hourly. The intervals between checks shall be progressively extended from the fifth day.

The **management of complications**. The management of the patient's blood flow, especially in the case of free tissue transplants or vascular reconstructions with deterioration of the visible circulation situation, requires rapid and consistent management. Any suspicion of deterioration should be checked personally by the surgeon and, in the least case of doubt, be subjected to a revision under anaesthesia and in the operating theatre. Often only postoperative haematomas are the cause of the deterioration. As soon as these are eliminated and the cause of the secondary bleeding is found, the blood circulation of the free graft also improves. Otherwise the anastomoses must be revised one after the other. In all cases of a surgical revision after complex interventions, it must always be considered whether a compartment release is necessary.

23.5.2 Long-Term Treatment

It has proved successful to continue the long-term clinical support with the same team of therapists. The surgeon's direct knowledge of the intraoperative findings and the procedure performed enables clear statements to be made about expected innervation times, possible complications and postoperative requirements.

As soon as all wounds have healed, there is a consistent **scar therapy** required. The parents can be instructed to integrate scar massages and local ointment therapeutics into the everyday life of the family and to make the time of care attractive for the child. In case of impending scar contractures, **compression garments** are recommended, whereby a second set of garments must be available to change for washing. Here a child-fair qualified support is necessary by the bandagists. The colour of the compression garment to be chosen, together with covered fasteners that facilitate putting on of the garment, often ensures that the garment is worn willingly and consistently. Children are sensitive to the fact that the compressing and decongestant effect of clothing improves hand mobility and function and reduces the feeling of heaviness.

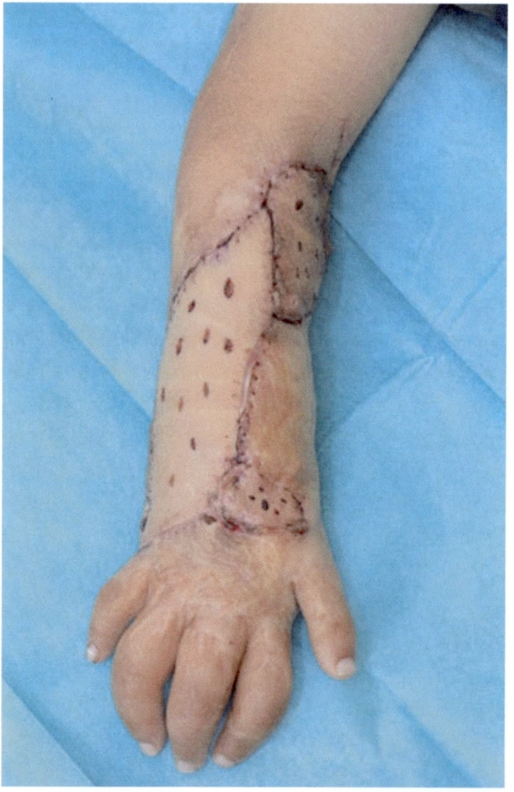

Fig. 23.5 Healed graft of a latissimus dorsi muscle of 12 cm × 6 cm with additional full skin coverage in a 2.5-year-old boy with neonatal compartment syndrome 15 days postoperatively, 2 smaller adjacent full skin grafts

23.6 Results

Only few and insufficient statistical statements are available on the results of microsurgical secondary interventions. Despite the small size of the vessels and nerves, surgical interventions are generally safer and more successful in children than in adults. Nevertheless, the underlying diseases cause permanent consequences and deteriorations which cannot be avoided despite the surgical effort. Figure 23.5 shows impressively that permanent consequences are unavoidable despite maximum surgical effort and a favourable course. In most of the clinical pictures described here, the microsurgical secondary interventions can only improve the consequences of the disease, but in no case lead to a complete cure.

References

1. Morris SF, Zuker RM. Functioning muscle transfers. In: Gupta M, Kay SPJ, Scheker LR, editors. The growing hand. London: Mosby; 2000. p. 1021–33.
2. Chim H, Kircher MF, Spinner RJ, Bishop AT, Shin AY. Free functioning gracilis transfer for traumatic brachial plexus injuries in children. J Hand Surg A. 2014;39:1959–66.
3. Hülsemann W, Böttcher R, Habenicht R. Kompartmentsyndrom der oberen Extremität beim Neugeborenen. Monatsschr Kinderheilkd. 2011;4:357–63.
4. Bjorklund KA, Venkatramani H, Venkateshwaran G, Boopathi V, Sabapathy RS. Regional anesthesia alone for pediatric free flaps. J Plast Recontr Aesthet Surg. 2015;68:705–8.
5. Wolff K-D, Hölzle R. Raising of microvascular flaps. 2nd ed. Berlin Heidelberg New York: Springer; 2011.
6. Erol B, Basci O, Topkar MO, Caypinar B, Basar H, Tetik C. Mid-term radiological and functional results of biological reconstructions of extremity-located bone sarcomas in children and young adults. J Pediatr Orthop B. 2015;24:469–78.
7. Kay SPJ, Lees VC. Free-tissue transfer in children. In: Gupta M, Kay SPJ, Scheker LR, editors. The growing hand. London: Mosby; 2000. p. 969–86.

Part VI

Follow-Up Treatment

Jörg Bahm

Each surgeon will initiate certain accompanying measures after an operation.

24.1 Post-operative Splinting

To protect nerve and tendon sutures, adjacent joints may be maintained for about 10–14 days for nerve sutures (interposition grafts for 3–4 weeks, without these periods being scientifically proven) and for tendon sutures, as a rule, 6 weeks (whereby interlaced sutures according to Pulvertaft may be moved earlier, e.g. after 2 weeks, without stress, and thus reduce the risk of post-operative adhesions). At the shoulder, limb-bearing orthoses must be used, which also allow progressive weaning after the 6 weeks have elapsed (Fig. 24.1). Soft tissue healing of superficial tissue layers takes 2–3 weeks; we use absorbable skin sutures that avoid anxiety-laden suture removal in children.

For the purpose of (nerve and tendon) suture protection, adjacent joints may be immobilised, but not the digits whose gentle active motion must be encouraged throughout the bandage.

24.1.1 Special Plaster Techniques for Small Children

In the case of extensive nerve reconstruction in the head and neck area (reconstruction of the brachial plexus), a so-called **Omega plaster** (named after its braces, Fig. 24.2) is applied for 3 weeks and checked weekly (the internal padding is renewed). Afterwards the operated arm should be protected in a sling for one additional week; and thereafter the physiotherapeutic treatment can be resumed.

24.2 Neurophysiologically Based Therapy

This serves to support or accompany nerve regeneration, integration of movements and sensory training and is the specific task of the therapist and overall the parents (Chap. 9). Likewise, after a tendon or muscle transfer, an appropriate muscle and function build-up must be accompanied by the therapist but also by the parents.

24.3 Occupational Therapy

It is aimed at older children who can and must accomplish specific tasks. Here, tasks of daily life can be addressed such as tying shoelaces, brushing teeth, buttoning shirts and doing hair or

J. Bahm (✉)
Plastic, Hand and Burn Surgery, Section for Plexus Surgery, University Hospital, Aachen, Germany
e-mail: jorg.bahm@belgacom.net,
jbahm@ukaachen.de

© Springer Nature Switzerland AG 2021
J. Bahm (ed.), *Movement Disorders of the Upper Extremities in Children*,
https://doi.org/10.1007/978-3-030-53622-0_24

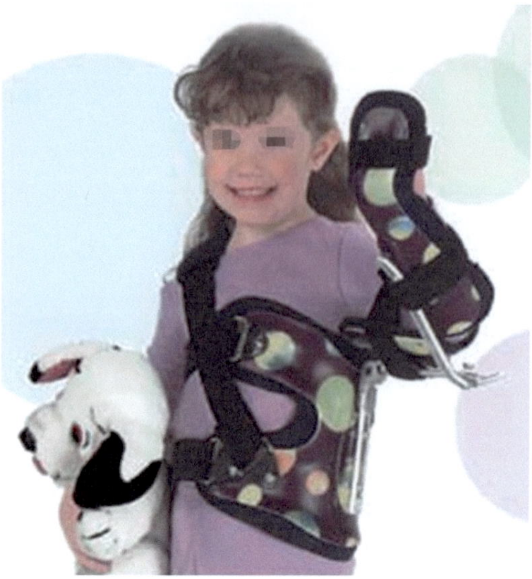

Fig. 24.1 Shoulder orthosis after tendon transfer to improve active external rotation

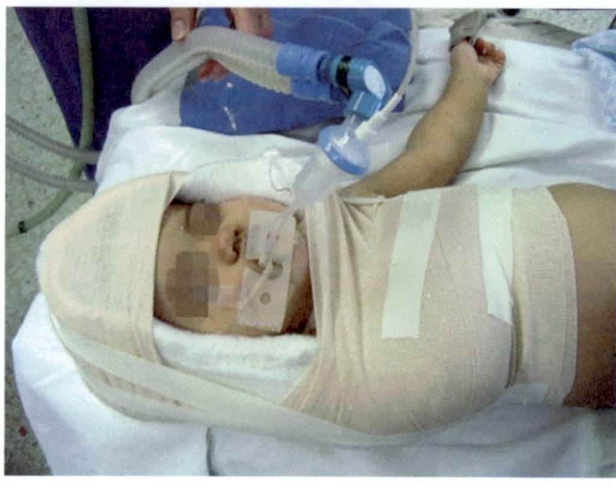

Fig. 24.2 Omega head and neck plaster for immobilisation after reconstruction of the brachial plexus

special handicrafts and games, but also sport movement patterns can be tackled. Sensory training is also very important. Complex movement patterns can be evaluated.

24.4 Sports

Sport is not a continuation of therapy and does not have to be "prescribed", but is designed to playfully support and strengthen the affected limb: Swimming is good for the shoulder, riding gives a straight back and enhances self-confidence, and ball games test fine motor skills and balance.

24.5 Fun Factor

Fun is very important for motivation in the long run. Therapy breaks are necessary. Children have to keep on exercising in their own way—in my opinion there are no "lazy" children. However, they use their resources and preferably the healthy arm with success logic and are less rationally oriented than we adults are. Therefore, exercises and games requiring **both** upper limbs are encouraged.

D. Schaakxs

25.1 Clinical Background: Nerve Injury and Muscular Atrophy

Peripheral nerve injuries affect about 300,000 people in Europe every year and therefore represent a considerable economic burden for society [1]. In most cases, peripheral nerve injuries are caused by road traffic or accidents at work in adult patients. The literature describes 1 in 2000 newborns with birth-associated plexus brachialis injuries [2, 3].

Peripheral nerve injuries are devastating to the affected limb and lead to reduced sensitive perception (sensitivity, sensation) and motor function and a lasting effect on the patient's life and ability to work if they cannot restore normal function. The peripheral nervous system, in contrast to the central nervous system, has a capacity for spontaneous regeneration after injury. Nevertheless, chronic muscular atrophy and fibrosis remain, in clinical practice, significant obstacles to optimal functional recovery if there is a longer delay in nerve regeneration and reinnervation of the target muscle.

In addition, traumatic peripheral nerve injuries are often associated with a *nerve tissue loss* and require a transplant to fill the gap. Although the autologous nerve graft is still the gold standard in reconstructive surgery, it has the serious disadvantage of sacrificing a functional donor nerve and leads to loss of sensation and scarring at the donor site (Fig. 25.1).

Although the focal point is on restoring the nerve at the site of injury, the denervated target muscle should not be overlooked to increase the chances for better functional results. The axotomy

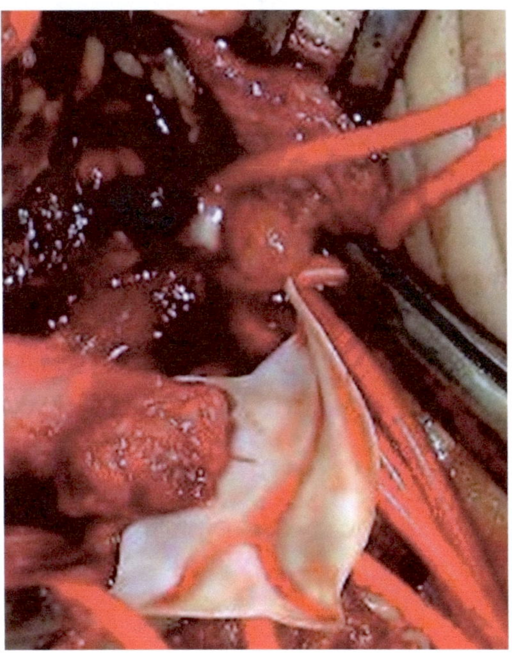

Fig. 25.1 Nerve lesion. There's no good nerve regeneration when the suture is under tension. Then a nerve graft is required to enable a good healing

D. Schaakxs (✉)
Plastic, Reconstructive and Aesthetic Surgery,
Galeries Benjamin-Constant 1,
1003 Lausanne, Switzerland

© Springer Nature Switzerland AG 2021
J. Bahm (ed.), *Movement Disorders of the Upper Extremities in Children*,
https://doi.org/10.1007/978-3-030-53622-0_25

of the peripheral nerves leads to a rapid decrease in target muscle mass, which can be reversible if there is a qualitative muscle reinnervation within about 2 months [4]. In the case of a sustainable denervation, *progressive muscle cell death* and *fibrosis* with irreversible muscle dysfunction occur [5–12]. Optimal functional recovery after peripheral nerve injury requires as follows:

– That the regenerating axons form functional connections with their original muscle fibers
– A restoration of the number and size of the motor units in these muscles [13].

In order to optimize clinical recovery after nerve lesion, it is important to treat at two levels: the *nerve lesion site* and the *neuromuscular junction*. Regenerative research involves treatments with stem cells and biomaterials as a new approach to treat the problems of peripheral nerve injury and associated muscular atrophy in two stages. It is believed that this global approach helps to optimize functional recovery after peripheral nerve lesion. It is also important to understand the possible mechanisms of an effect of fat tissue stem cells on nerve regeneration and neuromuscular synapse in order to understand the applications of new cell therapies. Human fat tissue stem cells are abundant and easily accessible and are an optimal source for regenerative medicine. In one study, different properties of human adult stem cells were shown depending on their localization [14].

Demanding nerve regeneration after a nerve lesion and keeping the motor unit "alive" through various stimulation mechanisms (electrostimulation, cell therapy) represent the key for later clinical application in peripheral nerve lesions.

25.2 Anatomy of Peripheral Nerves

The neuron with its accompanying Schwann cells can be seen as the smallest unit and functional basic structure of a peripheral nerve. *Neurons* consist of a cell body located in the dorsal root ganglion and its extensions, the dendrites on the one hand and the axon on the other hand. Dendrites transmit electrical impulses to the cell body, and the axon transmits electrical signals from the cell body [15].

The individual axons of a nerve are enclosed by a connective tissue sheath, which is called *endoneurium*. Several axons are grouped into bundles of nerve fibers, called fascicles, which in turn are enveloped by connective tissue *(perineurium)*. The connective tissue sheath around the entire nerve is called *epinurium*.

Glial cells are supporting cells and include in the peripheral nervous system the *Schwann cells*. Unlike neurons, glial cells can divide mitotically. Glial cells develop from the neural crest and are present in mature nerves as two different phenotypes, either myelinating or non-myelinating. The myelinating Schwann cells produce the *myelin sheath*, a greasy insolating layer that envelops the axon in several layers. About 70% of myelin is produced by lipids, and the rest is composed of different myelin-specific proteins. After myelinization has taken place, the Schwann cell is in an inactive stage and can be reactivated for myelinization if necessary.

There are gaps between the Schwann cells enveloping the axon, the nodes of *Ranvier*, along which the saltatoric conduction of action potentials is propagated. Each axon-Schwann cell is contained within an extracellular matrix of the peripheral nerve called basal lamina. After a nerve injury, peripheral nerve integrity is maintained by the close coordination and complex interactions between the two cellular and extracellular components (Fig. 25.2).

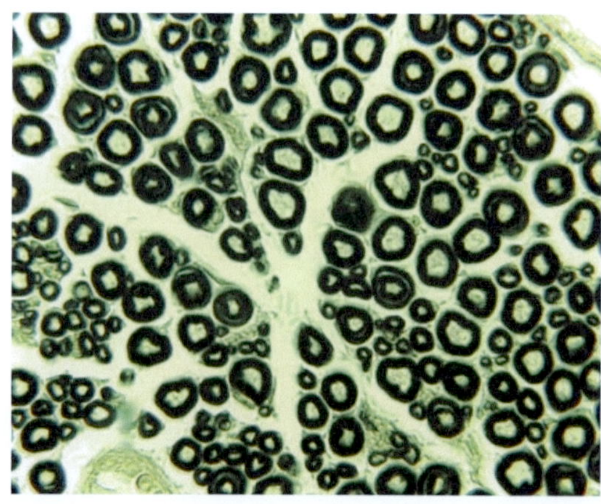

Fig. 25.2 Peripheral nerve with well-myelinized nerve fibers

25.3   Pathophysiology of Nerve Injury

25.3.1 Degeneration and Regeneration of Peripheral Nerves: Pathophysiology

Peripheral nerves can regenerate to a certain degree after injury, in contrast to the limited regeneration of nerves in the central nervous system (CNS). If a peripheral nerve is injured, this triggers the activation of Schwann cells (SCs) and macrophages [16]. The ability of peripheral nerves to regenerate is influenced by interactions between these cell elements and the extracellular matrix molecules of the basal lamina [17].

The pathophysiological changes of peripheral nerves after nerve transection affect both the cell body and the distal and proximal end of the affected axon. The cell body swells with chromatolysis, and the cell nucleus shifts to the periphery of the cell body. Degeneration occurs at the distal end of the nerve stump, the so-called nerve stump *Wallerian degeneration*. The proximal nerve axons degenerate retrogradely up to the nearest node of Ranvier, from which then form new axon sprouts.

Various *neurotransmitters* play a decisive role. They prevent the death of the nerve cell, are therefore neuroprotective, and regulate the outgrowth of the axon collaterals. If the distance between the nerve stumps remains small, cytokines originating from the distal nerve stump such as "tumor necrosis factor alpha" (TNF-α), growth factors such as "ciliary neurotrophic factor" (CNTF), and "neurotrophic growth factor" (NGF) as well as interferons can support the growth of axons. The axons sprouting out of the proximal nerve stump lose their orientation without a guiding structure and grow undirected into the resulting scar tissue. The result is a new scar, consisting of numerous minifascicles surrounded by a layer of perineural connective tissue.

Wallerian degeneration with its changes in the denervated distal nerve stump is completed approximately 5–8 weeks after the injury. Initially, macrophages are responsible for the phagocytosis of the degraded nerve components and promote the proliferation of Schwann cells.

After the decay of the myelin sheaths, the Schwann cells begin to dedifferentiate and divide. *Dedifferenciation* means that the Schwann cells change their phenotype from myelinating to non-myelinating. The newly formed Schwann cells arrange themselves in a longitudinal direction and form together with the basal lamina the *bands of Büngner*. These can serve as guide rails for proximal sprouting axons to grow over the lesion and reach the distal end [17, 18]. Numerous intracellular changes collectively regulate the subsequent regeneration of the axons and the restoration of the neuronal cytoskeleton [19]. Considering that the injury often occurs at a considerable distance from the target organ, the restoration of function often takes months and does not heal optimally [20].

25.3.2 Clinical Classification of Peripheral Nerve Injuries

The most common nerve lesions are caused by severing, compression, crushing, traction, and tearing mechanisms.

Seddon et al. [21] divided peripheral nerve injury into neurapraxia, axonotmesis, and neurotmesis. Sunderland further refined this classification and described five degrees of severity using histological analyses [22]:

– *Neurapraxia:* The continuity of the nerve is still preserved, but segmental demyelination reveals a conduction block. This injury is reversible, and regeneration takes place within a few months. Neurapraxia is caused by traction or light compression.
– *Axonotmesis*: Axonal lesion with myelin loss in which the perineurium is still preserved. In this case, regeneration may occur, which generally takes longer than in a neurapraxia.
– *Neurotmesis*: It describes a complete nerve transection with loss of function. The proximal axons do not reach the target organ, and neuroma is formed. There's no recovery. Microsurgical reconstructive surgery is necessary. Depending on the nerve injury, corresponding consecutive histopathological changes occur [1, 23].

25.4 Muscle Anatomy and Physiology of Muscle Contraction

Skeletal muscles are the arbitrarily controllable parts of the musculature and ensure mobility. The skeletal muscle consists of multinucleated, densely packed muscle fibers. The myofibril structures within the muscle fibers are divided into individual contractile units called the *sarcomeres*. The sarcomeres consist of thick filaments of *myosin* and thin filaments of *actin* associated with troponin and tropomyosin proteins. Together, these structures form the basic mechanism of muscle contraction.

Skeletal muscles are called striated muscles because their myofibrils, in contrast to smooth muscles, are arranged quite regularly and thus produce a recognizable ring pattern of red and white myosin filaments or actin filaments. The myosin protein determines the contraction speed of the muscle. Each myosin molecule consists of two heavy chains of myosin (MyHC) and four light chains with variable amino acid sequences [24]. Rapid myosin ("fast myosin") is found in particularly high numbers in the fast contracting muscle fibers; and slow myosin ("slow myosin") predominates in the slow contracting muscle fibers. Individual muscle fibers are classified into Type I and Type II fibers.

One *motor unit* comprises a single motoneuron with all of its innervated muscle fibers and thus represents the smallest functional unit for the control of arbitrary and involuntary motor function of a skeletal muscle. Several motor units work together to coordinate the contractions of a muscle. The neuromuscular synapse consists of a presynaptic axon terminal surrounded by terminal Schwann cells and the plasma membrane of postsynaptic muscle fibers containing *acetylcholine receptors* (AChRs). They are called motor end plates. If an action potential reaches the synapse, a change in the presynaptic membrane leads to an influx of calcium ions into the terminal nerve fiber. The calcium increase causes a release of acetylcholine (ACh) from the axon end into the synaptic cleft. The acetylcholine crosses the synaptic cleft and binds to ACh receptors in the postsynaptic membrane. This makes the muscle fiber membrane permeable for potassium and sodium, so that via the influx of sodium ions, an *action potential* in the muscle fiber can be triggered. The action potential is transferred and leads to contraction of the muscle fiber. The enzyme cholinesterase in the synaptic cleft cleaves the ACh so that the effect on the postsynaptic membrane is cancelled [25–27].

25.5 Pathophysiology of Denervated Muscle

Functional and structural maintenance of the target skeletal muscle depends on intact and effective innervation of peripheral nerves, which are important for muscle development, metabolism, and contractile properties. Denervation-induced pathological changes are closely related to the regeneration potential of the denervated skeletal muscle. The presence of intrinsic muscle satellite cells between a myofibril and the surrounding extracellular matrix helps to regenerate denervated muscles [28]. In response to injury, satellite cells are activated, replicated, and differentiated into myoblasts. The myoblasts can fuse with each other or with the mother muscle fiber to enable muscle repair. Prolonged denervation leads to reduced regeneration potential due to gradual muscle fiber atrophy and fibrosis and finally to irreversible pathological changes.

The time to reinnervation is one of the decisive factors for the functional recovery of the muscles after a nerve injury. Within 60 days after an axotomy, the muscle mass decreases by 70%.

This mass loss is initially reversible if there is a good quality of muscle reinnervation within 2 months. In cases of continuous denervation, progressive atrophy, muscle cell death, and fibrosis with irreversible muscle dysfunction are observed. After 6 months, the denervated muscle has 5–10% of its original weight and is mainly replaced by non-contractible connective tissue [4].

The *apoptosis* also plays a physiologically important role in the regulation of denervation-induced muscle atrophy with pro-apoptotic genes such as Bax and caspase 3 and 9, which are upregulated in the denervated muscle [4, 29, 30].

During this muscle remodeling process, various morphological changes occur at the muscle fiber and at the neuromuscular synapse. Muscular atrophy preferentially affects the fast muscle fiber type in the early stages of denervation, followed by atrophy of the slow fiber type. In the first 3–4 weeks after denervation, there is initially a myogenic reaction of the satellite cells followed by replacement of lost fibers; but later, between 7 and 20 weeks, the satellite cells decrease and fibrosis and fat cells increase [4, 31]. At the neuromuscular synapse, it was shown that after axotomy the denervation process affects the presynaptic nerve endings more than the postsynaptic acetylcholine receptors and muscle fibers, with a rapid degeneration of the presynaptic nerve endings compared to a relatively slow degeneration of the postsynaptic acetylcholine receptors and atrophy of the muscles.

The degeneration of the neuromuscular synapses (synaptophysin, a component of the presynaptic vesicle membrane) decreases after 18 h and disappears completely after 24 h. Acetylcholine receptors are fairly stable after denervation (no significant decrease after 4 weeks, still 70% of acetylcholine receptor reactivity after 10 weeks) [25–27].

In order to achieve optimal functional recovery after nerve lesion, the regenerating axons must form functional connections with their original muscle fibers, and the number and size of motor units in these muscles must be restored.

25.6 Nerve Transplantation

Peripheral nerve injuries without a defect or with a short gap can be treated with a simple *end-to-end epineurium suture technique* and lead to reasonable neurological recovery. If there is a longer defect (greater than 20 mm), as is the case with injuries to the brachial plexus, for example, direct nerve coaptation without tension is not possible, and an autologous nerve graft is required to fill the gap. *Autologous nerve transplants* contain Schwann cells, growth factors, and basal membrane components and are the current gold standard in reconstructive surgery of peripheral nerves. However, they currently have several disadvantages caused by the need to remove a donor nerve. This secondary procedure sacrifices some functional nerves and induces scarring, possible neuroma formation, and loss of sensation at the donor site [32].

25.7 Alternative Nerve Transplantation: Artificial Nerve Conduits

The development of *tissue-engineered alternatives* to replace autologous nerve grafts, which are still the gold standard in reconstructive surgery, remains a major challenge. The successful construction of a nerve gap is based on the formation of a new extracellular matrix scaffold via which blood vessels, fibroblasts, and Schwann cells can migrate in the direction of the distal nerve stump [33]. Alternatives to autologous grafts (venous and arterial conduction grafts) have been investigated, but these have shown no functional advantages over standard nerve grafts [34, 35].

Allografts have also been tested, but their usefulness is limited because they require unwanted long-term immunosuppressive therapy [36]. Today's surgical techniques have no satisfactory alternative to standard nerve transplants that allow good nerve regeneration. Therefore, an active field of research developed with the development of artificially constructed transplants or *conduits* which create a suitable environment for regenerating axons and represent a promising alternative therapy [37].

Various synthetic conduits of nondegradable materials such as silicone and others such as polytetrafluoroethylene and polypyrrole were tested, but these showed compression syndromes due to their nondegradable nature and their inability to adapt growth and maturation to the nerves [38–40]. Thus, research for other biomaterials was undertaken. The materials used should be highly biocompatible, ideally biodegradable, and permeable and show favorable biomechanical and surface properties such as flexibility and a predictable degradation rate. Among the materials commonly used in nerve regeneration studies are polyesters (e.g., poly-3-hydroxybutyrate [PHB], polycaprolactone, polyglycolide, and polylactide), proteins (e.g., fibrin, collagen, silk, and gelatin), and polysaccharides (e.g., PHB was used as scaffold material).

PHB is considered as a product for biotechnological research and as an exemple for clinical applications. It belongs to the class of polyhydroxyalkanoates, i.e., biodegradable and biocompatible synthetic thermoplastic polyesters produced by bacteria. PHB grafts offer several advantages such as soft moldable consistency, good tensile strength, and flexibility. PHB was first used as a wraparound in direct nerve repair [41] and then in tubular form in experimental animal models for bridging short [42] and long [43] nerve gaps. The fibrous composition of the PHB films can be aligned in the longitudinal direction of the cable, creating a directional, contact guide for the regenerating axons [43]. The regenerative potential of PHB can be improved by the incorporation of growth factors, molecules of the extracellular matrix, and cells. Recent clinical studies have shown that PHB has produced better results than epineural sutures without side effects (Fig. 25.3).

The use of *fibrin*, a naturally occurring molecule, mimics the physiological properties of nerve healing. Fibrin is a polypeptide formed from the plasma components fibrinogen and thrombin. Physiological fibrin formation takes place as the last step in the natural blood coagulation cascade, whereby a clot contributes to wound healing. Fibrin glues are commercially available, have good biocompatibility [44], are widely used, and are used in surgical practice [45], e.g., for hemostasis, nerve coaptation, and improvement of vascular anastomoses. Fibrin was also used in the construction of nerve fibers [44, 46, 47]. The short absorption time of fibrin glue makes it suitable for shorter distances and supports the early nerve regeneration process, while PHB can be used for longer nerve gaps. Fibrin can also be used as a matrix for cells. A short-term study showed the beneficial effect on nerve regeneration when using a fibrin matrix cell within/on PHB lines or strips (an open construction instead of tube). PHB strips showed better results and a faster nerve regeneration procedure compared to PHB conduits (Fig. 25.3) [47].

As a cell delivery vehicle, a fibrin tissue adhesive facilitates cell adhesion, proliferation, differentiation, and subsequent well-organized 3D tissue dressing and represents an important tool in biotechnological research for the treatment of peripheral nerve lesions.

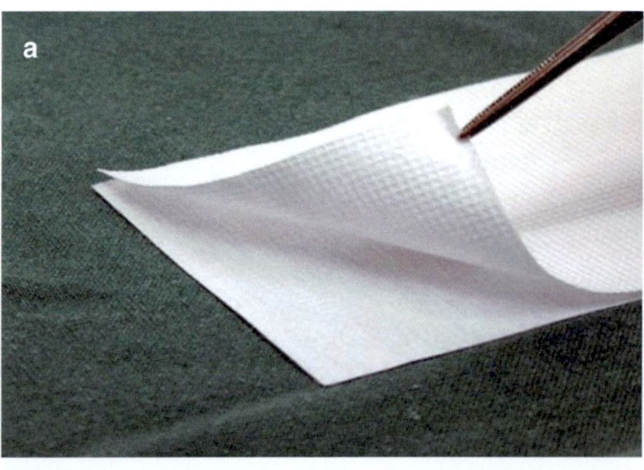
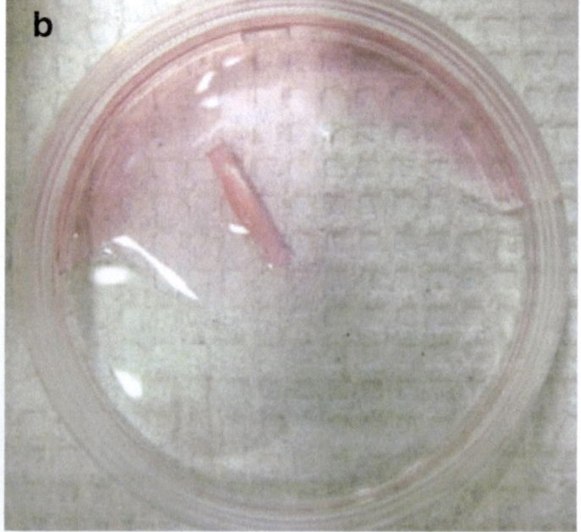

Fig. 25.3 (a, b) PHB strips with cells as an open system allow communication between the regenerating nerve fibers and the external neurotrophic and vascularization factors, which is an optimal medium for nerve regeneration. (a) PHB material. (b) Fibrin matrix cell on PHB strips in vitro

25.8 Cell Therapy: Regenerative Therapy Approaches in Plastic Surgery

25.8.1 Mesenchymal Stem Cells: Adipose Stem Cells

Mesenchymal stem cells (MSCs) play a central role in regenerative medicine. While the regenerative properties of MSC from bone marrow are well known, the finding that a population of cells with multipotential differentiation potential exists in fatty tissue alongside adipocytes, fibroblasts, blood vessels, and preadipocytes is relatively new [48]. Only in 2001 Zuk et al. recognized the potential of these adipose stem cells (ASCs) to differentiate into different terminal functional cells [49].

Most current regenerative therapy approaches in plastic surgery use mesenchymal stem cells from adipose tissue ("adipose-derived stem cells," ASC). They offer the advantage of being relatively easy to obtain (liposuction, abdominoplasty), unlike bone marrow MSCs, which require invasive and painful bone marrow punction. For a sufficiently large amount of ASC, only a liposuction of relatively small amounts of adipose tissue is required, since mesenchymal stem cells are found in adipose tissue in about 100 to 1000 times higher concentration than in bone marrow [50].

Interestingly, these ASCs can differentiate not only into different terminal cells of the mesenchymal lines, i.e., fibroblasts, osteoblasts, chondrocytes, and adipocytes, but also into neuron-like cells, pancreatic cells, and hematopoietic precursor cells. ASCs function as "secretomes" of growth factors that are angiogenetically effective or proliferation promoting, such as "vascular endothelial growth factor" (VEGF), "hepatocyte growth factor" (HGF), "fibroblast growth factor" (FGF), or "platelet-derived growth factor" (PDGF). This secretion can be further stimulated by hypoxia, which makes the use of ASC even more attractive [49].

Tissue replacement plays an important role in reconstructive surgery, as its task is to replace tissue lost through trauma or disease. In order to fulfill this task, replacement tissue is often removed from other parts of the body during operations, which in turn results in a lesion at the *donor site*. Through an improved understanding of the cell and molecular biological basis of healing, various regenerative therapy approaches have been developed in recent years.

Cell therapies that prefer to use autologous mesenchymal stem cells from adipose tissue show excellent healing results with minimal donor site defect. However, growth factor-based approaches or the use of platelet-rich plasma also leads to exceptionally good results in the field of wound or bone healing [49].

By using various cell or molecule therapies and biological mechanisms, the regenerative abilities of the adult organism can be improved. In both reconstructive and aesthetic surgery, many procedures are already being used clinically. However, the successes should not obscure the potential risk inherent in both cell- and growth factor-based approaches, and such therapy procedures should be carefully indicated until long-term experience is available [49].

25.8.2 Obtaining Fatty Tissue, Stem Cell Production, and Culture

Fat tissue is abundant and contains a higher concentration of multipotent stem cells compared to the bone marrow. The fat tissue obtained, at least in aesthetic surgery, is usually a "waste product." Two main techniques are used to obtain fatty tissue. One is *dermolipectomy*, excision of a complete flap of the skin including subcutaneous fat tissue, which is a method used when a tightening of the excess skin can no longer be expected. The other is the *liposuction,* a minimally invasive procedure with minimal scarring [51].

If liposuction is used as a procedure for obtaining fatty tissue, centrifugation can be started directly due to the suspension-like consistency. In dermolipectomies, the fat flap should be first removed in 1 cm^3 large lobules, which can be cut with a scalpel and then freed from skin parts.

Fatty tissue is digested enzymatically using 0, 15% (w/v) type I collagenase (Invitrogen, UK). The solution is filtered to remove undissociated tissue and then neutralized by addition of α-MEM and 10% (v/v) fetal bovine serum (FBS) and centrifuged. The oily supernatant consists of lipids and adipocytes, the middle layer of PBS, collagenase and erythrocyte lysis buffer, and the sediment of a mixed population of the stromal-vascular parts of the fatty tissue. At this point, it is possible to reinject the stromal cell pellet. If the ASCs need to be cultured before therapeutic application, the stromal cell pellets can be resuspended after filtration and incubated in growth medium DMEM (Dulbecco's Modified Eagle's Medium), additionally supplemented with 1% (v/v) antibiotic/antimycotic solution, in cell culture flasks. The cultures are maintained at sub-confluent levels in a 37 °C incubator with 5% CO_2 and passages with trypsin/EDTA (Invitrogen, UK) if needed (Figs. 25.4, 25.5, and 25.6).

25.8.3 Regenerative Therapy Approaches in Peripheral Nerve Surgery

25.8.3.1 Schwann Cells and ASC as an Alternative Therapy for Nerve Regeneration

The *Schwann cells* are responsible for the myelination of the peripheral nerves, which play an important role in nerve conduction. After a nerve injury, the Schwann cells produce neurotrophic factors and thus help nerve regeneration. However, the use of Schwann cells has several disadvantages: the use of an autologous nerve, which can cause neuropathic pain, and the long in vitro cultivation time.

Adipose stem cells, which are multipotent and have a neurotrophic potential, are a good alternative for nerve therapy. One study isolated ASC from the two subcutaneous abdominal fat layers (deep and superficial, i.e., under or above the fas-

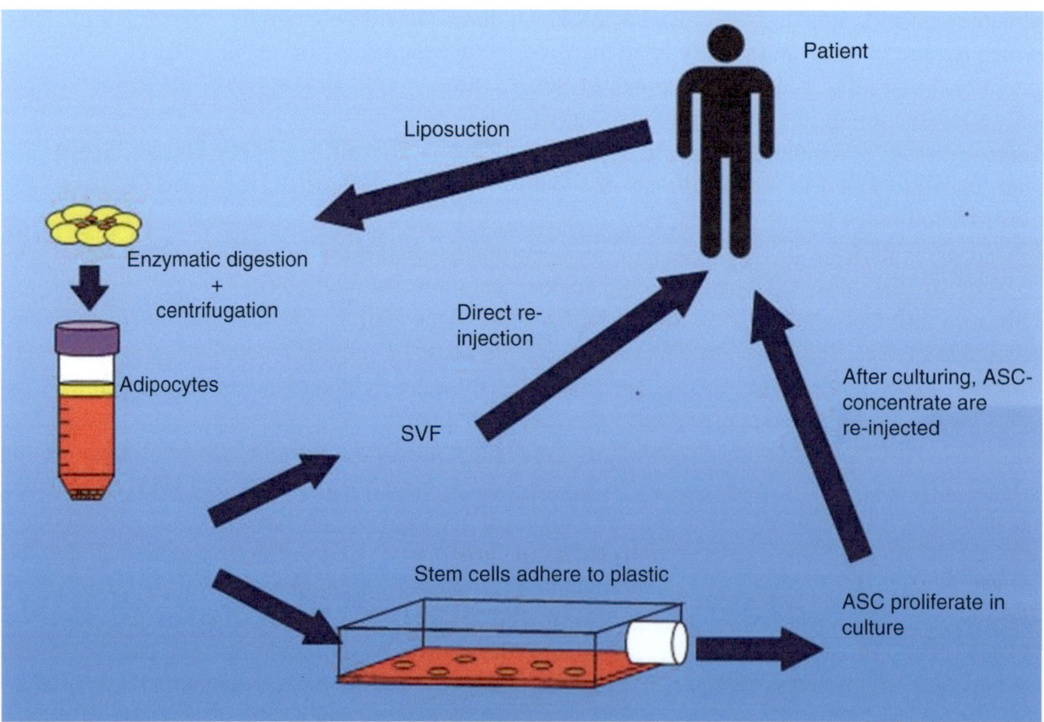

Fig. 25.4 Overview of the methodology of ASC culture and transplantation as cell-based therapy

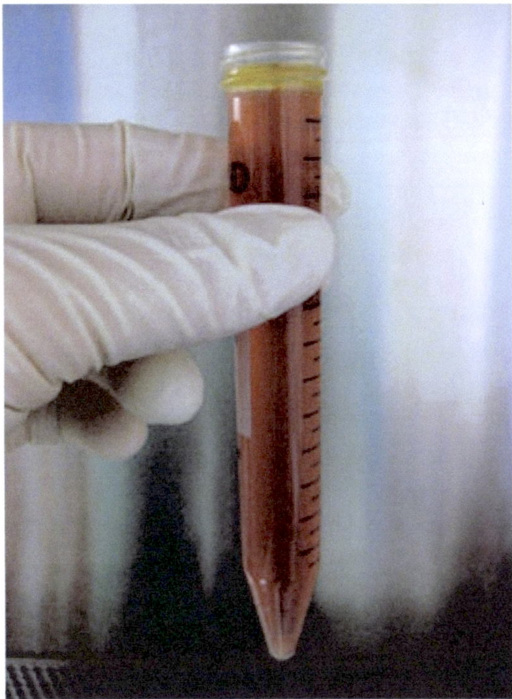

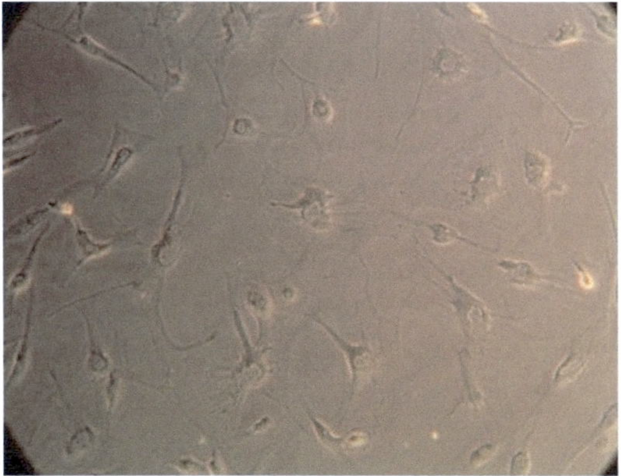

Fig. 25.6 Light microscope image of ASC in culture (magnification 10×)

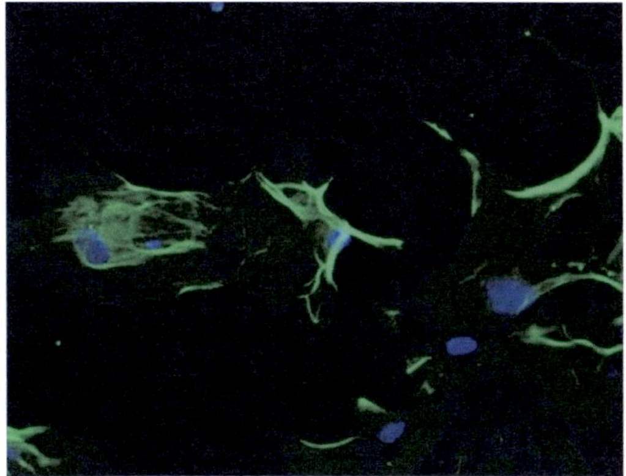

Fig. 25.5 Centrifugation tubes with fat typical three layers in oil fat emulsion (*at the top*), medium collagenase solution (*center*), and stromal-vascular fraction (*underneath*)

Fig 25.7 Stem cells express stem cell markers (positive for Stro 1)

cia of Scarpa) during abdominoplasty and studied the proliferation capacity of the cells and their respective neurotrophic profiles. The ability of cells to differentiate into multiple cell lines is also determined by the expression of various *stem cell markers*. Cells from both layers expressed different stem cell markers (Stro-1, Oct4, Nanog, CD54, β1-integrin, collagen type I and fibronectin) (Fig. 25.7). Cells cultured from the surface layer are a better source of ASC for possible use in nerve repair and other regenerative therapies. ASCs from the superficial fat layer show a significantly improved neurite growth compared to the cells of the deep layer. The RNA transcripts of neurotrophic factors showed similar levels of NGF, BDNF, GDNF, and NT3 expression in both deep and superficial ASCs. The superficial fat layer produced the largest number of cells, and they proliferated much faster than ASCs from the deep layer.

Another study has shown that there are significant differences in the concentration of cells from different parts of the body and that the lower abdomen is the best source of stem cells [52]. In contrast, another study showed no difference in the number of isolated viable cells from the abdomen, hip, or breast region but showed that cells removed after liposuction proliferated less than those obtained by fat tissue resection [53].

A study in rats [54] investigated the neurotrophic potential of fat tissue stem cells and found a protocol to differentiate fat tissue stem cells into Schwann cell-like cell types (DASC). These cells promote neurite growth in vitro [54].

25.8.3.2 Artificial Nerve Conduits and Cell Therapy

To improve a nerve conduit, several studies have combined conduits or strips with adipose stem cells or Schwann cells to promote peripheral nerve regeneration.

Several studies have shown an improvement in the early regeneration rate for conduits with undifferentiated and Schwann cell-like ASCs [55, 56]. A long-term study showed the survival of undifferentiated human adipose tissue progenitor cells in a polycaprolactone conduit up to 12 weeks after transplantation [57]. The addition of the cells to the conduit did not result in significantly improved long-term functional benefits [57].

A short-term study [47] has shown the advantage of using a PHB strip with Schwann cells as an open system compared to "closed" PHB conduits. This open system enables communication between the regenerating nerve fibers and the external neurotrophic and vascularization factors, which is an optimal medium for nerve regeneration.

A recent long-term study of 3 months [58] used a PHB strip with Schwann cells or adipose stem cells and found good nerve regeneration and low muscle atrophy.

The combination of well-biocompatible conduits or strips with adipose stem cells is a promising tool for the therapy of nerve lesions.

25.8.3.3 ASC for the Prevention of Muscular Atrophy

Various studies have also focused on cell therapy for the affected denervated muscle. A study has investigated the benefits of injecting satellite or myoblast cells into the injured muscle. In a rabbit model, it was shown that cell therapy can improve the properties of denervated muscles if they could be reinnervated [59]. Another study showed the positive effect of transplantation of embryonic stem cell-derived motor neurons on the prevention of muscle atrophy after a nerve lesion [13].

The neuromuscular junction consists of the presynaptic axon terminal, which is covered by terminal Schwann cells, and the postsynaptic structures such as the motor end plate and AChR, which are located on the muscle fibers [25, 26]. Studies have shown that after axotomy denervation has more severe effects on presynaptic nerve endings than on postsynaptic AChR and muscle fibers, leading to rapid regression of presynaptic nerve endings compared to relatively slow degeneration of postsynaptic AChR and muscle atrophy [25, 26].

In a recent study [60], adipose stem cells and Schwann cells were injected intramuscularly after nerve lesion, and the positive effects of these cells on the modulation of the myogenic response were shown. In this study, in one group, the nerve was repaired before intramuscular injection, and in the other group, the nerve was covered with a cap to assess only the effect of the cells on muscle maintenance. In both groups, the cells showed better nerve regeneration and less muscle atrophy compared to a control group (without cells).

The supplementation of neuromuscular junctions with exogenous Schwann cells or neurotrophic fat stem cells was used as a "babysitter" system to maintain the integrity of the motor unit. These cells could both influence the preservation of muscle fibers and increase their reinnervation after nerve repair. The exact mechanisms of action of these neurotrophic cells are not yet known, but they could potentially activate satellite cells, release angiogenic and neurotrophic factors that could attract regenerating nerve fibers, and thus support nerve regeneration and the prevention of muscular atrophy.

25.9 Outlook

Peripheral nerve lesion and the resulting muscular atrophy remain a challenge for research. Despite all investigations to replace nerve transplants, these still remain the gold standard for the therapy of nerve damage. Several studies have shown the benefits of adipose tissue stem cells, which have a neurotrophic potential. The fat tissue stem cells showed a positive effect in the treatment of nerve damage and in the prevention of muscular atrophy. The key to future clinical therapies would be to combine the treatment of nerve and corresponding denervated muscles to maximize the chances of functional recovery after nerve lesion. Fat tissue stem cells are promising and represent the future therapies in biotechnology.

References

1. Wiberg M, Terenghi G. Will it be possible to produce peripheral nerves? Surg Technol Int. 2003;11:303–10.
2. Bahm J, Noaman H, Becker M. The dorsal approach to the suprascapular nerve in neuromuscular reanimation for obstetric brachial plexus lesions. Plast Reconstr Surg. 2005;115:240–4.
3. Schaakxs D, Bahm J, Sellhaus B, Weis J. Clinical and neuropathological study about the neurotization of the suprascapular nerve in obstetric brachial plexus lesions. J Brachial Plexus Peripher Nerve Inj. 2009;4(15):1–11.
4. Batt J, Bain J, Goncalves J, Michalski B, Plant P, Fahnestock M, Woodgett J. Differential gene expression profiling of short and long term denervated muscle. FASEB J Express. 2005;20(1):115–7.
5. Bain JR, Veltri KL, Chamberlan D, Fahnestock M. Improved functional recovery of denervated skeletal muscle after temporary sensory nerve innervation. Neuroscience. 2001;103:503–10.
6. Borisov AB, Dedkov EI, Carlson BM. Interrelations of myogenic response, progressive atrophy of muscle fibers, and cell death in denervated skeletal muscle. Anat Rec. 2001;264:203–18.
7. Finkelstein DI, Dooley PC, Luff AR. Recovery of muscle after different periods of denervation and treatments. Muscle Nerve. 1993;16:769–77.
8. Fu SY, Gorton T. Contributing factors to poor functional recovery after delayed nerve repair: prolonged denervation. J Neurosci. 1995a;15:3886–95.
9. Fu SY, Gorton T. Contributing factors to poor functional recovery after delayed nerve repair: prolonged axotomy. J Neurosci. 1995b;15:3876–85.
10. Irintchev A, Draguhn A, Wernig A. Reinnervation and recovery of mouse soleus muscle after long-term denervation. Neuroscience. 1990;39:231–43.
11. Karpati G, Engel WK. Correlative histochemical study of skeletal muscle after suprasegmental denervation, peripheral nerve section, and skeletal fixation. Neurology. 1968;122(1):145–55.
12. Kobayashi JMS, Watanabe O, Ball DJ, Gu XM, Hunter DA, Kuzon WM. The effect of duration of muscle denervation on functional recovery in the rat model. Muscle Nerve. 1997;20:858–66.
13. Kubo T, Randolph MA, Gröger A, Winograd JM. Embryonic stem cell-derived motor neurons form neuromuscular junctions in vitro and enhance motor functional recovery in vivo. Plast Reconstr Surg. 2009;123:139S–8S.
14. Kalbermatten DF, Schaakxs D, Kingham PJ, Wiberg M. Neurotrophic activity of human adipose stem cells isolated from deep and superficial layers of abdominal fat. Cell Tissue Res. 2011;344:251–60.
15. Radtke C, Vogt PM. Nervenverletzungen und posttraumatische Versorgung. Unfallchirurg. 2014;117:539–56.
16. Burnett MG, Zager EL. Pathophysiology of peripheral nerve injury: a brief review. Neurosurg Focus. 2004;16:1–7.
17. Hall S. Axonal regeneration through acellular muscle grafts. J Anat. 1997;190:57–71.
18. Ide C. Peripheral nerve regeneration. Neurosci Res. 1996;25:101–21.
19. Schlaepfer WW, Bunge RP. Effects of calcium ion concentration on the degeneration of amputated axons in the tissue culture. J Cell Bio. 1973;59:456–70.
20. Kingham PJ, Terenghi G. Bioengineered nerve regeneration and muscle reinnervation. J Anat. 2006;209:511–26.
21. Seddon HJ, Medawar PB, Smith H. Rate of regeneration of peripheral nerves in man. J Physiol. 1943;102(2):191–215.
22. Sunderland S. A classification of peripheral nerve injuries producing loss of function. Brain Res. 1951;74:491–516.
23. Lundborg G. A 25-year perspective of peripheral nerve surgery: evolving neuroscientific concepts and clinical significance. J Hand Surg [Am]. 2000;25:391–414.
24. Schiaffino S, Reggiani C. Myosin isoforms in mammalian skeletal muscle. J Appl Physiol. 1985;77(2):493–501.
25. Kumai Y, Ito T, Matsukawa A, Yumoto E. Effects of denervation on neuromuscular junctions in the thyroarytenoid muscle. Laryngoscope. 2005;115:1869–72.
26. Lampa SJ, Potluri S, Norton AS, Laskowski MB. A morphological technique for exploring neuromuscular topography expressed in the mouse gluteus maximus muscle. J Neurosci Meth. 2004;138:51–6.
27. Monti RJ, Edgerton RR. Role of motor unit structure in defining function. Muscle Nerve. 2001;24:848–66.
28. Mauro A. Satellite cell of skeletal muscle fibers. J Biophys Biochem Cytol. 1961;9:493–5.
29. Siu PM, Alway SE. Mitochondria-associated apoptotic signalling in denervated rat skeletal muscle. J Physiol. 2005;565(1):309–23.
30. Siu PM, Always SE. Response and adaptation of skeletal muscle to denervation stress: the role of apoptosis in muscle loss. Front Biosci. 2009;14:432–52.
31. de Castro Rodrigues A, Andreo JC, Rosa GM Jr, dos Santos NB, Rapucci Moraes LH, Lauris JRP. Fat cell invasion in long-term denervated skeletal muscle. Microsurgery. 2007;27:664–7.
32. Millesi H. Factors affecting the outcome of peripheral nerve surgery. Microsurgery. 2006;26:295–302.
33. Rodriguez FJ, Verdu JE, Ceballos D, Navarro X. Nerve guides seeded with autologous Schwann cells improve nerve regeneration. Exp Neurol. 2000;161:571–84.

34. Battiston B, Geuna S, et al. Nerve repair by means of tubulization: literature review and personal clinical experience comparing biological and synthetic conduits for sensory nerve repair. Microsurgery. 2005;25(4):258–67.
35. Keskin M, Akbas H, et al. Enhancement of nerve regeneration and orientation across a gap with a nerve graft within a vein conduit graft: a functional stereological, and electrophysiological study. Plast Reconstr Surg. 2004;113(5):1372–9.
36. Evans PJ, Midha R, et al. The peripheral nerve allograft: a comprehensive review of regeneration and neuroimmunology. Prog Neurobiol. 1994;43(3):187–233.
37. Konofaos P, Ver Halen JP. Nerve repair by means of tubulization: past, present, future. J Reconstr Microsurg. 2013;29:149–64.
38. Konofaos P, Ver Halen JP. A comparison of nerve regeneration across a sural nerve graft and a vascularized pseudosheath. J Hand Surg. 1988;13:935–2.
39. Merle M, Dellon AL, et al. Complications from silicon-polymer intubulation of nerves. Microsurgery. 1989;10(2):130–3.
40. Mohanna PN, Terrenghi G, et al. Composite PHB-GGF conduit for long nerve gap repair: a long term evaluation. Scand J Plast Reconstr Surg Hand Surg. 2005;39(3):129–37.
41. Hazari A, Johansson-Ruden G, Junemo-Bostrom K, Ljungberg C, Terenghi G, Green C, Wiberg M. A new resorbable wrap-around implant as an alternative nerve repair technique. J Hand Surg. 1999a;24B:291–5.
42. Hazari A, Wiberg M, Johansson-Ruden G, Green C, Terenghi G. A resorbable nerve conduit as an alternative to nerve autograft in nerve gap repair. Br J Plast Surg. 1999b;52:653–7.
43. Young RC, Wiberg M, Terenghi G. Poly-3-hydroxybutyrate (PHB): a resorbable conduit for long-gap repair in peripheral nerves. Br J Plast Surg. 2002;55:235–40.
44. Albala DM, Lawson JH. Recent clinical and investigational applications of fibrin sealant in selected surgical specialties. J Am Coll Surg. 2006;202(4):685–97.
45. Fang H, Peng S, et al. Biocompatibility studies on fibrin glue cultured with bone marrow mesenchymal stem cells in vitro. J Huazhong Univ Sci Technolog Med Sci. 2004;24:272–4.
46. di Summa PG, Kalbermatten D, Pralong E, Raffoul W, Kingham PJ, Terenghi G. Long-term in vivo regeneration of peripheral nerves through bioengineered nerve grafts. Neuroscience. 2011;181:278–91.
47. Kalbermatten DF, Pettersson J, Kingham PJ, Pierer G, Wiberg M, Terenghi G. New fibrin conduit for peripheral nerve repair. J Reconstr Microsurg. 2008;25(1):27–33.
48. Zuk PA, Zhu M, Mizuno H, Huang J, Futrell JW, Katz AJ, Benhaim P, Lorenz HP, Hedrick MH. Multilineage cells from human adipose tissue: implications for cell-based therapies. Tissue Eng. 2001;7:211–28.
49. Kuhbier JW, Reimers K, Radtke C, Vogt PM. Regenerative Therapieansätze in der plastischen Chirurgie. Chirurg. 2015;86:214–22.
50. Strem BM, Hicok KC, et al. Multipotential differentiation of adipose tissue-derived stem cells. Keio J Med. 2005;54(3):132–41.
51. Kuhbier JW, Weyand B, Sorg H, Radtke C, Vogt PM, Reimers K. Stammzellen aus dem Fettgewebe: Eine neue Ressource für die regenerative Medizin? Chirurg. 2010;81:826–32.
52. Padoin AV, Braga-Silva J, Martins P, Rezende K, da Rosa Rezende AR, Grechi B, Gehlen D, Machado DC. Sources of processed lipoaspirate cells: influence of donor site on cell concentration. Plast Reconstr Surg. 2008;122(2):614–8.
53. Oedayrajsingh-Varma MJ, van Ham SM, et al. Adipose tissue derived mesenchymal stem cell yield and growth characteristics are affected by the tissue-harvesting procedure. Cytotherapy. 2006;8:166–77.
54. Kingham PJ, Kalbermatten DF, Mahay D, Armstrong SJ, Wiberg M, Terenghi GPJ. Adipose derived-stem cells differentiate into a Schwann cell phenotype and promote neurite outgrowth in vitro. Exp Neurol. 2007;207:267–74.
55. di Summa PG, Kingham PJ, Raffoul W, Wiberg M, Terenghi G, Kalbermatten DF. Adipose-derived stem cells enhance peripheral nerve regeneration. J Plast Reconstr Aesthet Surg. 2010;63:1544–52.
56. Erba P, Mantovani C, Kalbermatten DF, Pierer G, Terenghi G, Kingham PJ. Regeneration potential and survival of transplanted undifferentiated adipose tissue-derived stem cells in peripheral nerve conduits. J Plast Reconstr Aesthet Surg. 2010;63:e811–7.
57. Santiago LY, Clavijo-Alvarez J, Brayfield C, Rubin JP, Marra KG. Delivery of adipose-derived precursor cells for peripheral nerve repair. Cell Transplant. 2009;18:145–58.
58. Schaakxs D, Kalbermatten D, Pralong E, Raffoul W, Wiberg M, Kingham PJ. Poly-3-hydroxybutyrate strips seeded with regenerative cells are effective promoters of peripheral nerve repair. J Tissue Eng Regen Med. 2017;11(3):812–21.
59. Lazerges C, Daussin PA, Coulet B, El Andalousi RB, Micallef JP, Chammas M, et al. Transplantation of primary satellite cells improves properties of reinnervated skeletal muscles. Muscle Nerve. 2004;29:218–26.
60. Schaakxs D, Kalbermatten D, Raffoul W, Wiberg M, Kingham PJ. Regenerative cell injection in denervated muscle reduces atrophy and enhances recovery following nerve repair. Muscle Nerve. 2013;47:691–70.

Part VII

The Non-medical Concern

Jörg Bahm

26.1 Thomas

Hello, my name is Thomas. I am 29 years old and have a right Erb's palsy since birth. I am very grateful to my parents, because they did a lot of gymnastics with me, from an early age on; otherwise things would certainly look worse today. I would like to share my experiences and problems but also encourage those affected. My whole right arm is much thinner, I can't stretch the arm, and in my elbow the arm is angled at about 90°, I can't turn it, and I can't lift it far. This gives me some limitations in everyday life.

I can *drive*, but I prefer an automatic gearbox, because shifting into fifth gear is awkward. Also my sitting posture is not optimal, because due to my size (approx. 2 m). I would have to sit further back, but the seat is closer and closer to the steering wheel in order for me to be able to approach with my right arm. *Bicycling*—I can do it too, but I had to have a custom-made handlebar made in the meantime, because I had problems reaching the handlebars with my right hand. *Swimming*—I can do it, albeit a lot slower than someone without restriction. In the elementary school, I achieved the swimming badge silver at that time. I'm generally quite athletic. At the Federal Youth Games, I always had a winner's certificate. I only hated floor and apparatus gymnastics because of my handicap. I have always been one of the best at dodgeball and Brennball. Unfortunately I could never play volleyball, because I could not dig because of the missing rotation in my arm, and because of the stretch deficit, I could not splash. Then standing at the side and watching was stupid. But I was all the better at one-handed sports like badminton. Dressing, washing hair, and styling hair work so far without problems. Since I don't know any other way, I've come to terms with it well.

Apart from the constant physiotherapy, I had a normal childhood. On old photos, you can see the bad posture of the arm, but as a child, you didn't think about it as opposed to today. Only with puberty did it become more difficult when I realized that I had a disability. You want to belong and not be different. I never had any problems with teasing at school, but I do remember that someone had written "has a broken arm" about me in the Abibuch keyword list. I didn't want to read that there then and had it deleted; today I wouldn't care. As a teenager, I always tried to hide my handicap by putting my right hand in my pocket or by throwing my backpack over my right shoulder and holding it with my right hand on the way to school. So the disability didn't attract much attention. I had gotten used to this and kept it at university. Looking back, I know today that it was a mistake: I was dreading the

J. Bahm (✉)
Plastic, Hand and Burn Surgery, Section for Plexus Surgery, University Hospital, Aachen, Germany
e-mail: jorg.bahm@belgacom.net,
jbahm@ukaachen.de

© Springer Nature Switzerland AG 2021
J. Bahm (ed.), *Movement Disorders of the Upper Extremities in Children*,
https://doi.org/10.1007/978-3-030-53622-0_26

summer in a short T-shirt, because my disability was clearly visible after all. I simply didn't have enough self-confidence at that time (everyone deals with a disability differently and copes with it better or worse), so that I didn't have any success with women for a long time either. I can only recommend you to stand by it as you are, because as you are, you are unique!

Finding a job was a big problem after university: Despite professional experience through my training, top grades in my studies, a semester abroad, and further practical experience through an internship, it was very difficult to find a job that matched my qualifications. I have written over 200 applications but have hardly ever been invited for an interview. It couldn't be because of the professional qualifications or because of me, because the rejection always came without getting to know me better in a conversation. I therefore believe that the invitation did not take place due to the fact that I indicated my severely handicapped status. I have often heard in discussions that companies would have to pay a compensatory levy if they did not meet the statutory quota of severely disabled workers. In my opinion, however, many companies prefer to pay this levy rather than hire a severely disabled person, who is associated with many unknown variables for the company. Even the public service, which is actually required to invite severely disabled people with the same qualifications to an interview, has hardly ever fulfilled this obligation. You could say you don't have to declare the severely handicapped status. But I tell myself that if I should stand by it in life, why should I hide the severe disability at the interview; it is part of me. You can also only invoke this if your employer is aware of the severely disabled status (5 days more vacation, extended protection against dismissal, etc.). What is also worth mentioning with regard to the profession is that it is virtually impossible to get occupational disability insurance. I use a left-handed keyboard with the number pad on the left and a vertical mouse because I had problems with the tendon sheaths because of the one-sided strain on the left arm.

Even today I have some challenges: Whether it is buying clothes, where it is almost impossible to find tops that fit well due to the different arm lengths. While writing on the PC, I get cramps in the right hand relatively fast. I would love to attend dance classes, but dancing figures are difficult if you can't stretch and lift your arm.

But I am very proud of what I have achieved nevertheless: I graduated from high school, completed a bank apprenticeship, and studied and spent a semester abroad in South America. I have just successfully completed a trainee program at a large bank. In addition to my work, I have been volunteering for more than 1 year for a project of the Integrative Drogenhilfe e. V. (Integrative Drug Aid) at which one meets once a week with a drug addict for 1 year to show him a life outside the scene. I've seen a lot of the world, too: As a backpacker, I travelled around Thailand and Cambodia for a month and made a short trip to New York. Last year I spent my holidays in Colombia, Cuba, and Panama. The highlight last summer was definitely having crossed the Alps on foot.

There are also curious things that I would probably never have experienced without the severe disability and about which I can smile afterward: My orthopedist once sent me for a cure (due to the plexus paresis, I also have a scoliosis and also due to my height back problems and at that time just a herniated disc). Since I was unemployed after my studies, I did not go to an ordinary health resort but to one where only pensioners were accommodated (this had to do with the cost-bearer). On the first morning in the breakfast room with 200–300 pensioners, my jaw fell down when I felt like I was in an old people's home! Well, at least I know what it will feel like to play bingo later in life.

Often I thought, why me? Why must I have a disability? But there are much stronger restrictions in life; someone who is sitting in a wheelchair, for example, can do much less than I can. Since a meeting of the association Plexuskinder (registered association), I also know that quite a lot of children are affected by such a plexus paresis. On the one hand, it is good to know that you are not alone with it, and on the other hand, it is sad that nowadays so many children are still born with a plexus paresis. What the future holds? I don't know, I don't know, I don't know, I don't know. But I say to myself: It goes on and on. You have to believe in yourself. You can create so much, and life has so much beauty to offer!

26.2   Ronja

Hello, I am Ronja, 18 years old, and this year I am graduating from high school. In my spare time, I like to play handball and meet up with friends. You might think playing handball with a plexus paresis is difficult or even impossible.

My plexus paresis was caused by birth, so I don't know any other way. It's part of my life and part of me. In my life so far, I have always found a way for myself and have rarely reached my limits. Of course I have already experienced them and had to learn how to deal with them. But my family and friends always helped me.

My parents were always there for me and always supported me. So in my childhood, they went with me to physiotherapy/occupational therapy and regularly to the doctor. Especially during puberty, they had to motivate me. I still do regular physiotherapy for 18 years now. It is important for me to go there regularly because I often have back pain and the special exercises in my arm make me feel good.

In *everyday life,* I have virtually no problems with my disability and have never had the experience of being bullied. Many daily routines I do differently than my two siblings, but I have found my way to master my day without any problems. So I have a special technique to open bottles or to catch the ball when playing handball.

At *handball* I rarely notice a difference to my teammates. Even my coaches don't make a difference between me and others. That's important to me too, because I don't want special treatment. There are also some movement preparation exercises that I can't do correctly, but my coaches always think of a substitute for me.

I get a lot of support from my teachers and trainers, and I am happy when I notice that they are worried about my disability and are thinking about ways to replace me. For many, a disabled student is also a new situation. I am open to them

and try to answer their questions. Under no circumstances should misunderstandings arise.

Last year, I made my own *driving license* with only very minor limitations. For example, I can only drive automatic cars because I don't have enough power in my left arm to hold the steering wheel when I shift gears. It may sound like a disadvantage, but I think that in a few years' time, most cars will have an automatic transmission anyway and there will be fewer manual cars, so an automatic driving license won't be a restriction. I also need a button on the steering wheel, which is in no way a limitation, as my sister has also got used to riding with it, as it is more comfortable on long distances.

In my environment, everyone is informed about my disability and can always approach me with open questions. But many people didn't notice my disability, because you don't see it directly if you don't know that I have it. I can be open-minded about that disability and talk about it, but it is not the first thing I tell when I meet new people. But I believe that this is normal, and I also want to be defined personally not only through that.

26.3   Katja

My name is Katja. I am 35 years old and have a complete plexus paresis on the right side (shoulder to hand) since birth.

From stories and pictures, I know that after my birth, my arm was first immobilized. When I was a baby and toddler, I got gymnastics, which my parents told me was very tedious.

In the first class, I had my first difficulties with other people. I can consciously remember that the class teacher did not get involved in supporting me in manual work. It was difficult for me to think that I could adapt the tasks shown for myself. Today I can do this very well, so that I don't have to buy special books for my hobby and can simply work with my left hand.

Also *sports* was a difficult subject. My parents had some laborious conversations with the teachers and partly also with the school management. So my sports teacher didn't want to let me join the swimmers, although I had completed a swimming course and I was just before the seahorse certificate. I got a bad grade because I couldn't play volleyball because I couldn't lift my arm.

At the age of 10, an orthopedist was recommended to me. There I was confronted with the topic of surgery for the first time. Also, the paralysis in my right arm got the name Erb's palsy. My parents and I decided against the operation because of concerns that it might get worse.

Treatment with physiotherapy was started. Therefore we were recommended a practice using Bobath and Vojta. I went there weekly until I was 21 years old. The therapist had become like a big sister. My best friend often accompanied me. This was part of it and was then combined with a stroll through the city.

During my *career choice*, there were also difficulties. My decisions, which I had made, were influenced by teachers, parents, and employees of the employment agency. Although I wanted to do an apprenticeship as an educator, I first completed a vocational baccalaureate. Then I completed my training as a curative education nurse. It turned out that I could never pursue this profession until I retired. It was also very difficult to get a job after my apprenticeship, so I subsequently completed a degree in social pedagogy.

I don't need any support at work today. I make my documentation with the one-finger system with support of the right index finger for capitalization.

I can never use the company cars with my employers. Therefore I offer that I make business trips with the private car. I'm driving in *automatic* and I need a power steering. As far as the car is concerned, it is always an adventure when it comes to registration and acceptance of the steering aid. You never know which information is right and which is wrong. In addition, additional costs are always incurred.

I have always tried everything to get along in my environment, which was not always easy, but since 2 years I am in the Plexuskinder association, and it feels very good to exchange with other affected people.

At Home and at School

27

M. Mahler

27.1 Parents Need Support and Guidance: Children Need Strong Parents

27.1.1 Congratulations on the Birth of Your Child?

The baby is finally here. Family and friends, acquaintances, and neighbors congratulate the young parents and pester them with questions: "Boy or girl? How big? Mother and child are well? Everything OK?"

The parents have trouble forming the reply which does not come as easily or joyfully as expected: "A boy, 51 cm 3,800 g, but…," they pause, because everything is not OK. What's the decorum? What do you say when "everything isn't fine"? "There were complications." "Our baby is mostly healthy, but there's this thing with his arm."

The expectant smile of the counterpart turns into a puzzled facial expression. He didn't expect this kind of answer. His stammered "Oh, but it will all be fine" feels like a slap in the face for the new parents. They don't know if it will all be fine, and they don't know exactly why this injury happened, how it can be treated, and how it will affect their child's life as well as their own.

27.1.2 "Your Child Has…"

The illness or disability of a child is always difficult for parents, regardless of whether they already know during pregnancy, whether there were complications at birth, or whether an accident or illness is the cause.

The manner in which parents are informed about their child's health is of enormous importance to them. Even if a doctor invests a lot of time and explains with empathy, factually and clearly using simple words of what exactly has happened and what the next steps are, it is difficult.

Due to the lack of specialist knowledge or communication skills, uncertainty, fear of consequences under labor or liability law, lack of empathy, or even for their own consternation, parents experience interlocutors who brutally confront them with the situation ("Your son will neither be a pilot nor a pianist, but there are other professions out there.") or downplay the situation ("You will soon see a physical therapist who will explain everything to you, there are worse things.").

In the first few days after birth, parents interact with many people. Some support and understand them, but others often act in a careless and hurtful manner. Parents of a child with a disability would also like to be congratulated on the birth. One mother reports that she never received the hospital's "Welcome to the World" package with bibs, diapers, and samples. "A breastfeeding

M. Mahler (✉)
Plexuskinder e.V., Ulm, Germany
e-mail: info@plexuskinder.de

© Springer Nature Switzerland AG 2021
J. Bahm (ed.), *Movement Disorders of the Upper Extremities in Children*,
https://doi.org/10.1007/978-3-030-53622-0_27

consultant and a translator rushed straight to the mother, who still had problems breastfeeding after her fifth child and nobody came to me," she says, still agitated years later by the memory of the first days in her child's life.

Parents often report how traumatic these conversations and encounters were for them and how negatively they influenced their trust in conventional medicine.

27.2 Information and Education: What Parents Want and What Parents Need

First of all, parents want to turn back time, undo "it." They want the nightmare "our child is not healthy" to end. Now this nightmare has become a reality. The parents are shocked, angry, desperate, and completely overwhelmed by the situation.

"The birth was terrible, panic broke out in the delivery room and my husband was thrown out of the room. Then the child was there, but something was wrong. No one said what was going on," reports a mother after complications during delivery.

27.2.1 Who Informs and Educates the Parents?

Parents must be informed immediately and comprehensively about the diagnosis and its causes and consequences. Parents don't want a doctor rattling down a prepared text, they want (some more, some less) to be taken by the hand and to be carefully confronted with this new and unknown situation, and above all they want to know how things are going to proceed in concrete clear terms and how and where they can get more information.

They want answers to their questions and expect them from the obstetrician, midwife, and pediatrician. In the case of a birth injury, in most cases, the delivering doctor or midwife will no longer look after the family and will never know what happened to the "emergency in the delivery room."

In many cases, professionals do not feel "responsible" for the time-consuming and demanding task of educating and accompanying the family. Some don't want to or are not allowed to be responsible. They do not have enough information, background knowledge, training, and experience and have no time, no authority, or no desire or simply fear to inform and educate the parents. "I understand the parents," says a pediatrician, "but there is so much time spent on research and counseling with no possibility of billing this time and my waiting room is full."

It is often the physical therapists who see the child and the families regularly over the years, who explain to the parents in simple words what is going on and who often take (mostly unpaid) time for conversations.

27.2.2 Empathy

For the doctor, it may be a moderate impairment, but for the parents, it is a catastrophe, because suddenly nothing is as it was supposed to be. A succinct "the physical therapist explains everything else to you" is just as wrong as a "you can have a good life with such a disability."

27.2.3 Admit: I Am Not Familiar with This Injury

Obstetricians, pediatricians, and therapists are rarely experts in the extremely versatile field of upper extremity impairments. In the case of a rare disease or disability, it is essential that a physician openly admits that he does not have the necessary expertise to adequately educate and comprehensively advise the family. The reference to corresponding experts, specialist literature, and support groups offers should therefore be made promptly and unconditionally.

27.2.4 Always to the Specialist

In all cases, it is essential to consult a specialist in the field. Again and again, families report that they rely on their inexperienced doctor in this field ("wait and see, your child will outgrow this") and have lost valuable time as a result. Many treatments and therapies only have a limited time window.

27.2.5 Support the Parents' Research

The young father rushes home from the obstetrical clinic and researches the technical terms that previously buzzed through the room. Lonely in front of the computer, he reads about prognosis, therapies, operations, aids, legal consequences, degrees of disability, and other things that are difficult to understand and digest.

Parents need to become experts in the disease and treatment of their child and should receive as much help as possible. They should be supported in their search for diagnosis, treatment, therapies, and support services and, if possible, accompanied. For this purpose, a list of medical terms used in diagnosis (in the relevant language) or a reference to literature that is understandable for laypersons (e.g., Wikipedia, a medical textbook for students) can be very helpful.

The publications or website of a support group (e.g. Plexuskinder e.V., Section 27.6) can be a very good source of information for parents. This source should provide medical layperson with understandable, objective, neutral, and as complete information as possible. Many support groups have their own section "For newcomers" which summarizes the most important information.

In addition to the specialist information, the exchange with other affected persons is a great help.

27.2.6 Understanding the Exceptional Circumstances

Even if comprehensive information takes place, parents in this situation are not able to understand and process the information. Besides the complicated medical facts, the difficult to understand language, and the possibly still unclear diagnosis, the thought "my child is disabled" floats over the parents. The parents should be shown understanding.

Instead of asking "Do you have questions?", it is often better for the parents if they are visited or called a few days after the first discussion, if tangible help is given in the form of a brochure or a reference book and if they are introduced to other affected families or experienced therapists.

27.3 The Question of Guilt

Why is this happening to our child? Why is this happening to us? Who is to blame? What have we done wrong? What have the doctor, the midwife, and the hospital done wrong? How could this have been avoided?

Some of these questions are on the mind of and torment the affected families for years and are also burdensome for the medical staff.

First, the diagnosis and treatment of the child has top priority. The processing of the causes of the impairment, whether by force majeure or unfortunate human errors, must also take place. The exchange with other affected families can be of great help to the parents.

27.4 Coping

Parents should get professional support to cope with the situation.

The sometimes highly dramatic and traumatic birth, the feelings of guilt, reproaches, anger, dismay, disappointment, and powerlessness of the affected family should be discussed and dealt with immediately by a suitable specialist, a "professional" (midwife, doctors, psychologists, therapist, counselor).

The birth of a child with a disability can be very stressful for the couple and for the whole family.

27.5 The Role of Support Groups

For many impairments and chronic and rare diseases, there are support groups that operate regionally or even nationwide and internationally.

Not only the exchange of information and experience and tips from everyday life is an important component of self-help but also mutual emotional support. "We are not alone, there are others like us, and they are there for us."

In support groups, affected families find other families who have already gained a lot of experience with the impairment, who are experts in this special field and who like to take "new" parents by the hand, advise, and support them.

In conversation with affected parents with older or already adult children, affected parents experience hope and confidence. Life goes on.

The exchange also helps the affected families to shift their focus from the affected arm to the child attached to the arm.

In the coming months and years, the family will encounter people again and again who will want to know what happened. Parents are very burdened by this duty to inform and educate the public. They relive the stressful experiences with each narration. The reference to a publication, brochure, or website of a support group that explains the details in laymen's terms can be very helpful.

27.6 Guidance for Parental Contacts and Educational Conversations

A guide can help healthcare professionals prepare and conduct interviews and deal with affected parents. The guide should also be used by caregivers.

Possible components are:

- Who's talking to the parents?
- Choice of words
- When and where does the conversation take place?
- Is the conversation recorded in writing?
- Who participates?

- What is communicated?
- Which documents can support and supplement the clarification? (see Sect. 27.7)
- References to further information, support group offers?
- Offers for follow-up talks?

27.7 Annex: Plexuskinder e.V.

27.7.1 Publication

Plexuskinder e.V. has published a booklet the *Plexusfibel* in which the clinical picture, its causes, and treatment options are described from the point of view of all those involved: *Der geburtstraumatische Plexus brachialis Schaden* — Information für Betroffene, interessierte Laien und Fachleute; Dr. Jörg Bahm, Dr. Roland Uphoff, Mirjam Mahler [Hrsg.]

27.7.2 Herbie Children's Book Series

In a three-part children's book series, Herbie, a child with a brachial plexus injury, talks about his arm, his operation, and his exercises. With the help of Herbie, affected children and their siblings, family, and friends can understand what a brachial plexus injury is and what children who have a brachial plexus injury do differently.

- *Herbie and His Special Arm*
- *Herbie Has an Operation*
- *Herbie and His Exercises*

The books are available in German through https://www.plexuskinder.de *and in English through* https://www.erbspalsygroup.co.uk. *They were written and published by The Erb's Palsy Group and translated and adapted for the German group by Mirjam Mahler.*

A fourth book A Child Like Herbie written by Mirjam Mahler and directed at the parents is also available in German.

Herbie is a positive identification figure. Happy and self-confident, he tells of his life with a brachial plexus injury. With the help of the books, affected children and siblings can be informed about the brachial plexus injury and its consequences in a child-friendly and clear way. In the surrounding of the affected children, in the kindergarten and in the school, during activities, or in the sports with the help of the Herbie books, small and big people can understand better how life is different for a child with this injury.

On the website of the German support group https://www.plexuskinder.de, there are not only medical topics but also advice and ideas which can help to achieve a good quality of life.

A short video about the brachi al plexus injury designed for children and adults is also available on https://www.plexuskinder.de

Reference of the Plexusfibel and the Herbie books:
- Plexuskinder e. V.
- Georgstrasse 3
- 89077 Ulm, Germany
- Phone: (0731) 96427575
- Fax: (0731) 96429626
- https://plexuskinder.de
- info@plexuskinder.de

Jörg Bahm

28.1 Sports

In general swimming is beneficial for the development of muscle strength and riding for a good alignment of the axial posture; but many boys want to play football first, which will certainly improve the general health condition. No sport is forbidden or contraindicated, unless the fun factor is completely lost or severe stress pain occurs again and again.

Sport also means social integration!

How this can appear in everyday life can be read in the personal experience reports in Chap. 26.

Even over long periods of time, sports muscle training in patients with nerve damage does not lead to unlimited muscle buildup and the attainment of normality, the unconscious desire of all parents to reverse the initial damage, but it does help to bring general physical fitness together with weight control into health care.

There is also much dynamism in disabled sports; we are currently running a nationwide swimming campaign with the self-help group "Plexuskinder" (www.plexuskinder.de).

28.2 Occupation

The choice and practice of a profession imply a long-term perspective, which must take into particular account the continuing physical strain on the upper extremity: I do not recommend heavy, repeated, often one-sided and two-sided physical strain as encountered when one works, for example, as a heating installer. In addition, counselling and classification by the national compensation office can also help here (Chap. 29). Considering the disablement degree, controversies often arise regarding an alleged undervaluation, and especially in the case of a slight degree of movement restriction, the question must be asked whether one wants the "stamp" related to disability or wants to enter adulthood without any mark.

Every one-sided affected person will be able to cope in our working world, which is so rich in aids—this is my first message to parents and children at the first consultation. But of course it is a long process of learning, adaptation, and sometimes even renunciation until then.

The choice of profession and the world of careers are another chapter of probation, where all therapists should, of course, be available for advice.

Prudent courage, taking into account the specific limitations, socialization, and a good acceptance of the body image and limitation, coupled with a healthy self-esteem, are important and universal prerequisites for a balanced adult life in the midst of our society.

The term "disability" should be avoided!

J. Bahm (✉)
Plastic, Hand and Burn Surgery, Section for Plexus Surgery, University Hospital, Aachen, Germany
e-mail: jorg.bahm@belgacom.net,
jbahm@ukaachen.de

© Springer Nature Switzerland AG 2021
J. Bahm (ed.), *Movement Disorders of the Upper Extremities in Children*,
https://doi.org/10.1007/978-3-030-53622-0_28

Legal Benefits for the Severely Disabled: The Process for Filing an Eligibility Claim with the Pension and Benefits Office

A. Kaiser

29.1 Introduction

In cases dealing with movement disorders in children of the upper extremities, e.g. where fine and gross motor skills are performed with the arms and hands, more specifically when tasks are required to be performed ambidextrously, movement is restricted or impossible indicating that a disability could be present. In such cases, the affected individuals or their parents are eligible to file claims for the corresponding compensatory benefit payments according to the Severely Disabled Persons Act. Specifically, it is possible to have a degree of disability (DoD) recognised when certain prerequisites are met due to movement restrictions of the upper extremities. In addition, in such cases people are also eligible to apply for a severely disabled identity card, and when applicable disabled individuals can claim certain rights and concessions depending on the degree of disability. These disabilities are then indicated on the disabled identity card with coded letter identifiers, each identifying a specific disability.

Here, a disability does not merely represent the existence of a physical (or mental) condition deviating from the norm, but is always solely based on the effects of an abnormal physical (or mental) functional impairment that is not temporary. A period of more than 6 months is no longer considered temporary.

29.2 Individual and Total DoD

The DoD is determined on the basis of the effects of the impairments in their entirety while taking into account their reciprocal relationships based on degree increments of 10, which are graded from 20 to 100. Individual impairments are taken into account when viewed alone; they would amount to a DoD of at least 10. If several impairments exist simultaneously, for example, arm plexus paralysis together with spinal damage, metabolic diseases or diseases of the respiratory tract, a single DoD must first be determined for each functional impairment. Therefore, the total DoD for several dysfunctions depends on how these affect different areas of an individual's life.

These are referred to as **functional systems**, e.g. the brain including psyche, eyes, ears, respiration, cardiovascular system, digestion, urinary system, skin, blood, metabolism, arms, legs, etc. A total DoD is then calculated from the individual or partial DoDs. Here, the individual DoDs are not added together, but rather the functional impairment that is the most plausible to cause the highest individual DoD. Then with regard to all further functional impairments, it must be exam-

A. Kaiser (✉)
Halle, Germany
e-mail: mail@kaiser-koepke.de,
mail@rechtsanwalt-halle.de

© Springer Nature Switzerland AG 2021
J. Bahm (ed.), *Movement Disorders of the Upper Extremities in Children*,
https://doi.org/10.1007/978-3-030-53622-0_29

ined if they increase the extent of the disability and if so to what extent. Therefore, the DoD calculation as a whole must be based on how much an individual's life and participation in society is restricted; in other words which activities the disabilities lead to impairments and what are the impairments. Minor health disorders that cause a DoD of 10 are not taken into account when calculating the DoD.

29.3 Process

In the following, a description of the process applying for and claiming benefits with the agencies responsible for disability laws will be presented. Depending on the federal state, responsibility for these services lies with the pension and benefits offices, the regional agencies or municipal councils.

The process that a person must go through to have a degree of disability (DoD) determined and to obtain a severely disabled ID card and when applicable any disability concessions coded on the ID card begins, as with all laws pertaining to social security statutes, with the **application**. The application first requests all pertinent personal information on the child in question and the child's current medical history listing the disorders in order to determine the disability. These impairments will have to be indicated, as far as possible with their respective functional losses. Additionally, information must be provided regarding the doctors, therapists and rehabilitation centres where the child was or is still being treated for the disabilities that have caused movement restrictions in the arms and hands.

In such cases, it is advisable to provide detailed information obtained from physicians and therapists involved in the treatment of the child, in accordance with the instructions provided in the application form, because the child's entire medical history documentation will be requested later by the pension and benefits office. However, the initial application does not necessarily have to include the patient's complete medical history documentation.

In cases where a formal decision has already been determined regarding a particular DoD and additional functional impairments or restrictions now have to be added, an application must also be submitted to the appropriate agencies for a decision to be made regarding a change in the status of the DoD. However, a change is only essential if the DoD changes upwards by at least 10 as a result of the disability worsening or if any additional letter code identifiers have to be added to disabled ID card.

Once the agency has compiled all the information and documentation, the office for medical services working on behalf of the pension and benefits office, regional agencies and municipal councils will in almost all cases be advised by a medical consultant to provide an **expert opinion** on the applicant's behalf. The consultant will examine and base his/her expert opinion on the medical documents available and determine whether or not and to what degree a disability can be ascertained.

> The evaluation of each individual case regarding disabilities is based on the medical care ordinance, where an individual DoD is specified for each of the disabilities and diseases according to their severity and extent.

In the case of an amendment request, the responsible agency checks the conditions in a similar way to an initial request using the most current medical documents. However, this review could also lead to a conclusion that the DoD will be reduced, e.g. when contrary to the applicant's assumption, the disability has not worsened but has improved or the previous assessment was incorrect.

Once the medical opinion has been issued, the responsible agency will issue a **notification indicating** a specific DoD, which must be at least 20. At this time, the exact designation of the disability is also listed in the decision.

When a DoD of at least 50 has been established, the individual concerned will be deemed severely **handicapped** and a disabled ID card will be issued.

> Only with a DoD of at least 50 will the ID card have any codes regarding compensation for the disabilities and this information will also be stated in the decision.

In the case of children with movement disorders of the upper extremities, the disability letter code identifiers H and B may be considered in individual cases and under certain conditions.

The **Letter Code Identifier concession H** stands for "helpless". According to (*Versorgungsmedizinischen Grundsätzen*) basic law on medical compensation, an individual is deemed helpless when due to a health disorder he/she needs continual daily external help and, not only on a temporary basis, to perform a series of frequently and regularly recurring tasks in order to secure his/her personal existence during the course of a day. Here, too, a period of more than 6 months is not considered temporary. The tasks that are frequently and regularly performed to secure an individual's existence are in accordance with the decisive criteria for assessing the need for long-term care, namely, dressing and undressing, eating and drinking, personal hygiene (washing, hair care, shaving), performing bodily functions (bowel movements, urinating) and mobility (getting up, going to bed, moving around inside and outside the home). In addition, the time required for mental stimulation and communication, i.e. seeing, hearing, speaking and the ability to interact, is also taken into account.

> According to the jurisprudence of the Federal Social Court, at least three of the aforementioned tasks must take at least 2 hours a day to meet the requirements for the letter code identifier concession **H.**

The **Letter Code Identifier concession B** is obtained when a person is regularly and permanently dependent on outside help when using public transport, for example, when getting on and off public transportation. The disability identifier code **B** concession can only be granted according to the law for severely disabled persons for whom the disability letter code identifier concession **H** has also been determined. This entitles severely handicapped people to take along a companion free of charge on public transport without any limitations on the number of kilometres travelled.

With regard to the assessment of infants and children, a comparison to children of the same age is not used as a standard, but it will be investigated whether or not the health disorders identified in adults would justify granting the disability identifier letter code **B** concession. In other words, the assessment of infants and children is not based on a comparison to children of the same age. In children with movement disorders of the upper extremities, the letter code identifier B concession can only be used for very severe plexus paralysis.

In cases where the decision does not correspond to the claimant's expectations regarding the degree level of the DoD or the identifier code determinant, because the child's disability and its associated effects on the child's daily life can be assessed differently or higher, the claimant has the right to make an **objection**, in writing, to the decision made by the responsible agency within 1 month of receipt of this decision.

The objection letter does not have to include the reasons for objecting to the decision, but it would be advisable to indicate to the pension and benefits office which points made in the decision are considered unlawful. The entire administrative process is then submitted again to the medical service for its opinion. The responsible agency then issues its **ruling on the objection** including the entire objection proceedings and the out-of-court procedure. Either the agency has complied or has not complied with the claimant's objection.

If the objection was rejected, the claimant now has the possibility to file a **Lawsuit in the social court** in order to receive what the claimant considers a rightful benefit. As with the letter of objection, the lawsuit must be filed within 1 month after receiving notification that the objection was rejected.

It is advisable to contact the attending physician or therapist and, if necessary, a lawyer in good time within procedural time limits for making an objection and/or filing a lawsuit in order to discuss the chances of success. In this context, a claimant or his/her parents may at any time at the responsible agency inspect the case files of his/her administrative process.

Once the proceedings have been brought to the social court, an external independent expert medical opinion is once again frequently requested to determine if the requested DoD and/or the disability letter code of concession should be retained or not, in order to determine if the legal action should proceed through the social court. The legal action before the social court usually ends with a judgement. In principle the judgement can be challenged with an appeal, which in turn means each individual case is then carefully reviewed.

Forensic and Legal Issues

Legal Issues and Forensic Problems in Obstetrical Brachial Plexus Paresis

R. Uphoff

OBPP is a different story; this common childbirth complication has often been the subject of litigation and legal opinion in Germany.

No precise statistical surveys have been made on the incidence of OBPP, and the literature on the subject has answered this question in different ways. According to Berle et al., who surveyed the data in the Hessian Perinatal Survey and the Horst Schmidt Clinics in Wiesbaden, Germany, the incidence of shoulder dystocia is 0.82% and of plexus paresis 0.2% of all vaginal births with cephalic presentation. The estimates below are based on those figures.

The total number of births in the Federal Republic of Germany in 2014 was 714,927. This number includes caesarian section and other birth presentations; based on the commonly used statistics, the number of vaginal births with cephalic presentation was approximately 470,000. Using Berle et al.'s figures:

- The annual incidence of obstetric dystocia is 3854.
- The annual incidence of OBPP is 940.

From the forensic point of view, OBPP is a mass phenomenon.

The number of legal disputes resulting from OBPP is not clearly known; here too no statistics are available.

It has been said (although without much further detail) that almost every case of obstetric brachial plexus injury in the United States leads to a lawsuit. Although this is certainly not the case in Germany, the number of lawsuits is likely to be very high here as well.

Parents of injured children often suspect that brachial plexus paresis after shoulder dystocia in the final stages of birth might have been prevented by another medical procedure, such as a prophylactic c-section, in cases where risk factors for shoulder dystocia are known before birth, such as another medical procedure after a known shoulder dystocia. Although courts have repeatedly stated that an occurrence of OBPP alone is not sufficient to show medical malpractice, medical laypersons ask themselves if, when in approximately 75% of all cases of shoulder dystocia brachial plexus paresis can be prevented, it could have been prevented in their specific case.

Plexus paresis can have major effect on the future life of an affected child. Permanent plexus paresis typically leads to a child being a priori excluded from a number of careers, such as craftsperson or doctor. It is almost impossible to learn to play traditional musical instruments. Plexus paresis makes it extremely difficult to participate in sport and drastically diminishes the chance of marrying and starting a family. With

R. Uphoff (✉)
Dr. Roland Uphoff Rechtsanwälte, Bonn, Germany
e-mail: mail@uphoff.de

© Springer Nature Switzerland AG 2021
J. Bahm (ed.), *Movement Disorders of the Upper Extremities in Children*,
https://doi.org/10.1007/978-3-030-53622-0_30

this in mind, it is understandable that a great number of cases of OBPP lead to legal action. From the point of view of legal practice, OBPP is by far one of the most common forensically significant birth complications.

Lawsuits concerning OBPP as well as the pareses themselves are mass phenomena.

30.1 Failure to Inform

For a patient to prove a medical liability case in Germany, either medical malpractice or a failure to inform must be established. Failure to inform plays a very large role in medical liability cases, including cases where medical liability in shoulder dystocia is at stake.

30.2 German Federal Court of Justice Decisions on Failure to Inform

The German Federal Court of Justice (BGH) has stated in a number of decisions that a doctor is fundamentally not required in a normal childbirth situation to discuss the possibility of delivery by caesarian section with the woman who will give birth. Information about alternative treatments is nevertheless required when concrete signs of a high-risk birth become apparent or the child would be subject to serious risks if vaginal birth is carried out or continued and a c-section in that concrete case, the mother's condition and situation being considered, would be a medically responsible alternative (BGH Decision of 13.5.2011, VersR 2011, 1146, 1147). The doctor must in such cases offer to perform a c-section; the final decision must in this case be left to the mother.

This legal decision applies as well and especially in cases where there is an increased risk of obstetric shoulder dystocia that could result in the child suffering a plexus paresis (BGH VersR 1993, 835, 836).

It is not yet settled in medical circles whether caesarian section delivery can be considered a suitable prophylactic procedure against OBPP. The primary argument against prophylactic c-section is that, if c-section were offered as an alternative treatment in case of higher risk of shoulder dystocia to all women, the number of c-sections would increase to an intolerable level. Various attempts have been made to estimate the number of c-section deliveries that would be necessary to eliminate brachial plexus paresis completely, with great variation in the estimates. It has also been claimed that shoulder dystocia in the late stages of labor often occurs in cases where no increased prepartal risk factors were seen.

Case law has as yet not accepted these arguments. The BGH has taken the position that the statistical risk density for a specific woman is not legally significant; in all cases where a treatment alternative is available because of higher risks associated with vaginal delivery, the woman about to give birth must herself be allowed to decide whether to accept or avoid a particular risk. Generally, case law assumes that a significant alternative treatment in the sense intended by the BGH must only be considered after a significant increase in the risk of vaginal delivery has been established. Cut-off values must be set. The setting of these values in specific cases has been left by the BGH to medical science, specifically to the court-appointed experts in any specific case. If a court follows the opinion of the appointed expert, its judgment is as a rule not subject to overturning by the BGH. It thus follows that the reported opinions of lower courts who are charged with deciding on the basis of the facts of a case cannot be entirely uniform.

30.3 Cut-Off Values

Although shoulder dystocia also occurs in infants whose birthrate is clearly within the normal range, it is generally recognized that **fetal macrosomia** is the most significant risk factor for shoulder dystocia. It greatly outweighs all other predisposing factors. The risk of shoulder dystocia rises steeply with birth weight. The risk is 3% with birth weights greater than 4 kg, 11% with birth weights greater than 4.5 kg, and 40% with birthweights greater than 5 kg.

There are a large number of other risk factors besides birth weight. As a rule, courts have generally referred to these collectively as "other risk factors."

The tendency in existing case law, as inferred from a large number of decisions, leans towards recognizing a duty to inform in the absence of other risk factors when birth weight has been estimated by means of sonographic examination to be 4.5 kg or greater, because of the significantly higher general risk of shoulder dystocia in such cases (examination of written opinions in). Case law focuses on the birth weight as estimated from sonographic images using certain formulas, without considering any supplementary risk analysis. This method is problematic to the extent that, as is generally known, sonographic weight estimation is relatively inexact and, particularly as actual weight rises, often too low.

Case law is not consistent in its treatment of other risk factors. A number of risk factors are referred to by some experts as "non-independent," because they are basically additional indications that a macrosomic baby is expected. These include:

- Obesity of the mother
- Higher than normal weight gain during pregnancy
- The prior birth of a macrosomic baby
- Overdue pregnancy

In the opinion of most court-appointed experts, these non-independent factors need not be considered separately.

This is not the case for maternal diabetes, in particular for gestational diabetes. Particularly in the many cases where it has not been detected or treated, it can lead to disproportional growth of the fetus particularly in the body and not head of the baby, which is particularly relevant. For this reason, macrosomic babies of diabetic mothers are particularly at risk, as the relation between the circumference of the head and the width of the shoulders is particularly adverse. The risk of shoulder dystocia is raised in such cases by a factor of 5.

For these reasons, a majority of the experts most often appointed by courts agree that in these cases, a lower cut-off of 4 kg should be set.

The **risk of recurrence** has a special position among the risk factors. If shoulder dystocia has occurred in a prior birth, the risk of recurrence is between 7.3 and 25%. In these cases, the majority opinion tends to be that caesarian section must always be discussed as an alternative treatment, particularly as experience has shown that birth weight tends to increase with repeated pregnancies.

30.4 Legal Consequences of Failure to Inform

In settled case law, the BGH considers vaginal delivery management as not legally justifiable when a caesarian section would be a reasonable alternative treatment about which the patient must be informed, with the result that treating professionals must bear responsibility for all negative effects of the vaginal birth, particularly OBPP. If information is determined to have been necessary, the doctor has the burden of proving that information was in fact given.

In defense, a doctor may argue that the patient, if she had been properly informed about an alternative treatment, would have herself chosen the standard mode of labor. This hypothetical consent argument has been specifically allowed by the BGH (BGH Ruling of 17.04.2007, VersR 2007, 999). If this defense is raised, the Court must take testimony from the mother. She can counter the argument that she would have consented to vaginal labor if she had been properly informed by credibly stating that proper information would have confronted her with a difficult decision. This is nearly always the case, as a mother can generally convincingly testify that she would have chosen the physical risk to herself resulting from a c-section over the risk of damage to her baby if she had been informed that vaginal labor brought with it the risk of OBPP.

It is often the case that a doctor or hospital involved in litigation raises the defense that, even if a c-section had been performed, damage to the brachial plexus could not be completely ruled out. It has been argued that brachial plexus injury to a baby can occur, if rarely, in the case of a c-section, as the removal of the baby from the uterus occasionally requires the use of not-insignificant force that can work on the baby's brachial plexus.

This argument is not relevant. The correct legal position is that if liability is based on a failure to inform, the plaintiff must prove that the damage resulted from the treatment for which no alternatives were discussed, in this, vaginal birth. The mere statement of the possibility that a brachial plexus injury can occur in a c-section is not relevant evidence of the lack of a causal connection between the injury and the vaginal birth.

When a brachial plexus injury that could only have been caused by physical force has been determined to have occurred after a shoulder dystocia in the last stages of labor, this is considered prima facie evidence that the brachial plexus injury is a direct result of the shoulder dystocia.

The mere suggestion that another process *might* have led to a brachial plexus injury of the baby would only mitigate against the causal connection between the actual treatment and the injury when caesarian section always or at least usually resulted in brachial plexus injury to the baby, which is in fact not the case. Arguments of hypothetical causes do not help the doctor who has not properly informed his patient.

However, the argument that there is in a particular case no causal connection between the actual method of delivery and the shoulder dystocia is one that courts have taken seriously. A doctor can argue in a specific case that the brachial plexus had already been damaged intrauterine and thus with no causal connection to the method of delivery. This argument is derived from a number of American studies that have investigated the possibility of intrauterine injuries of this kind. It has become almost standard procedure to raise this argument in litigation; thus court-appointed medical experts must consider the possibility of intrauterine injury.

Even in cases where it is not clearly established that the baby's brachial plexus injury was the result of a shoulder dystocia, this argument does not prevail. We do not here discuss the discussion within the medical field on the possibility of intrauterine brachial plexus injury; this is not a legal question. However, it is clear that a large majority of court-appointed medical experts today do believe that intrauterine injuries of this kind are possible based on the findings of the afore-mentioned American studies. It is fair to say that the current state of discussion in the medical field is not to rule out the possibility of such injury.

Whether in a specific birth case it can be seriously considered that a brachial plexus injury established immediately after birth is of **intrauterine origin**, particularly when shoulder dystocia has occurred in the last stages of labor, is a completely different question. Experience has shown that this is seldom the case.

Cases in which intrauterine injury can be seriously considered can be clearly distinguished from shoulder dystocia cases. According to relevant studies, intrauterine injury only occurs in very specific cases, namely:

- Malformation of the uterus, e.g., in the case of uterus bicornis
- The presence of uterine septum tissue or large myomas that can exert intrauterine pressure on the fetus
- Intrauterine malposition, particularly transverse presentation

In such cases, it is plausible occurring to contemporary medical science that physical forces could come to bear on the brachial plexus intrauterine. However, in births of such babies, which are rarely macrosomic and usually notably under average size, shoulder dystocia does not occur in the last stages of labor. Brachial plexus paresis generally comes as something of a surprise after the birth of such babies.

When the baby is closely examined after birth, particularly in the course of surgical treatment of the brachial plexus paresis, it is possible to determine exactly how the injury to the brachial plexus occurred. If, as is often the case, a pull or tear in the spinal nerves c5 to t1 or if nerve root avulsion has occurred, traction damage, which is not caused by persistent intrauterine pressure, is present.

30.5 Secondary Caesarian Section as an Alternative Treatment

Often, a delivery that begins as vaginal delivery encounters complications, such as stalled labor. It is generally known that macrosomia in babies can increase the risk of stalled labor.

In these cases, the doctor managing the delivery must quickly make a decision.

If the baby's head is still engaged in the birth canal, vacuum extraction (ventouse) is considered in addition to caesarian section. Many labor assistants also use the Kristeller maneuver. All of these delivery methods increase the risk of shoulder dystocia significantly: "Forceps and vacuum extraction, particularly the Kristeller maneuver, present secondary risk factors for a shoulder dystocia".

There are occasions where there are no alternative treatments to these sorts of extraction. If, for example, the baby is suffering from an acute lack of oxygen, which as a rule can be observed on CTG, and the baby's head is in a good position for the use of forceps or suction, instrumented vaginal delivery is to be preferred because it is faster.

The reverse is also true: if the baby's head is not yet in position for the use of forceps or suction, instrumented vaginal delivery is too dangerous; in these cases, c-section is preferable.

Cases in which both c-section and instrumented vaginal delivery can be seriously considered are more difficult. In these cases, there is an alternative treatment of which the mother must be informed.

In this situation, the BGH has ruled that, to the extent that such a situation could be or could have been predicted before labor begins, the mother must be informed and asked how she would decide to proceed.

If the situation was not predictable, the question is raised if a woman can and should be informed of alternative treatments during labor. Many doctors answer this question in the negative. A woman in labor, such doctors argue, is not in a position to engage in conversation with a doctor. In such cases, the obstetrician must make the decision on further procedures alone.

In fact, experience has shown that it is not the case that women in labor cannot communicate with doctors. Considering that the question in such cases is the simple choice between a c-section and instrumented vaginal delivery, it is reasonable to say that such a discussion can take place with a woman in labor, particularly when epidural or spinal anesthesia has been used.

It is also important to note here that, according to current case law, even in this stage of birth the mother must be informed about appropriate alternative treatments; the doctor bears the burden of proof that even a brief and direct exchange on the subject was not possible.

In cases where the obstetric doctor single-handedly, without asking for any opinion or reaction from the mother, has decided for instrumented vaginal delivery, these doctors have been found liable when the use of suction or forceps (and particularly where the Kristeller maneuver has been used) has led to shoulder dystocia resulting in arm plexus paresis.

Doctors have objected to these rulings, calling them a violation of practitioners' therapeutic freedom based on a lack of medical knowledge.

This objection is not justified; practitioners' therapeutic freedom is limited by the bounds of the law. Every medical therapy must respect patients' freedom to decide and human dignity. To the extent that in any particular situation the patient's freedom of choice has been infringed upon when there is an alternative treatment of which the patient must be informed, sanction by the court is not an infringement on medical therapeutic freedom.

30.6 Malpractice

30.6.1 General

When a plaintiff claims that OBPP is the result of medical malpractice, the burden of proof appears at first to be much greater than in the case of a failure to inform.

In cases where liability is based on failure to inform, the plaintiff need argue only the existence of a situation in which information about an alternative treatment was required (and prove this). Where there is no stipulation in such a case that proper information was properly given, the burden of proof is upon the medical defendant.

A plaintiff must prove much more in a case where it is argued that the injuries to the child are a result of medical malpractice. The mere fact that brachial plexus paresis following shoulder dystocia during its birth occurs in a child does not, as case law has repeatedly found, in itself justify the finding of medical malpractice and does not give rise to a presumption of malpractice.

Although in the great majority of cases of shoulder dystocia (according to Beirle, more than 75% of cases) OBPP can be avoided, the medical consensus is that even optimal medical treatment cannot always prevent OBPP.

The patient must not only prove medical malpractice itself but also a causal relationship between this malpractice and the primary injury, i.e., the occurrence of OBPP. According to settled BGH case law, the burden of proof on the question of causality is only reversed if the treating defendant has committed "gross" malpractice as the BGH has defined this concept in its settled case law.

Gross malpractice has occurred when, according to this somewhat inexact definition, a doctor has clearly acted against established rules of medical treatment or settled medical knowledge and thus committed an error that from the objective medical point of view is no longer understandable because such a mistake absolutely must not be made by a doctor (BGH, Judgement of 19.06.2012, NJW 2012, 2653). Such malpractice can be established when from an objective point of view elementary medical treatment standards have been violated or basic medical knowledge is ignored (Greiß/Greiner 2014, p. 211 and references).

This disadvantage to the plaintiff in terms of evidentiary burden is relativized by the fact that, in practice, obstetric standards are largely settled and in essence entirely uncontroversial. Where there is a good deal of controversy in the question of informing on alternative treatments, there is no argument about the correct method of treatment for shoulder dystocia; courts, experts,

and parties are not casting about in the dark when investing such matters. This explains why the large majority of legal rulings in favor of plaintiffs are based upon findings of malpractice. The types of malpractice can be divided into groups.

30.7 Standardized Procedure

If labor suddenly stalls in its final phase, i.e., as the baby's head has partially emerged from the birth canal, this is a prima facie indication that shoulder dystocia has occurred.

In this phase of labor, it is important first to distinguish between the two forms of shoulder dystocia, i.e., the high or the low dystocia, as the latter is much more easily dealt with and brings far fewer obstetric complications with it. The dangerous form of shoulder dystocia, the high dystocia (the anterior shoulder of the baby is pressed against the maternal symphysis), is recognizable when the baby's head retracts partially back into the vagina (the so-called turtle sign). The turtle sign is unmistakable.

There are clearly defined obstetric measures to avoid injury to a baby after shoulder dystocia (OLG Karlsruhe, Judgement of 15.08.2001, AHRS III, 2500/317). They were described in a relevant judgment of the Higher Regional Court (OLG) of Düsseldorf as follows:

> Proper practice is to medically stop labor; subsequently, a substantial episiotomy is to be performed to limit soft tissue resistance and, especially, to insure an optimal vaginal entryway. After these preparatory procedures, it can and should be attempted to free the impacted shoulder through appropriate maneuvers; it is often possible to continue the childbirth through repeated bending and stretching of the mother's legs; it is also possible to remove other obstacles through the application of external pressure above the symphysis; finally, manipulation in the birth canal can bring about a rotation of the baby's shoulder.

The medically correct procedure is described in entirely the same fashion in relevant German textbooks and in the relevant Treatment Guidelines (Recommendations for Treatment,

Diagnosis, Prevention, and Management of Shoulder Dystocia) first published in 1998.

In this context, it is important to note that very little time to decide is available when a shoulder dystocia occurs. The obstetrician must therefore be able to do the procedure blindfolded, as it were. Regular practice of the treatment procedure for shoulder dystocia on dummies is generally recommended. If the proper procedure has been adhered to, the doctor cannot be found to have committed medical malpractice in this regard, even when the delivery does result in plexus paresis.

It is thus all the more shocking that, to this day, litigation practice shows that cases continually occur where the settled standard practice is deviated from without explanation. Forgetting to take measures to stop the labor is a particularly common occurrence. Episiotomies are also commonly forgotten, resulting in complications and delays when Woods or Rubin maneuvers become necessary in the course of treatment.

30.8 Failure to Meet Specialist Standards

According to settled case law, every patient—and thus every pregnant woman—is entitled to conformity with specialist standards in their medical treatment. This does not rule out the possibility that a labor can begin under the sole care of a midwife. Midwives are authorized to give care in the course of labor that proceeds without complications even without the presence of a doctor and in this connection to perform a number of procedures as delegated to them by a doctor.

A pregnant woman may nevertheless expect, unless she explicitly waives this entitlement, that as of a certain point in the process, labor care will be performed with the presence and under the responsibility of a doctor (compare the treatment guidelines published in 1999 entitled *Empfehlungen zur Zusammenarbeit von Arzt und Hebamme in der Geburtshilfe*). In any event, a doctor should be present during a normal labor from the beginning of the expulsive stage, as the same standards state. This is important because

shoulder dystocia always occurs after the beginning of the expulsive stage. In any case, the midwife's responsibility ends with the determination of shoulder dystocia (OLG Karlsruhe, Judgement of 26.10.2005, AHRS Part III, 3210/311).

In practice, however, midwives are very often left alone after shoulder dystocia has occurred. Midwives are only authorized to perform procedures to treat shoulder dystocia when a doctor is not available. If this is the case, the midwife is not to be held liable. In most cases where a midwife has no possibility to bring in a doctor to treat the shoulder dystocia, there has been an improper organization. This is also the case when the midwife can only rely on the assistance of a junior doctor without the qualifications of a specialist.

In such cases, the failure to meet required specialist standards speaks in favor of a presumption that injuries to the baby are a result of this failure, i.e., the insufficient qualifications of the person treating the shoulder dystocia.

30.9 Absent or Insufficient Documentation

Today, it is generally understood that the procedure to treat shoulder dystocia requires precise chronological and material documentation (compare the treatment guidelines *Empfehlungen zur Schulterdystokie – Erkennung, Prävention und Management*). All measures that have been taken must be chronologically documented. The names of all active medical personnel present and which medical procedures they performed must also be recorded.

This rule is often broken. Case law has repeatedly criticized, for example, medical reports on the birth contain only the phrase "shoulder-related complications." Less terse documentation is also objectionable whenever it makes a reconstruction of the procedures taken to treat the shoulder dystocia impossible.

According to settled case law, documentation problems are not an independent basis of liability. They can nevertheless give rise to certain presumptions, particularly the presumption that procedures that require documentation were omitted. Failure to perform such procedures can suffice to show malpractice.

The BGH allows more conclusions to be drawn from completely absent documentation. It is generally understood in obstetrics that the complete absence of documentation on treatment procedures for shoulder dystocia gives rise to a presumption of improper treatment (OLG Saarbrücken, VersR 1988, 916; OLG Stuttgart VersR 1999, 582; OLG Köln, VersR 1994, 1425; overview of the relevant cases) Thus, if a court-appointed obstetric expert concludes that birth documentation is such that no determination of which procedures were used to treat the shoulder dystocia is possible, this generally leads to a finding of liability for the treating doctor.

30.10 Measures Generally Considered Improper in the Treatment of Shoulder Dystocia

It has widely been recognized in medical literature, and thus regularly emphasized by court-appointed experts, that the use of the **Kristeller maneuver** in the treatment of shoulder dystocia, i.e., in order to release the impaction of the anterior shoulder, is generally considered improper. Generally speaking, the Kristeller maneuver is unsuitable in the treatment of shoulder dystocia because it results in the shoulder being pressed even more firmly against the impacting symphysis.

Pulling the baby's head in order to correct the malposition of the anterior shoulder is another strictly forbidden maneuver. According to O'Leary, pulling in this way with the head pushed away to the side, so-called oblique traction, is by far the most common source of injury. This maneuver is not only grossly negligent when the anterior shoulder is still blocked by the symphysis. Oblique traction on the baby's head is, on the contrary, also not appropriate after the shoulder dystocia has been eliminated, i.e., as soon as the baby's anterior shoulder has passed the symphysis, as in cases of fetal macrosomia the baby's

body may still be stuck in the birth canal after the shoulder dystocia has been eliminated.

Among the procedures generally considered impermissible is, finally, the external pivoting of the baby's head with the goal of bringing the shoulder girdle along with it.

This was not always the case. External pivoting of the head was indeed once recommended as a treatment for shoulder dystocia; the recommendation was conditioned on the external pivoting only being used prophylactically, i.e., only so long as the baby's anterior shoulder was not pressed firmly against the symphysis. It has been a firmly established rule since at least 2004, however, that external pivoting of the baby's head is extremely dangerous:

> External pivoting of the head, which is still somewhat present, has been increasingly criticized in the last ten years and can now no longer be recommended, as in the case of a blocked shoulder it favours the overstretching of the arm plexus. There are safer and more efficient methods available to treat shoulder dystocia (the treatment guidelines *Empfehlungen zur Schulterdystokie – Erkennung, Prävention und Management*, edition of 2004).

As testimony about actual procedures during delivery has shown, the use of these strictly forbidden procedures is not uncommonly the result of the medical personal panicking when shoulder dystocia occurs.

This is why the American literature refers to the "3 Ps" ("panic, pushing, pulling") in discussing the main causes of OBPP. The Feige textbook discusses this point thus:

> Once the pathological event of shoulder dystocia does occur, the general successful McRoberts maneuver is not actually performed. Instead, there is random, haphazard reaction and doing exactly what absolutely must not be done: powerful pulling on the baby's head with oblique traction and the Kristeller maneuver.

Whether the baby's head was indeed pulled in an improper way to treat the shoulder dystocia is regularly subject to dispute. Even when the mother herself or the father present at the birth testifies in litigation that the baby's head was pulled in this critical situation, the treating persons deny it; this becomes a case of one word against the other, which usually works against the plaintiff with the burden of proof.

Things have changed here, however, as a result of the increase in brachial plexus surgery. When brachial plexus injury is treated surgically, signs of powerful pulling on the baby's head are regularly recognizable. Particularly in cases where a complete avulsion of nerve fibers or even spinal cord avulsion has occurred, powerful pulling on the baby's head is generally considered a proven cause. How strong the pulling was can be at least approximately reconstructed by the nature of the injury. Accordingly, there have been in recent years a number of legal decisions that have found the cause of obstetric brachial plexus injury to be an impermissible tug on the baby's head, based solely on expert analysis of the injury related to the brachial plexus paresis.

30.11 Damage Awards

When judgments have been made in favor of plaintiffs, damage awards for pain and suffering (*Schmerzensgelder*) have been—depending on the severity of the brachial plexus injury—around €70,000. Material damages due to a disability-related increase of need (B*ehinderungsbedingten Vermehrung der Bedürfnisse;* § 843 BGB) are routinely added to this. In OBPP cases, this refers to extremely high cost of support and care, in particular time and costs associated with reflex loco-motion therapy (the Vojta method), ergotherapy, and manual therapy. These costs are calculated according to standard general medical liability rules; in this regard, litigation concerning OBPP is not particularly remarkable.

30.12 Summary

The legal issues and forensic problems involved in cases of OBPP in Germany are complex and require exact medical and medical liability-related research.

OBPP challenges and changes the lives of affected children and their families drastically. Thus, legal practitioners must be prepared to supply good medical and medical liability information and advice to parents.

Jörg Bahm

31.1 Forensics of the Plexus Lesion

Regarding the brachial plexus damage associated with childbirth, the question arises about the correlation between the tensile forces acting on the neck region during birth and the injury patterns found intraoperatively within the brachial plexus, including the typical root ruptures and their biological consequence, the **neuroma**. Typically, the injury zone is located above and behind the collarbone, and therefore the tears are found either at the level of the spinal nerves and trunks or more central to the radicles or ventral and dorsal roots from the spinal cord.

31.2 Causes of Root Avulsion(s)

The root rupture is found either representing the maximum of traction damage to the supraclavicular plexus. Instead of a rupture within the plexus with remaining proximal root stumps, the traction forces are transferred into the foramen to the transition zone between the central and peripheral nervous system at the level of the rootlets leaving the spinal cord.

J. Bahm (✉)
Plastic, Hand and Burn Surgery, Section for Plexus Surgery, University Hospital, Aachen, Germany
e-mail: jorg.bahm@belgacom.net,
jbahm@ukaachen.de

The only other known cause of a very proximal root rupture or even avulsion, this time due to shearing of the radicles, occurs during a breech presentation, when excessive axial tension occurs in line with the head, onto the spinal cord with the cervical spine fixed, shearing the rootlets or the roots within the spinal canal or within the foramina (Fig. 31.1).

31.3 Pathophysiological Assessment During Surgery

During operation, supraclavicular nerve damage can be visually and photographically documented. We have been working for years with a sketch on solid cardboard. This shows evidence of a traction force which only damages the nerve tissue. In case of pressure the surrounding tissue layers should be injured and stigmata on skin and subcutaneous tissue, on muscles and vessels appearing like scars and strictures should be visible—but this is never the case.

Furthermore, we cannot make a forensic statement, neither what traction force has injured the plexus during the course of birth, nor whether there is anything defective or avoidable related to these forces.

Only an obstetrician knows the movements of the foetus and the forces applied during a natural foetal development or during birth-promoting

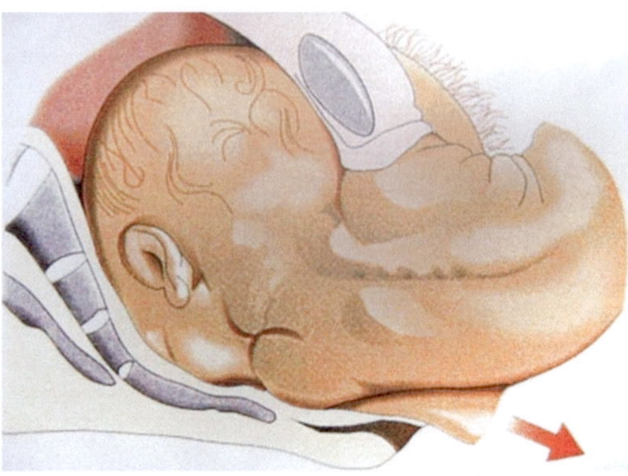

Fig. 31.1 Special pathophysiology of breech birth and axial shearing of radicles

movements; only he or she can advise about the amount of force acting on the child during birth or on the simulation model in the exercise situation (and this in both normal and emergency cases) and thus establish a reference to the pathophysiology of the documented nerve damage.

31.4 Basic Knowledge

An important research contribution is the repeatedly cited work of Metaizeau, a French orthopaedic surgeon who measured and documented the forces required for nerve rupture in stillborn infants [1].

All further discussions must be left to the obstetricians and lawyers. The reconstructive surgeon, who is familiar with the severe and most severe plexus damage in the field of operation, inevitably wonders what must have happened during birth in order to achieve this extent of damage.

Reference

1. Métaizeau JP, Gayet C, Plenary F. Les lésions obstétricales du plexus brachial. Chir Pédiatr. 1979;20:159–63.

Index

© Springer Nature Switzerland AG 2021
J. Bahm (ed.), *Movement Disorders of the Upper Extremities in Children*,
https://doi.org/10.1007/978-3-030-53622-0